PURPLE CANARY

The Girl Who Was Allergic to School

The true story of how school chemicals unleashed
a "rare" illness that devastated a young girl's life

By Joyce Gould

with

Jill Gould

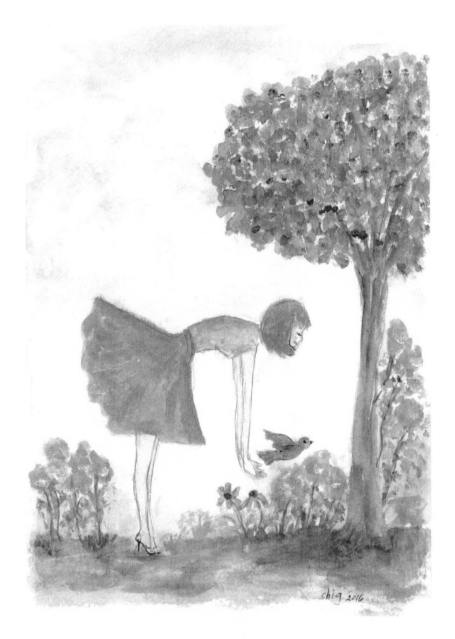

"Being Free" painted, contributed and used with permission
by R.D. Bruno, AIPoprhyric, of Images

TABLE OF CONTENTS

DEDICATION

Purple Canary is dedicated to all purple canaries—particularly those diagnosed and yet to be diagnosed with manifest acute intermittent porphyria (MAIP); the memory of Paula Frias Allende whose story is seared into my heart and soul; the generations of AIPorphyrics whose battle with porphyria has ended and now rest in peace; victims of academic, medical and societal bullying; those who suffer extraordinary physical and/or neurological reactions due to environmental chemical exposure and to those whose medical diagnoses remain elusive.

ACKNOWLEDGEMENTS

What began as a simple quest for medical answers mushroomed into a long-term, many-trailed odyssey. As we tumbled and stumbled along an unmapped route, we encountered many people who were helpful, kind and empathetic about the predicament our family found itself in and offered whatever support they could— general advice, a sympathetic ear, words of comfort and prayer. We are grateful to have encountered each and every one. And we are most grateful for the wonderful wizards who created the World Wide Web. Had it not been for this magnificent tool, we would *never* have connected so many dots that in the end *will* make a difference.

Special thanks go to phlebotomist Vladamir who drew the crucial blood sample that started the porphyria identification ball rolling; Dr. Nathan Hagstrom, Connecticut Children's Medical Center's former chief of hematology and the first medical professional to join us when Jill and I squared off against acute intermit-tent porphyria; Dr. Lisa Alonso of Middlesex Pediatrics who bravely entered our AIP medical loop; Dr. Eva Perdahl-Wallace, then pediatric hematologist at the Children's Center for Cancer and Blood Disorders of Northern Virginia for giving us hope and guidance when things turned so precipitously downward, then as we barreled along, facing frustrations aplenty; to Laura Pieper LCSW, for support through the many ups and downs and to Lloyd Cloud LCSW for helping to pick up the pieces left in the DNA debacle's wake. Thanks too, are extended to the many doctors we encountered throughout this odyssey for their attempts to help us reach a diagnosis.

Sincerest appreciation goes to the caring CCMC Hem/Onc nurses, APRNs and medical team for their much needed support and particularly to Yale/NH Children's Hospital's ER APRN Brian, whose observation helped reverse a critical downhill trend for Jill. We extend special thanks to our town's first response team who always held strong, particularly during the terrifying and confusing early times when Jill was experiencing frequent fainting/neurological spells.

Loving praises are reserved for acclaimed novelist Isabel Allende whose auto-biographical memoir and tribute to her daughter Paula is seared forever into my heart and soul. Thanks go to Diana Deats-O'Reilly who suffers with AIP *and* PCT and authored *Porphyria: The Unknown Disease* and founded the online Porphyria Educational Service (PES) and Desiree Lyon Howe, AIPorphyric author of *Porphyria, A Lyon's Share of Trouble* and co-founder of the American Porphyria Foundation. Their willingness to tell their stories helped me better understand and gear up for the full potential of what Jill was up against.

Other writers/authors provided insight and motivation, too. Lisa Sanderson, MD, *Every Patient Tells a Story* approaches the most daunting medical dilemmas with a humble and open mind, especially when differential diagnoses run amok. Rosalind Wiseman, author of *Queen Bees and Wannabees* described how the cliques that glide easily beneath the school adult radar impact school life and author Philip Zimbardo's *The Lucifer Effect: Understanding How Good People Turn Evil* profoundly altered my understanding of how individual *and* group behavior can be affected by situational circumstances, granting me insight to bullying operatives. After reading how rare it is for adults to speak out against wrongful behavior they not only witnessed but also *contributed* to, I better understood why depravity is so readily inculcated into the layers of our society. At Toxicologist Dr. Marc Bayer's suggestion, I read Rachel Carson's book *Silent Spring* which is recognized for launching the "Environmental Movement" and exposing the chemical/environmental debacle. It is interesting to note that more than five decades after her book's publication, our society in general continues to sanction an ever-escalating use of chemicals designed to make our lives easier, cleaner, softer, smell better, etc. yet questions why rogue illnesses plague humankind at alarming rates.

Gratitude goes to blogger Jonathan Morrow for his recollection about how his mother fought relentlessly for her Spinal Muscular Atrophy-affected child and encouraged him in the face of phenomenal odds and unpopular expectations because "…that's [a mother's] job." Those words encouraged me to stay on track, square off and forge ahead when pursuing outrageous school and medical situations in the face of Jill's challenging diagnosis and treatment programs.

Thanks go to the many individuals we tapped for special help including those who shared memories about childhood health issues and/or war stories: Alan, Amanda, Barbara, Bill, Cathy, Cheyenne, Claire, Danielle, Deborah, Dee, Dorothy, Ed, Elizabeth, Jane, Jessica, Jim, Joyce, Karen, Kristen, Lauren, Lisa, Lynda, Morgan, Patricia, Patrick, Rev. R. Lee, Shery and William. Loving thanks also go to the many individuals and families, especially the Clarks, the Confers, the Eccles, the Hannas, the Lords, the Wyllis's, the Wrobel-Mancinis, the "Bear Ladies," and the Vogts who comforted our troubled hearts.

Special appreciation is reserved for beta readers Megan Collins, Joanna Gerolami, Cyndee Spilker-Jacobson, Amanda Hanna, Sarah Hanna, Desiree Howe (very early draft), Maureen M. O'Brien, Danielle Pelton, Marietta Shlien and Barbara Bradbury Wilcox. And, for helping to make the *Purple Canary* manuscript readable and presentable, thank you to fabulous copyeditor Roberta Buland!

Our eternal gratitude and love remains with husband/dad Ed and son/brother Kevin who bumped along this calamitous road with us. And, in spite of a generation or more's worth of social awareness programs aimed at preaching respect for others and tolerance for those with differences, we thank those who hurled hurtful attitudes, words and deeds our way as they spurred us onward, outward and upward. One can only hope that these individuals will come to understand that God sees and hears *everything*.

AUTHOR'S NOTES

Purple Canary tells of our unintended journey that was initiated and underpinned by the genetic metabolic disorder known as acute intermittent porphyria (AIP). My "mom" observations and thoughts provide the book's narrative; Jill's writings are in italics as journal entries and songs, interspersed throughout the book to emphasize her anxiety, pain and desperation. We are a mother and daughter with no formal scientific, medical, legal or educational teaching or administrative school position training. To that end, nothing in *Purple Canary* should be construed as being personal, medical, legal, educational or similar professional advice. Readers are advised to seek guidance for his/her specific physical or emotional health, academic, legal or similar concerns from certified and/or licensed professionals. Many names of people and places have been changed and are so denoted by an asterisk (*) at the initial mention. The Internet's ongoing dynamics have sometimes resulted in URLs having been changed from the time of initial writing; in most instances, titles of books and/or articles are provided in the endnotes so the reader can search online if they wish.

It was disconcerting early on when multiple scientific, medical and educational specialists seemed unable or unwilling to answer questions Jill and I had about AIP, particularly as it related to children presenting with extremely alarming symptoms. So I decided to ask those who were most likely to know about juvenile AIP—adult AIPorphyrics. These wonderful people imparted childhood recollections that corroborated many of Jill's odd symptomology and reactions and helped to hatch *Purple Canary*. Realizing that domestic knowledge of AIP had at most two, possibly three generations of documented exposure, I cast my net to the World Wide Internet for answers. And as twigs of information came from those who have known AIP for multiple generations, the true essence of the book began to emerge.

Purple Canary's intent is not to teach about acute intermittent porphyria (AIP), the exhaustive lists of chemicals that are toxic to humans nor the formidable social condition known as bullying. Rather, by exposing the seemingly fantastical yet very real problems that made every day challenging, we hope *Purple Canary* will encourage discussion and action directed toward better identification and understanding of juvenile-onset AIPorphyria. Too many U.S. AIPorphyrics remember childhood symptoms up to and including bouts of paralysis and coma for which many were subjected to indifferent and/or unfair punitive responses. Discussions should also help improve the odds of AIP being added to doctors' differential diagnoses, to challenge the status quo of hard and fast U.S. MAIP diagnostic measures and to encourage experts to look into ambiguous, atypical presentations. After all, this is the United States of America where generations of genes have mingled and mutated since the first European settlers arrived. *Purple Canary's* intent is also to demonstrate the grave impact that human indifference, cynicism and cruel judgment has on people for things over which they have no control

U.S. AIP prevalence is unknown but it is likely underestimated and under-reported. Meanwhile, schools cope with the highest prevalence and escalating incidences of the 4As (asthma, ADHD, allergies, autism) even as the use of toxic chemicals, though increasingly under suspicion for possible connection to many conditions, continues to permeate everyday life. In addition to some concerning environmental conditions, school bullying remains pervasive throughout the U.S. and other countries. In fact, experts across the globe have drawn a connection between school social problems and bullying-related suicides.[1]

Purple Canary is our story—one that will undoubtedly generate cheers and jeers. But in the end, God willing, it will inspire conversation and eventually, a better understanding of acute porphyrias, particularly AIP; chemical toxicity in schools and a truism that Philip Zimbardo made society aware of: the pervasive human character flaw of bullying.

---

1 No identified author. *Bullying Statistics: Bullying and Suicide.* http://www.bullyingstatistics.org/content/bullying-and-suicide.html. 2013.

PROLOGUE

Changing Winds

The universe is always speaking to us…causing coincidences and serendipities, reminding us to stop, to look around, to believe in something else, something more.
— NANCY THAYER

Given that my daughter, Jill survived serious chemical, alcohol and physical inutero abuse, was born drug affected and removed at birth from her biological mother whose own health was severely compromised then relegated to the foster care system for the better part of her first year, it was understandable why most people, doctors included, attributed her delays and behavioral quirks as she grew to any or all of these reasons. As time went on, so many different medical concerns were bandied about but never confirmed that I just ministered to her changing idiosyncrasies as she grew. By the time she was in first grade, my own medical challenges and other close family members' severe health issues had cropped up. In today's parlance the word journey is used to describe medical predicaments one contends with. I did not know it at the time, but managing these different health-related crises afforded me knowledge of, experience with, and insight into the amazing awe inspiring, divinely interconnected human body as well as the complexities associated with medical caregiving. So when Jill began to exhibit bizarre symptoms at school shortly after starting sixth grade I was fairly adept at patient advocacy and unafraid to press for explanations or to research information myself.

*I need help! Is anybody out there? Is anyone listening? I have no idea what's happening to me. Something's happening to my body. I'm scared! Am I going crazy? If anyone is out there that believes me, **I need help!**[2]*

---

2 Jill's journal. Circa November 2007.

No one knew how to understand the peculiar physical and neurological symptoms Jill had begun experiencing at school which had within a matter of weeks intensified to fainting/convulsive spells accompanied by very challenging breathing problems. As weeks turned into months, the symptoms not only persisted; they also were joined by horrific, incapacitating abdominal pain. School officials labeled her an "attention-seeking faker." Skeptical medical professionals cautioned, "When you hear hoof beats, look for horses, not zebras" and pointed to biological inheritance and then to a mental illness. My mom-gut disagreed with all of them.

All staring faces, all these blank pages. I gotta get up. Don't understand it. My head is spinning round. I keep falling down… It's a warning. I'm calling for help but it's like an empty, silver screen… And nobody hears my screams.[3]

I attribute my unwavering surety that there was a physical reason for the odd symptoms Jill kept having at school and not that she was faking, looking for attention or attempting to avoid work, to mother's intuition—*knowing* my daughter as any mother knows her child. Eventually, the DNA testing that I kept insisting on revealed that the itty-bitty gene associated with AIP is harbored in Jill's liver. A zebra had been found after all. A life-threatening disease rooted in an ancient Nordic people seldom identified in U.S. adults never mind kids had been identified in my adopted child and no one but me seemed to be interested in it. But when that door closed, others opened and Jill's, and therefore our family's life, became a confluence of surrealism. With Jill in tow, I set out with a mother's vengeance to get help for her. I researched AIP, talked with AIPorphyrics and/or their caregivers and realized that Jill was essentially stuck in a child-version of adult-onset AIPorphyria. What was happening to her mirrored what generations of adult U.S. AIPorphyrics have known: the physical aspects of the disease are routinely trivialized; the neurological aspects may be tolerated, but the psychiatric components are almost always amplified and patients are too often accused of being hypochondriacs, whiners, malingerers or drug seekers.

Once upon a time I was one of those career for life women who truly enjoyed business challenges, took great pleasure in fast paced multitasking and was noted for my fierce loyalty to the commercial real estate company where I started as a temporary clerk typist and ultimately became a partner. But that all changed when my husband Ed and I committed to a long-term foster/pre-adoptive teenager. Though the placement disrupted in less than a year, the experience had changed me—it was time to move on to a more purposeful life. We built a home on a bucolic country road in Littleton,* Connecticut where Ed and I joked about raising miniature goats with the strange characteristic of fainting when startled, because they were so darned cute. As it turned out, the future would indeed bring us a fainting kid—cute, yes—but not of the bleating, furry four-legged variety.

Within a few months of having moved into our new home, a social worker from the State of Connecticut's Department of Children and Families contacted us about a toddler in need of a forever family and then again two years later when his infant sister entered the picture. It was not long before I realized that compared to

3 Lyrics to the song "Warning" written by Jill. 2009.

parenting these two neurologically and emotionally affected special needs children, my business career had been a cakewalk.

Fear, anger, embarrassment, humiliation, desperation, resignation and isolation are among the many feelings that permeate the men and women who live with the rare, hard-to-diagnose and disease-imitating genetic enzyme deficiency disorder known as manifest acute intermittent porphyria (MAIP) that is interchangeably referred to as AIP throughout this book. For the most part, fear underpins each symptomatic phase: fear of the incapacitating pain ripping through one's innards; fear another attack is around the corner; fear a reason for the weird symptoms will never be explained; fear that those who matter to the AIP patient, be they loved ones, friends, co-workers or doctors, will not believe the complaints; that he or she will be labeled as having exaggerating symptoms, seeking attention, a psycho-nutcase or any such qualifier and be written off by family members, friends, the medical community and society. And then comes the realization that life as he or she knows it is no longer. By the time of this realization, it is not unusual for eventually diagnosed porphyrics to end up with fewer internal organs; gallbladders and appendixes, in particular, seem prone to disappear when a surgeon's knife is wielded. When AIP is finally identified, relief may be short-lived as it was for Jill because the reality is there is no cure, and no sure path to long-term liberation from recurrent symptoms. When a porphyric's unpredictable liver with its mutant gene detects a trigger strong enough to activate a potentially perilous AIP attack, debilitating fear and accompanying anguish can return at any time.

As the mother of a juvenile porphyric, I know of these fears and how the range of emotions can grab hold of one's heart and soul, squeezing to the very core. I also know in my heart though it will never be proven, that Jill's peculiar symptoms likely started right at birth—actually at conception—which probably contributed to her having been pushed through two foster homes before coming home to our family.

In retrospect, getting to the medical diagnosis was relatively easy compared to the years-long dot connection puzzle of trying to figure out why Jill's neurological symptoms not only continued but also worsened at school in spite of frequent AIP treatments. She bounced between homebound tutoring and returns to regular school where AIP continued to ravage her body and brain, at times robbing her of the ability to speak, walk, think or even breathe.

My dot connection pursuit led me to Rachel Carson's book, *Silent Spring*, credited for having launched the Environmental Movement more than fifty years ago. Following its publication, U.S. laws were passed and society as a whole was required to adhere to legal requirements aimed at making the earth's living space safer and better fit to support human, plant and animal life. Then, about a decade after *Silent Spring* was published, an increasing number of people and groups zeroed in on internal environmental toxin exposure as being problematic for a growing number of building occupants. Thanks to a group led by former educators with illnesses directly linked to poor environmental conditions in school buildings, Connecticut enacted "An Act Concerning Indoor Air Quality in Schools" in 2003, making it one of the more progressive states. Laws directed at maintaining and improving indoor air quality (IAQ) in Connecticut schools were passed but as

[handwritten note in right margin: When I was teaching I going out to my car only air...]

was found out, not necessarily regularly or fully adhered to by school districts nor enforced by state agencies. One particular State mandate requires school districts to conduct a "uniform inspection and evaluation program" of fourteen separate IAQ points including "heating, ventilation and air conditioning systems…radon levels in the air; potential for exposure to fungi, mold, bacteria and other microbiological airborne particles…the degree of pest infestation and chemical compounds of concern to IAQ including, but not limited to volatile organic compounds [VOCs]."[4] In the end, I found the latter point to be a significant contributor to most of Jill's troubles while in Littleton's schools and warned, to no avail, that allegedly safe chemicals should be investigated further because the next generation of school IAQ issues with the potential to harm some school occupants would likely increase. Unfortunately, no one was interested in reviewing my information about the specific chemicals connected to Jill's AIP activity even though an IAQ report produced by the school district hired state agency documented excessive levels of those toxins. And still, the Environmental Protection Agency (EAP) continues to rank indoor air pollution among the top five environmental risks to public health.[5] Families and schools contend with the highest prevalence ever seen of asthma, ADHD, allergies and autism (known as the 4 As) with incidence increasing exponentially every year. More and more medical professionals are beginning to, if not agree then at least suspect, that exposure to internal environmental toxins bears some causal or contributing responsibility for some medically-affected patients' unexplainable physical and/or neurological symptoms.

As the medical professionals came around to support Jill, school problems really heated up. Having found a diagnosis, my attention turned to investigating my suspicion of a connection between Jill's AIP and chemicals used within the school buildings, why Jill's medical condition was being ignored by administrators charged by federal law with identifying and protecting students with special needs and why peer bullying and administrator persecution of a child with a serious illness were allowed. School administrators ignored, scoffed at and/or ridiculed my attempts to engage them in discussion about AIP, school chemicals or the ongoing bullying of the weird child, Jill. In fact, it was clear that Jill was considered the common denominator—she was trouble so trouble she would get. I witnessed my once smiling, beautifully resilient daughter's attempts to maintain dignity as she struggled with relentless harassment and routinely inhaled/ingested low levels of toxic chemicals all while embroiled in AIP's tormenting symptom/treatment circus. The district won a reprieve when it shunted her to out of district schools. Yet that was when dots finally began to connect for me and I figured out that Jill, AIP and certain "safe" chemicals permeating Littleton's school buildings were inextricably linked. A lonely, isolated schoolgirl's life blew up amid a range of professional adults' "misspeaks," "misconceptions," hidden agendas and blatant lies.

---

4 Connecticut General Assembly. *Chapter 170 Boards of Education.* Cite. 182 C.93 Sec.10-220 and Sec. 220(d); www.cag.gov/2011/pub/chap170.htm.
5 Connecticut Foundation for Environmentally Safe Schools. http://pollutionfreeschools.org/connfess/about/.

Coincidentally, a *Smart Brief*, an online business marketing social networking site, message appeared in my email box. "You have to attack with the madness of a mother whose child is surrounded by predators," blogger Jonathan Morrow wrote as he urged marketing professionals to fight for their ideas. His statement galvanized me—and jogged a memory: several years earlier, my sister and I had attended a metaphysical fair and came upon a woman reading totem animal cards. I paid her fee and hoped for something along the lines of the feline family but a few card turns later revealed that my total animal was—a badger. Unimpressed, I pushed the thought to the back of my mind. But Morrow's blog post inspired me to revisit what I knew about badgers. The description of the animal's protectiveness of their young sure seemed to fit now that I was a mother and my young 'un was being threatened with a rare disease. As peers and adults harassed and assaulted her with their GOTCHAJill! and WHACK-A-Jill! exploits, I abandoned my stalwart pre-parenting position of expecting children to fight their own battles, especially during the tween and teen years.

She is a special one, my Jill. Strong-willed and good-hearted, with both traits worn on *both* sleeves, she has been a formidable combatant against AIP, which has ravaged her physically, neurologically and mentally since she was eleven. Aspects of her story parallel many, if not most, adult AIPorphyrics' struggles. But her story is unique. After a few years of relentless and fruitless searching for another case of juvenile AIP that required infusion treatments of a human, blood based medical product, I steadied my nerves and asked recognized U.S. porphyria experts if they knew of any other such case of juvenile porphyria. The answer was "no" but should have been, "not yet" because my research had already begun to prove that children are not and have never been simply little adults.

When I first suggested to Jill that we write a book about her and our AIP and school chemical trials, she was adamant about titling it *Caught in a Nightmare* because, she said, "I am" and came back with: *"A medical mystery is hard for anyone, but imagine an 11-year-old kid fighting every which way and fighting a sickness that no one knew about. Especially if that disease is not known to happen in children because kids are not supposed to get it. Well, my name is Jill Gould, I am 12 years old and I have Acute Intermittent Porphyria."[6]*

That was all I would get. So I developed logs for tracking my observations and complaints made by or about her. Then I began to write the story that raised eyebrows, elicited numerous exclamations or expletives and prompted uncounted prayers from those who empathized with a young girl and her family.

Considered to be an adult-onset disease and still largely unknown to too many U.S. medical practitioners, I believe God gave Jill these challenges because He knew she would help bring light to the subject of AIP in general and to advocate for juvenile-onset MAIP patients in particular. He further knew that her challenging journey could expose the next generation of school IAQ toxicities, unmask contemporary bullying of sick or disabled people and, in the end, question the information that U.S. porphyria patients and their doctors have relied on for years.

---

6 Jill's journal. January 2009.

Sometimes it seems all any of us have are hopes, dreams and prayers. Porphyria does not define the essence of who Jill is but it sure made a mess of her growing years. Her dream is to become a singer/songwriter. Too often, AIP "purple days" put that dream on hold. Writer Langston Hughes said, "Hold fast to dreams, for if dreams die life is a broken winged bird that cannot fly."[7] Jill continues to hold onto her dreams, and that purple canary *so* wants to fly!

---

7 Hughes, Langston. http://www.poemhunter.com/poem/dreams-2/. "Dreams."

PART I

Before the Storm

If I can stop one heart from breaking,
I shall not live in vain.
If I can ease one life the aching,
Or cool one pain,
Or help one fainting robin
Unto his nest again,
I shall not live in vain.

— EMILY ELIZABETH DICKINSON[8]

8 Dickenson, Emily Elizabeth. "If I Can Stop One Heart From Breaking." www.bartleby.com/113/1006. html. Emily Dickinson Complete Poems, Part One: Life.

CHAPTER 1

The Calm

*You made all the delicate, inner parts of my body and
knit them together in my mother's womb.*

— PSALM 139:13-14

In 1939, Swedish physician Einar Wallquist wrote, "...There were some cases that more than others aroused my curiosity and interest, since their violent acute abdominal pains again and again prompted surgical intervention which never resulted in a diagnosis. So was the case with the pale housewife who one day fell ill in severe pains. When I arrived she lay in her bed agonized and twisting, agitated and in confusion. But I could not find any fault with her body. After a few difficult days her crisis was over and she continued her work as usual. But there came new attacks and my suspicions were directed to virtually all internal organs in her body. She was sent to hospital and its specialists, she was x-rayed, operated and treated. One time her appendix was removed, the other the gall bladder, and a third time a renal calculous was suspected. But no changes pointing to any specific disease were found. In this way she passed her life a number of years, but her tranquility of mind was disturbed by the recurrent attacks of pain and perhaps even more by anxiety about what kind of illness ravaged her body. Her strength fell off, her pulse grew rapid even if her heart was healthy. Her gait became tottering, her hands fumbling and her mind nervous, irritable, gloomy and anxious. I was sometimes called to her and sat at her bedside talking with her, supporting and comforting, pondering and prescribing—the latter into the blue.

Another woman went through the same history of suffering. Whenever I choose I can see before me her distorted features where she lay there in exceptional pain but otherwise obviously healthy without any temperature

9

and without abdominal tenderness or muscular defence. I remember her gradual decay, her hopelessness when in spite of the many journeys to the hospital never could get her health back between the attacks, her increasing nervousness and so the tottering gait, the ascending paralysis, the sloppy hands, the rigid facial expressions, and finally the resignation when she after a final try had again been sent home from hospital without any other diagnosis than—only nervousness. Now she had not any attacks anymore, she just deteriorated and got more and more dependent on help from her surroundings. At last she stayed silent and immovable in her bed, tired of living and probably welcoming death when he one late afternoon came in disguise of respiratory paralysis.

Which was this curious disease that ravaged in case after case? I phoned a colleague who had helped in her care. Respiratory paralysis pointed to some kind of organic nerve disease, but which? We talked for a long time without coming up with any ideas."

The next morning he phoned me back. 'I have not been able to let her go from my thoughts. Can it be porphyrinuria?'"[9]

Nearly sixty years after doctor Wallquist's recount of a medical conundrum that could neither be resolved nor released from his memory appeared in his book, another female porphyric entered this world. She was an American infant born of a substance- and alcohol-abusing woman who had lost three children to the children's welfare system. The Connecticut Department of Children and Families (DCF) took immediate custody of the drug-affected baby girl and placed her in foster care. By then, the peculiar group of symptoms suffered by Dr. Wallquist's female patient had long before been given a name—Acute Intermittent Porphyria (AIP), also known as "Swedish Porphyria" due to its original identification and sustained high prevalence in that country. The patient described in Dr. Wallquist's medical account lived with and, ultimately died from, acute intermittent porphyria.

Also by that time two forward-thinking American porphyrics had established a U.S. organization intent on increasing not only awareness of, but also providing to the nation's medical community, education about the porphyrias. The American Porphyria Foundation opened its doors for business in 1982 and began reaching out to U.S. porphyrics and the doctors who treated them.

None of this was known or mattered to me in the early fall of 1996 as Ed and I made plans for Kevin's adoption party; we were unaware of a phone call that would change our lives.

---

9 Thunell, S. et al. *Porphyria in Sweden*. Excerpted from the chapter *"Arv" (Inheritence)* in *Få mans land"* (*A land of few*) by Einar Wallquist, 1939. At biomed.cas.cz/physiolres/pdf/55%20Suppl%202/55_S109.pdf. or www.ncbi.nlm.nih.gov/pubmed/17298215 (free full text). Porphyria Centre Sweden. 2005.

CHAPTER 2

Clouds

*A child will fill a spot in your heart you
never knew you had.*
— ANONYMOUS

One warm fall day, the DCF social worker who had matched Kevin with us called
to say birth mother Kathy* had delivered another child and asked if we were interested in adding to our family. My immediate response was, "A baby? *No way!*" For
the five years following Kevin's birth, Kathy had maintained a risky lifestyle of drug
and alcohol abuse, poor nutrition and little or no medical attention. Adding to the
consternation, the social worker reported the baby girl had been born early because
Kathy had been physically abused by the birth father in the waning days of her pregnancy. I was more than a little ambivalent. Kevin had just started sleeping through
the night, was working with a new therapist and had started to improve. Besides, I
had never been one of those women who felt the need to give birth to and care for
an infant. But DCF is persistent, and within a couple of days Karolina* paid the
obligatory visit to our home. As she explained about the baby, Kevin sat on the floor
drawing. I said, "Kevin, did you hear what Karolina said? Mommy Kathy had a baby.
We have a lot to think about." At that, Kevin jumped up, grabbed my hands and said
urgently, "We *have* to take that baby away from Mommy Kathy! She does bad things
to people." We agreed to meet the baby named Melissa Ann.

Five weeks later, the social worker assigned to the baby brought her to a DCF
office where Ed, Kevin and I nervously waited to meet Kevin's sister. As Nedra*
opened the conference room door and entered the room, she slid the car seat containing the infant across the long, polished table and hissed, "This is a nasty baby!"
Ed picked the baby up and put her on his shoulder. She promptly threw up all over
his leather jacket. Kevin was ecstatic about meeting this "Mommy Kathy Tummy

Baby" and looked closely and carefully at her before softly murmuring, "She's not brown," then, abruptly said, "I already have a sister Melissa (a foster sister to whom he had become close). I can't have another one!" I was struck by how intently the baby watched Kevin as he moved around the room and thought, "There's someone special in there." After an hour, we left to give thought to baby Melissa's—and our—fate. After a discussion about skin color variations with Kevin (Kathy is fair-skinned Caucasian, he is biracial with light brown skin and baby Melissa Ann was pale white and very drawn-looking), I gave serious thought to how our lives could change. Everything was pretty much decided when Ed said, "Here's your chance to get your 'Jill,' my favorite girl's name. It seemed the child had been destined for us. We decided her first name would be Jill, her middle name Melissa. Another life-altering adventure had begun.

CHAPTER 3

Rumbles of Thunder

Not flesh of my flesh nor bone of my bone but still
miraculously my own. Never forget for a single minute
you didn't grow under my heart, but in it.
— AUTHOR UNKNOWN

Baby Jill Melissa was moved through two foster families before finally arriving home at almost eight months of age. It had taken so long because our foster care license had lapsed and once I found that out, I was adamant about delaying her homecoming until we received an updated one. DCF wanted us to retake foster/adoptive care classes, but that did not make sense to us. Kevin had lived happily and safely in our home for two years. We were well-known to the agency, and since this was a sibling arrangement, it seemed reasonable that DCF should provide us with an updated license. Another reason I was resolute about getting the license in hand before Jill came home was more poignant; several years earlier, Kathy's first infant had died in foster care. I felt *if*, God forbid, something tragic happened to this baby without our having an updated license, not only would our family be devastated, but also the potential for adverse media attention announcing "DCF baby dies in unlicensed foster home" was almost a given and I was not willing to chance that. So we visited Jill frequently in her foster home so she could become familiar and comfortable with us and we would get to know her schedule and personality.

The social worker's introductory remark about baby Melissa/Jill proved to be prophetic. She was a baby of dichotomies. I initially wrote most if not all of her problems off to having been born substance-affected with poor prenatal nutrition, the stress and inutero physical abuse she had been subjected to, her recent introduction to baby food or the number of homes she had been moved through during her short life. She was difficult to soothe, could not self-console, had frequent nasty vomiting episodes and suffered chronic diarrhea. She had difficulty swallowing thin liquids and would go from crying to screeching howls long and loud enough to threaten the household's sanity. Without rhyme or reason, her full-body muscle tone ranged from stiff and rigid to unusually pliant or flaccid. When seated alone she flopped forward like a folded taco and when placed in a baby walker or bouncer, her legs hung as though wasted. She drooled nonstop in excessive amounts, even for babies; I thought it was because she was teething but her foster mother said that she had done that for as long as she had known the child. Jill's reaction to sensory input was downright intimidating to witness. Attempting to dress her was a nightmare and as a result she spent much of the time in only a diaper.

Being rocked in a rocking chair or pushed along in a stroller prompted screaming fits and episodes of projectile vomiting. In fact, she sometimes would scream in panic mode for hours at a time. Her bowel movements were frighteningly frequent and copious. She would pull her legs up so often and tight, I guessed she had colic and assumed I would have to get through it like generations of mothers have done. Her sleep pattern was drastically off. After weeks of not being able to regulate her nightly slumber in the crib, I relented and put a low inflatable mattress on her bedroom floor, covered it with a Velux blanket, the only bedding she tolerated, and tried her out on it for naps. As soon as it became apparent the air mattress/blanket helped her sleep, the crib was pushed against a wall. I never knew why she could not sleep in that crib, but something about it distressed her deeply and I was glad to give up that battle.

Prior to Jill's arrival, several neighborhood women graced me with a baby shower and with a baby girl only a year older than Jill, Nadine* provided bags of soft, used clothing that Jill allowed me to dress her in. Claire,* skilled in pediatric physical therapy, offered helpful suggestions, one of which was to contact the local Birth-to-Three (Bt3) early intervention program to ask that Jill be evaluated. She taught me several therapeutic techniques to help improve Jill's obvious physical development dysfunctions. By the time the Bt3 evaluation team arrived a couple of weeks later, Jill had improved so much she no longer met the program's requirements.

Ed nicknamed her "chaos." Her pediatrician called her quirky. She was both. Within a month, Kevin asked if we could return her—somewhere, anywhere. Baby Jill had flipped our world upside down. Yet she could turn on a dime and her sweet nature would come shining through. Unlike Kevin, who had been labeled failure to thrive from birth until his salvation arrived in the form of foster care placement, Jill's special personality came blazing through her myriad discomforts from the start. It was clear this child would fight for the life God had given her. However, as time went on, developmental problems pointed to the effects of prenatal drug, alcohol and health-neglecting lifestyle during pregnancy. Throw in the oddball environmental toxins that birth mom may have been exposed to and the importance of Jill's problems shriveled. The real wonder was that she had made it out of the womb alive.

CHAPTER 4

Lightning Flashes

And though she be but little, she is fierce.[10]
— SHAKESPEARE

With two children not sleeping for nights on end and varying health and special needs crises cropping up on a daily basis, our family life skittered erratically. The consulting business that had been bopping along fairly well and the real estate marketing book I had been writing came to screeching halts as priorities realigned. Over the years, I had held a host of business titles: supervisor, manager, marketer, researcher, vice president, chief operating officer, business partner. I realized that I now held the most important job and title of all: mom to two neurologically challenged, special needs children. I gave up trying to figure out if daily issues ignited because of developmental stage; age appropriateness; lack of sleep; a multitude of physical, neurological or psychological issues or genetic predisposition. In the end, the reasons were irrelevant; the confluence had to be managed. What I had thought was stress in the business world was made abundantly clear—*this* was honest-to-God *stress*—twenty four hours a day, seven days a week, 365 days a year.

Though cheerful, cute and loving, Jill could be challenging. She was prone to outbursts and tantrums, sometimes multiple times a day, when things did not go her way, especially when things changed unexpectedly. Never a lightweight, she grew full- and able-bodied—not to mention strong-willed and headstrong. She was our "Little girl with a little curl right in the middle of her forehead," and like the nursery rhyme says, "when she was good, she was very good but when she was bad" her behavior could be "horrid." But she wasn't "bad" or "mean" in that she was not malicious. As time went on it became clear she had some developmental

---

10 Shakespeare, W. "A Midsummer Night's Dream." Act 3, Scene 2.

issues; she began walking on schedule, but was woefully behind in speech development. She was susceptible to one communicable illness after another, so much so that I wondered about the state of her immune system. Just before the age of two, worries about speech progress, inconsistent behavior and ongoing equilibrium issues prompted me to re-contact Bt3. This time, they determined that cognitively, she was fine, in fact she was on the intelligent side, but her expressive speech was severely delayed and her neurological issues were concerning. Soon, multiple therapists were coming to our home to provide a variety of developmental therapies.

It was not unusual for Jill to occasionally fall asleep during her Bt3 session, and she regularly slept for hours as soon as the daily morning program was finished. One day the speech pathologist recorded a particularly odd occurrence, "… [Jill] was receiving candy as a motivator, put a piece in her mouth and became nonresponsive. She sat very still, staring straight out. At first I thought she didn't like the candy but after she did not respond to continued prompts, her father put her on his lap and tried to 'snap her out of it.' [T]he episode…lasted for a good 2 minutes."[11] Per Bt3 recommendation, we pursued a neurological evaluation for Jill who was pronounced "in the range neurologically for her age group." She continued to have frequent bouts of diarrhea and difficulty swallowing thin liquids so doctors ordered a breath test for malabsorption of sugars or lactase intolerance, a barium swallow test, an endoscopy and a sigmoidoscopy to attempt to find if/how the conditions were connected. I asked if Jill should undergo an MRI or CT scan to rule out evidence of head trauma, but the specialists did not see any reason for doing so. We were told she had an aversion to food textures and toddler diarrhea and that she would grow out of both. She suffered frequent, arbitrary episodes of loss of gait which did not seem to be associated with the surface she was attempting to navigate or even whether or not she was in motion. In fact, there were times when she would be standing still and suddenly end up on the floor or ground.

From a very early age, she suffered vicious nosebleeds, especially when she was upset but also when sleeping. It became oddly routine for us to be awakened by her panicked screaming in the middle of the night and to find her pillow and pajamas saturated with blood. Ultimately, blood tests detected she had thalassemia, and we were told she would always present with a low iron count on clinical tests. We were assured there was nothing to be concerned about even as the nosebleeds persisted. As time went on and she became more ambulatory, it was not unusual for one or both of us to find independent little Jill standing at the bathroom sink in the middle of the night holding a wad of tissues to her nose trying to handle the latest nosebleed herself, determined not to wake anyone.

Her erratic sensory and neurological issues, recurrent diarrhea and vomiting episodes made for tough daily living. Desperate for answers and with preschool attendance looming (and her doctor continually advising me to "be patient"), I sought a naturopathic doctor's (ND) advice. Dr. Rice* listened to my description of Jill's disturbingly frequent and plentiful bowel movements and behavioral issues and suggested she be tested for a systemic yeast infection. Within a week, the results

11 Bt3 Speech-Language pathologist. Letter to Dr. Garner.* July 13, 1999

were back. Candida or yeast measurements reflected an overgrowth condition with severely elevated gut flora. Dr. Rice explained not only could this cause the diarrhea and vomiting Jill endured, but it also quite possibly was associated with some of the neurological and emotional issues she was noted for. Furthermore, he said, Jill most likely had had the problem since birth. Besides eliminating juice and sweets from her diet he recommended an oral fungicide medication to cure the exceedingly high level of yeast. I said a prayer and agreed to try the incredibly expensive treatment for a chance to give Jill relief from a condition that was clearly draining her. When told the ND had treated Jill for the condition, her pediatrician angrily voiced displeasure, which I ignored—for months she had offered nothing better. Within a matter of weeks Jill's diarrhea was much improved and her irritation had calmed considerably. Most startling, but very welcome was that she had begun to articulate words and started potty training in earnest so I looked ahead to the prospect of preschool for her.

Bt3 warned that because of her high cognition level, Jill might not be accepted into Littleton's preschool program. But the school district acknowledged she was an at-risk child and admitted her to the program under the Special Education (SE), Speech & Language (S&L) category. At the time she ranked in the ninety-fifth percentile for speech comprehension but only in the eighteenth percentile of her age group for articulation. She eagerly applied herself to the routine and was drawn to helping other students, particularly those with noticeable physical challenges. Her empathetic response was duly noted; however, preschool faculty and staff reported frequent episodes of irritability, obstinacy and at times, defiance, from Jill. The assertions perplexed me; she enjoyed being around other children and from what I'd observed and had been told by other adults, did well at mixing and playing with children in various programs, playgrounds, children's museums, etc. She had a tendency at times to become overly attached to one or another child, especially those who were kind to her, but not enough to be truly concerning. I could understand Jill's speech fairly well but I wondered if maybe she was frustrated about not being able to communicate as easily with the children and adults at school. Since she still had some developmental deficiencies, I kept hoping school professionals would offer insight and clues about what her problem might be. They obviously thought communication was part of the problem so suggested that Jill learn sign language, but she wanted to speak like everyone else and would have none of it. Without Jill's buy in, the lessons were discontinued.

With summer coming, it was determined that Jill would benefit from attending summer school prior to starting kindergarten. She enjoyed the experience and made considerable progress, but another medical surprise appeared when she tested positive for TB exposure, which required that the entire family be tested, too. Fortunately, the results for the rest of us were negative. While not contagious, Jill's case was registered with the Connecticut State Department of Public Health and she had to take daily medication for months. The medication's side effects brought back the discomfort she had known for most of her life: irritability, diarrhea, bloating and upset stomach. Still, kindergarten turned out to be a relatively good year for her.

Kevin had benefited greatly from neurofeedback therapy, and I wondered if the same could happen for Jill. So during the summer after kindergarten I signed her up for sessions. She applied herself diligently and, by the start of first grade, her speech was much improved. However, once in school for a full day, she spent a good amount of time in the health room because of upper respiratory problems often accompanied by long-lasting nosebleeds. Jill and her first grade teacher connected well; peer socialization, however, was not much better; she was clearly the odd one out. Her teacher and I communicated daily through notebook messages. It was plain that something was wrong. Having moved on from preschool temper tantrums and kindergarten spells of irritability, now she was prone to inexplicable crying spells. And her visual-spatial abilities were problematic. It was not unusual for her to lean over to retrieve something she had dropped on the floor only to smack her head on a neighboring desk on the way up. Judging distances for something so slight did not come naturally to her and contributed to the impression she was a clumsy child. When I questioned her about school, Jill said kids sometimes said bad things to her. I assumed they still had trouble understanding her speech and that her sporadic crying and/or clumsiness prompted ostracizing. I explained the Golden Rule to her as I had done with Kevin at that age. Jill replied, "If they be nice to me, I be nice to them." I could not argue with that; I would hear something very similar to that credo several years later which would, I suppose, confirm the "leopard doesn't change its spots" theory. Not wanting Jill to capitulate to meanness directed her way, I suggested she tell the children she felt were truly being unkind, "That is rude and mean, please don't say that to me," and I advised her teacher I had encouraged her to respond as such. Apparently, the stage had already been set for bullying of the student who was "different."

CHAPTER 5

High Pressure Systems

Do not worry about tomorrow for tomorrow will worry about itself. Each day has enough trouble of its own.
— MATTHEW 6:34

My dad's health began to decline when Jill started first grade. By late January it was time for the family to assemble. My sister, niece and I headed to Florida; Ed stayed behind with Kevin and Jill. We returned to frigid Connecticut a week later, I with nasty flu/cold symptoms acquired during the trip south that stayed with me for weeks. Dad hung on until early March when the Lord welcomed him home. Then on Easter Sunday, I felt a sharp spasm in my head. Concluding another migraine was coming, I took aspirin, but as the week slogged on, my condition worsened until I ended up in an emergency clinic. It was determined that my normally low blood pressure had spiked dramatically. I was transferred to a full service hospital where a CT scan detected a brain anomaly. The doctors were mystified as to what it could be. Ed and I were terrified; the children were young and doctors were unsure about what the something in my brain was. A couple of days later, a neurologist said I had either a "teensy brain tumor" or had suffered a small stroke. I rhetorically thought, "Oh great! Which would I rather have, a brain tumor or a stroke?" Later, an MRI confirmed I had suffered a small stroke. Less than a month later the source of that stroke was revealed with the diagnosis of an uncommon genetic kidney condition that caused a narrowing of the renal arteries, producing a blood clot that had traveled to my brain. I barely had time to absorb that information when I had a second, more severe attack. I was diagnosed with an inner ear infection and released from the ER with a prescription for antibiotics and instructions to "take it easy." It was later discovered I actually had had another, stronger stroke and was put on a strict medication regimen.

By summer, I was able to drive again so began taking Jill to see Iris* for therapy. Within a month of starting second grade her teacher reported she was having fun at recess and was more relaxed with a lot less frustration and crying. But during the winter, despite three nose cauterizations, her nosebleeds were back. The school nurse described one as "the most severe I've witnessed. [Jill] was weak from blood loss and vomiting due to swallowing so much blood."[12] The season brought frequent respiratory ailments, earaches and sinus infections to both children which only exacerbated Jill's nosebleeds. Humidifiers and nebulizers became mainstays in our home. Jill was diagnosed with intermittent asthma attributed to unknown irritants. Since schools are notorious germ generators, who could say what affected her when? She was prescribed an inhaler and clung to it like a lifeline. As time went on, Jill began to complain frequently of stomachaches, that her head felt warm, that her legs ached, her arms hurt and other ailments. Then, after a particularly horrific late-night nosebleed during which blood oozed from her tear ducts, Ed insisted on bringing her blood-saturated pillowcase and the trash bin filled with bloodied tissues to the pediatrician. Tests were ordered and a couple of days later Dr. Wade* called to say a clotting abnormality had been found. She referred us to Nutmeg Hospital for Children* (NHC) where Dr. O'Connor* diagnosed Jill with, in addition to thalassemia, a form of hemophilia known as von Willebrand disease. We had not been overreacting after all.

Jill was thrilled to move on to third grade at the Main Street Elementary School* (MSES) but soon found that the student social cliques had developed stronger alliances, and she did not seem to fit into any of them. Oddly, her abdomen had become noticeably distended but she did not complain. I attributed it to the propensity for fast food we had all acquired with our tight schedules. Dr. Wade had noted she was somewhat overweight, but did not seem concerned about it. Third grade brought weird mood and behavior changes and some children circled, poking her with sharpened words, looks and attitudes. Always an "old soul" with a comprehension peers did not necessarily relate to and adults did not often appreciate, Jill stuck up for herself and did not always take the jabs and gibes quietly, endearing herself neither to bullies nor teachers. She sometimes went over the top with meltdowns because "someone rolled her eyes at me like I'm stupid or something." More often than not, that someone happened to be Camerin,* an outspoken classmate who slammed her way into Jill's psyche. For an unknown reason, Jill wanted her for a friend so I arranged a couple of play dates between the girls. Camerin did not display any of the behaviors while in our home that Jill complained she did at school but oddly, she had to be returned home both times because she developed severe anxiety about being "in the woods."

Then, my mother began to mention extraordinarily painful headaches and to exhibit odd memory lapses. The diagnosis of terminal, aggressive brain cancer sent us reeling and we trekked to Florida. Mom opted for chemotherapy and radiation treatments that offered the prognosis of surviving "a year at most." The oncologist neglected to tell her and us that her quality of life for much of that year would be

---

12 Littleton* elementary school nurse. Letter to NCH otolaryngologist. January 30, 2002

severely compromised. After enduring eight nerve-wracking months of cobbled long-distance caregiver coordination for Mom's deteriorating condition, my sister Linda and I came to the conclusion we would have to share on-site caregiving responsibilities until it was time for Mom to join Dad. Jill and I took the summer shift where her empathetic nature blossomed as she ferried drinks, snacks, meals and medications to her grandmother, pushed her wheelchair whenever she could and sat by her side overlooking the flora-lined canal Mom loved so much. Shortly after Jill began fourth grade, Mom's cognitive ability plummeted and with nothing more to be done, nursing home arrangements were made. Back in Connecticut, I was putting final touches on a belated seventh birthday party for Jill, because she and I had been in Florida during her August birthday. We were awaiting her guests when I experienced my third stroke. That time, I lost my ability to speak and spent several days in the hospital.

Having undergone years of speech and language therapy, Jill took it upon herself to augment my outpatient speech therapy sessions. She began with recitations from a calendar and insisted I repeat letters, numbers, days of the week and the months over and over again. "Oh, come on! I know you can do better than that!" she would chide. I quickly gained insight and better empathy for what baby/toddler Jill must have felt when she had had something to say but no one but me could figure out what she was saying. Thankfully, Ed became my voice and spoke on my behalf with the nursing home staff, hospice personnel, attorneys and other professionals in Florida. When it was time to say final good-byes to my mother, we climbed into the van and headed to the Sunshine State to prepare my parents' house for sale. We had not been back home in Connecticut for more than an hour or two when the nursing home staff called to say that Mom and Dad were together again. The memorial service had to wait because I experienced yet another stroke. This time, my cognitive abilities were severely impacted and my entire left side was paralyzed; I was relegated to the stroke rehab clinic. My days were filled with fatiguing cognitive evaluations, draining neurological testing and exhausting strength and balance training. Prior to my discharge, the doctor called a family meeting to which Jill brought a notebook on which she'd written: *"JILL's Inportin stuff to help MOM."* She took notes as the neurologist spoke: "Medacine–take by herself. Travel to Florida— NO. Physical therapy. Stairs—WITH HELP. Outside—WALK WITH someone. Speech—Talk with someone. NO DRIVING. Practice COOKING, MATH, Reading, Counting." I had figured that I would not be able to attend mom's service but still, my heart hurt. Fortunately, Ed and I had already coordinated the details and though I could not be there, relatives told me the service turned out fine. Mom was laid to rest beside Dad in their beloved Florida.

That fall, Kevin was diagnosed with Type 1 diabetes and spent a weekend in the hospital as he and we received training to care for this life-changing challenge. On the first anniversary of my mom's death, my mother-in-law's funeral was held. As sad as the loss was, by this time I was able to deliver a heartfelt eulogy to the woman who had been so dear to so many.

As our household routine pitched and rolled, Jill and Kevin went to school, did homework, took tests and stoically carried on. Jill's rotund middle drew chortles and daily references about her being fat. Her abdominal girth *was* concerning. Still, she seemed healthy, rarely complained of stomachaches anymore, and her diarrhea and reflux problems appeared to have resolved. She looked forward to attending the Benton* School as a fifth grader. There had been plenty of talk in the community about high levels of mold/allergens in the building so Jill's moving to the antiquated facility admittedly raised a few alarms in my head. However, Kevin, who had more allergies than anyone I knew had been fine there so I pushed my discomfort away. But within a few months, complaints about Jill's irritability and stubbornness flared up. As Jill herself described it, "... *my behavior was VERY odd.*" Therapist Iris was baffled by my reports of Jill's ill temperament at school. Since arriving home as an infant, various conditions had been raised as possibilities to explain different behaviors: potential infant stroke (inutero, neonatal, at birth), fetal alcohol affect; attachment disorder; dyslexia; seizure disorder; attention deficit disorder (ADD); obsessive compulsive disorder (OCD); oppositional defiant disorder (ODD); pervasive development disorder (PDD); autism spectrum; pervasive anxiety disorder; social comprehension and boundaries deficits; sensory deficits; gait, spatial, balance and visual processing deficits. Except for the visual processing problem and her obvious speech and language deficit, none had actually been diagnosed. Still, she maintained a stable self-image and almost as if in testimony to that, one day I happened upon a note she had written, "*Hi! I'm Jill Gould. I am nine years old. I am funny, fun and smart. I want to be a chef when I grow up. Yep. That's me. Jill.*" Seeing the note confirmed that in spite of everything our family had been through, Jill was okay. But why she was oddly touchy sometimes at school was perplexing.

As fifth grade wound down, Iris suggested Jill might benefit from a psychiatric workup. Because Kevin had been struggling with his fragile Type 1 diabetes and depression, I had already located a "new" child psychiatrist for Kevin so made an appointment for Jill, too. Dr. Bludonowitz* had diagnosed Kevin with bipolar disorder—not entirely surprising because the diagnosis was in their biological family medical history. In short order, Dr. Bludonowitz diagnosed Jill with bipolar disorder and prescribed Lamictal, Abilify and Risperdal. With my own and my parents' neurological health issues still reverberating through my mind, I really wanted to rule out organic problems before starting Jill on the medications so I asked the psychiatrist to order an MRI of Jill's brain. Dr. Bludonowitz readily approved the request and I made an appointment. The equipment produced quick results. No brain tumor. No stroke(s). No seizure activity. A few weeks later Jill eagerly planned for sixth grade. She was almost at the optimum dosage of her medications. She had had a great summer; her behavior had been steady and very well managed but my trepidation grew as school time approached. I prayed the coming school year would be a good one for both children, but especially for Jill. Kevin's middle school experience had not been great and with Jill's propensity to speak out, I was doubly ambivalent about her entry into preteen turmoil. Little did we know, we were about to be plunged into something none of us was remotely ready for: Purple Days.

PART II

Storm's A Comin'

God grant me the serenity
to accept the things I cannot change;
courage to change those things I can;
and wisdom to know the difference.

— **REINHOLD NIEBUHR**

CHAPTER 6
Warning Winds

In school, you're taught lessons and then given a test. In life, you're given a test that teaches you a lesson.
—TOM BODETT, AMERICAN AUTHOR, VOICE ACTOR, RADIO HOST

I usually arranged to meet with Jill's teachers and administrators early in the school year so we could become familiar with each other and I could update them about her summer's progress. This time I shared that Jill had recently been diagnosed with bipolar disorder and was on increasing doses of medications. I asked them to let me know of anything, no matter how slight, that might seem out-of-the-ordinary with her during school hours. At that, a few of the teachers said Jill tended to frequent the school nurse's office with complaints of nausea, headaches, stomachaches and other ailments and then asked if I knew why her arms and torso sometimes shook. Surprised, I said I had no idea why she would be visibly shaking to the point it was noticeable. I thanked them for telling me and said I would meet with the nurse to hear her thoughts on the matter. The school nurse produced a report that showed since the start of school Jill had visited the health room up to three times a day with complaints of nausea, vomiting, headache, stomachache, "shaking," pain in her left ankle and nosebleeds. In each case, she had been given crackers, fluid and/or time to rest, then was sent back to class. Regarding the "shaking," Nurse Williams* had written, "Hands appear very shaky." [13] Neither of us understood what was going on.

Things worsened in October when phone calls from school started. "Jill has suffered some sort of fainting/possible seizure activity, the ambulance has been called and she is on her way to the ER"; "Jill fainted, can you come right away?" "Jill is

---

13 Benton* school nurse. Daily health complaint register. October 23, 2007

non-responsive, 911 has been called!" and then simply, "Jill's down again!" When a call came in, I'd spring into action.

I turned eleven and was really excited about going back to school as a sixth grader. I got some new clothes and my first pair of Etnies [sneakers]. I loved them and couldn't wait to show them off. There was a new principal and I was kind of excited about changing classes and not having to go up and down stairs anymore like we did in fifth grade. My friend, Sarenah,* moved away during the summer so I started hanging around with Camerin, Tammy,* Nellie* and Miranda.* They were kind of nasty to me sometimes. Other times they acted like they were my friends. The first week was kind of fun but then my arms started shaking. I started getting nauseous like on the first day. And pretty soon I was getting nauseous a lot and got some nosebleeds, too. I had to go to the nurse's office almost every day for something.

My mom had a meeting with my teachers and the principal like she does every year. The teachers told her that they could see my arms shaking and asked if she knew why I did that. She thought maybe I was reacting to some medicines that a new doctor gave me. But I told her, no, they always shake like that in school. She was surprised about that.

After that meeting, I was still getting nauseous and a couple of times I threw up. It was gross and embarrassing. Then something even weirder started happening. I would get light-headed and pass out. I honestly don't remember what really happened the first time or two. But I got nervous because I was afraid I would hit my head on something and then really have problems. Once I was outside shooting baskets with Geoffrey.* I got a cramp in my leg, then my legs gave out and bam, the next thing I knew I was laying on the ground looking up at all the people standing around looking at me. Another time I was sitting with my friends at lunch and I was starting not to feel good when all of a sudden everything went black and I passed out. That time I woke up in an ambulance. The school principal went with me and then my mom came to the hospital. By then I was ok, so they let me go home.[14]

Jill passed out while walking through the hallway, collapsed while sitting in the cafeteria, fainted when sitting on gymnasium bleachers and blacked out seated in a classroom chair. I soon despised the ringing of the home phone. When the caller ID screen registered Benton School, my heart revved, my stomach clenched and my blood pressure shot up. I would answer the phone and sure enough, off to the hospital I would go. I reported each episode to Dr. Wade and then to Dr. Bludonowitz who wrote a note indicating that Jill should have a snack in her backpack to eat any time she began to feel shaky. The school nurse kept juice, yogurt and crackers on hand but that did not help. As the fainting spells continued, odd seizure type activity accompanied them. My days were filled with anxiety; my nights spent worrying about this bizarre set of circumstances and all the time, I prayed for answers.

As I drove the three-mile route from home to the Benton School and then continued on to MedCity* Hospital for the third time in a nine day period, I realized I was not panicked as I had been the first few times I had followed the same pattern— still nervous and worried, but not panicked. After having dealt with the strokes, my parents' terminal illnesses and Kevin's diabetes, I had no energy for ongoing panic. Instead, I developed an almost clinical approach to what was happening with Jill.

---

14 Jill's journal. November 2007

When I arrived at the school, the ambulance had already whisked her off to the hospital, and by the time I got to the emergency department (ED) she was alert, awake and after a time, able to get up and walk out of the hospital with me. After several more episodes, Jill told me she had been experiencing almost daily stomachaches, headaches, nausea, vomiting and ongoing shakiness in her arms and torso since the start of the school year. She said her eyes would become blurry, her heart would start racing (she described it as "my heart was bumping really hard"), she would have difficulty breathing and then she would lose consciousness. She also had some nosebleeds, but because of her von Willebrand diagnosis that was not unusual for Jill being in school so it was not overly worrisome. Besides, Mrs. Williams routinely treated other students' nosebleeds, particularly in the dry fall and winter months. In addition, Jill had recently developed the unusual habit of not being able to eat breakfast, and as I soon found out, she had been skipping lunch, too. I attributed this to a comment about weight gain that Dr. Wade made during her last physical exam. But Jill said she had simply lost her appetite. Traveling from ED visits, we had plenty of time to talk about what she remembered had happened prior to each medical emergency. Her recollections matched what witnesses reported. I looked for possible causes: Was she worried about a test or particular class content? Had she not finished her homework? Had she been hungry, thirsty, overtired? Had anyone bothered her? Were the books she carried too heavy? What?

At one point, fleeting thoughts of the days Ed and I had talked about a fainting goat came to mind, "Now I have a different kind of fainting kid!" I tried to make myself smile, but it was not funny. I knew God had something in mind for us but I could not imagine what.

CHAPTER 7

Cloudbursts

Trust your instincts. Intuition doesn't lie.
— OPRAH WINFREY

*I was sitting with my class in the gym on the bleachers. I started getting nauseous again and passed out. When I woke up, I found out I threw up on myself. My mom came to get me. I just wanted to stay in school. But no. They said I **had** to go home. Every day I went to school but I was worried. What was the matter with me? Some of the kids started making fun of me and staring at me like I was a freak or something. My mom was really worried. The doctors kept saying everything checked out ok. But I didn't feel ok. I was mad because the doctors said I was fine. I was nauseous, throwing up and falling down. What's so fine about that? I just wanted to be in school. Why didn't anyone get that?"*[15]

Jill's fainting spells began to be preceded or followed by nasty outbursts, and her frustration at not being allowed to stay in school became more than she could bear. She was terrified and embarrassed about what was happening to her. Her inability to control behavioral issues around those times troubled her greatly. All she wanted was to be part of daily school activities, yet school administrators only wanted her off the premises. A contingent of peers routinely smirked and fixed loathsome looks on her. Between the aggressors and the bystanders who stared but wouldn't talk to her, Jill felt isolated. Looking at the big picture, I could understand the other students' perspective; watching a fellow student faint then be carried off to the hospital only to have her return the next day had to be unnerving. Added to that was the negative attitude being thrown her way by Benton administrators. Jill confided, "Don't be fooled by their niceness, Mom. They end up getting nastier and nastier to me every time I faint." At a time when she desperately needed adult guidance

---

15 Jill's journal. December 2007.

and peer interaction and support, *no one* at school was there for her. Benton school psychologist, Debbie* was the first to challenge Jill's episodes with me. She asked if I thought Jill might be seeking attention through the fainting spells, complaints of nausea, stomachaches and such. I answered, "No, I honestly don't." I said I did not know what was going on, but I *knew* whatever was happening was for real. Then the ED doctors' attitudes about Jill's recurring spells abruptly changed; it became apparent that they thought she might be either looking for attention or attempting to avoid school work—or both. That she was being treated for bipolar disorder only added to the problem. Jill underwent several diagnostic tests: head CT scan, EEG, EKG, numerous blood and urine tests. Nothing was out of the ordinary. It was bad enough she was besieged by an unseen medical assailant, but the addition of overtly skeptical adults who suggested she was faking proved disheartening for both of us.

Every diagnostic test result for weeks showed no abnormalities. I was really concerned and scared because Jill's blackouts were *not* ordinary. What started out as fainting spells of a few seconds worked up to several minutes in duration accompanied with seizure type activity until Jill was out for up to twenty minutes at a time. In fact, sometimes it seemed as though she had fallen into a deep sleep. On occasion, just before collapsing, the school nurse was able to get her into a wheelchair where her head would loll from side to side and she exhibited jerky arm, limb and body motions. She was missing significant amounts of learning time and became notorious within the school community. Students and teachers were curious—and nervous, too. The situation became oddly routine. Jill would faint and I would be called by someone at the school, the ambulance team would cart her off to MedCity Hospital ED and I would go directly there. By the time I arrived, she would be alert. Within about an hour she would be fit enough to walk and I would take her home. After a few weeks of this, doctors introduced the hospital's psych team to us. They recommended I consider an Immediate Mobile Psychiatric Adolescent and Child Crisis Team (IMPACCT) consultation. However, after a lengthy telephone conversation with an administrator from that group, it was clear to me and them they had nothing better or different to offer us. In addition to keeping in touch with Dr. Wade following each fainting episode, I again sought Dr. Rice's advice. But nothing seemed to make sense about what could possibly be causing Jill's frequent fainting spells at school with him either.

Dr. Bludonowitz asked if it might be possible to record one of Jill's fainting episodes so the principal videotaped the next episode. After viewing it, she announced that Jill was suffering from temporal lobe seizures. She was certain, she said, because another patient she had treated had the seizure disorder and Jill's seizure activity was "just like that."

I wasn't convinced, "Wouldn't seizures have shown up on the MRI?" No, she said, that would only happen if the seizures were taking place when she was actually undergoing the MRI. That made sense to me and was good information to know going forward. By this time, Jill was taking the highest dosage of Abilify and Lamictal recommended for adults. I also had Risperdal capsules to administer to her if or when behavioral problems crept up.

Dr. Wade was confounded by Jill's presentations and, since the ED visits were proving fruitless, she approved my sitting with her during episodes as the school nurse monitored vital signs until the spell had subsided. The doctor reasoned we should just keep her safe until she recovered. I suspected she, too, probably felt Jill was somehow manifesting them. Soon the behavioral problems following her spells expanded to include obstinate refusal to follow directions, talking back to teachers and administrators and running through the corridors to seek refuge in stairwells—because she was determined to stay in school no matter what. That is when the Risperdal came into play. I would be called to administer a dose and hope for the best. One time as I entered the nurse's office yet again, Principal Anne* announced excitedly, "I got to see that bipolar change thing myself!" Her comment sparked a light bulb in my head. "*If* Jill really has bipolar disorder, shouldn't there be improvement by now? She isn't getting better—she's getting *worse!*" When I got home, I pulled out the medication information sheets I had gotten from the pharmacy and scrutinized them line by line. What I read made me sick. Lamictal's side effects included "dizziness, headache, blurred/double vision, shaking (tremor), muscle weakness, drowsiness, nausea, vomiting, diarrhea, difficulty sleeping, and lower stomach/abdominal discomfort. Unlikely but serious side effects: unusual mental/mood changes such as agitation."[16] Side effects of Abilify included "dizziness, lightheadedness, vomiting, blurred vision, weight gain, and drowsiness. Serious side effects: fast/pounding heartbeat, fainting, mental/mood changes, weakness, feelings of restlessness, shakiness (tremors); rare but very serious side effect: seizures (requiring immediate notification to "your doctor"). [Finally]... seek immediate medical attention for any of these very serious side effects: confusion, fast heartbeat...severe dizziness, trouble breathing."[17] Next, Risperdal's side effects: "dizziness, drowsiness, fatigue, nausea, weight gain, nervousness, difficulty concentrating; serious side effects: fainting, rapid/pounding/irregular heartbeat, mental/mood changes...seizures."[18]

My guilt about addressing Jill's behavioral quirks at school with medication was boundless. She was exhibiting too many of the side effects to think nothing of it. "Is it just a coincidence, or is something else going on?" I worried. I called my sister Linda, billing manager for a mental health treatment agency to ask what the billing code of DSM-IV-296.90 meant.

"Mood disorder—NOS (non-specified)," she answered.

"Not biplolar disorder?" I wanted to clarify.

"No."

I went back to Google and researched the DSM-IV bipolar disorder symptoms. The list was very specific. Jill had never matched any of the depressive symptoms. It seemed as though Dr. Bludonowitz was hoping one or more medications would

---

16 Medication guide. Lamictal (lamotrigine) tablets. Manufactured by DSM Pharmaceuticals, Inc. Registered trademark of GlaxoSmithKline.

17 Dosing guide, Abilify (Aripiprazole). Manufactured by Otsuka Pharmaceutical Co., Japan or Bristol-Myers Squibb Company, New Jersey. As of December 2007.

18 Medication guide, Risperdal (Risperidone). Manufactured by Janssen Pharmaceuticals division of Johnson & Johnson. As of December 2007.

work. "That's it," I decided, "I'm taking Jill *and* Kevin, who had been on them longer than Jill, off these medications. *Right now.*" I immediately set about reversing the dosing pattern we had followed. If nothing else, I figured we would be back to the behaviors we had seen by both kids over the years and somehow, some other time, we would get to the bottom of their individual idiosyncrasies.

But one day the school nurse presented me with a printed "Nursing Care Plan" for Jill's "anxiety, ineffective individual coping, and noncompliance" and requested that Jill and I both sign it. I guess the thinking was if we both signed a "contract" the "episodes of unresponsiveness, elevated blood pressure, apprehension, nervousness, tension; blocking of thoughts, hyper-attentiveness and no more non-compliance"[19] would simply disappear. "This is ridiculous." I fumed, "What if she really *can't* control any of it? What then?" It would not have mattered if I had said it aloud. In the school's mind Jill was trouble. I was so discouraged but did not know where else to turn. The "contract" would be only another thing for them to remind Jill that when she fainted she had not done what she had *promised* in writing to do. We signed the paper. The GOTCHAJill! game had begun. In their eyes, every time Jill collapsed, they had more ammunition. Intuitively, I knew she could no more control the fainting episodes and related outbursts than she could control a sneeze. I did not know when or how, but I *knew* someday they would be proved wrong. The school people might be familiar with children in general through their jobs and past work experience, but they didn't *know* Jill. Yes, she could be headstrong, but I also knew she was a diligent worker who tried her best, loved being in school, the band, chorus and playing basketball. Something was definitely not right. Anne asked if I would consider contacting the State's DCF Voluntary Services program for assistance. I said, "What the heck; maybe *they'll* be able to help figure out what was going on," and I made the call.

---

19 Benton* school nurse. Nursing Care Plan for Jill. November 26, 2007

CHAPTER 8

Stationary Front

For He will command His angels concerning
you to guard you in all your ways.
— **PSALM 91:11**

It was clear that school administrators would not acquiesce to Jill, the troublemaker, and knowing that school leaders did not believe she could not control her fainting episodes did not help matters.

One day, Jill was standing in front of Principal Anne's desk arguing her position about something when she suddenly fell "straight as a board" backward. But this time a new dimension to the mysterious set of circumstances was at play and no one but Jill, who was experiencing it, knew. Unnerved, she said nothing about it then but the occurrence prompted what happened next. Anne reported when Jill recovered she had become confrontational and attempted to run out of the office. Anne said she'd thrust her arm in front of Jill to stop her, but it had not. Jill ran through the halls to a stairwell where she sat down and would not budge. I was called to the school. Upon arrival, I learned the police had been called, too, and two officers had Jill engaged in conversation. After trying without success to get runaway Jill to come with me, I left her to the officers and made my way to the main office where the superintendent happened to be visiting the school. Clearly, Anne had already filled her in on what was going on. Exhausted, I looked at Maria* and shrugged; there was nothing more I felt I could do. The police officers were talking to Jill and all I could hope for was that she would eventually calm down and come with me. Maria haughtily snapped that Jill was to leave the school and not return "until she can get herself together" or something to that effect. About half an hour later, Jill and I left the school. I was pondering Maria's cryptic message and wishing to God that Jill could just stop fainting. Before too long I received a notice in the mail to attend a "Request for Parent to Attend a Section 504 Student Review Meeting" to be held in early December. I was confused. The last time I had received an "official" meeting request concerning Jill had been a special education (SE) meeting notice. Why the change? I wondered what was up, but I was not able to focus on it with all that was going on. I noted the meeting on the calendar and planned to be there.

By this time, both Kevin and Jill had finished the bipolar medication reduction. Kevin had improved, but not Jill. As had recently been evidenced, she continued fainting and having outbursts at school. I continued to bring her to see Dr. Wade after every episode. She did what most general practitioners do when seeking reasons for symptoms—order more tests and refer the patient to a specialist. Another electroencephalogram (EEG) test was arranged and this time Jill would be expected to sleep during the session, so she had to wake very early that morning to ensure she would be tired when it was time for the test. Then because Jill had complained about rapid or erratic heartbeat prior to every school episode, Dr. Wade ordered a cardio loop monitor for her to wear every day and night for a month. A technician came to our house and taught us how to use the monitor and gave us information for the school nurse about recording and transmitting information during school hours. Once again, we saw Dr. Garner,* the neurologist who had seen Jill as a toddler years before, once again she reported that Jill was in the neurological range for her age.

At about the same time, I began to wonder if anything in the school building might have something to do with Jill's fainting spells. After all, though kept scrupulously clean, the building itself *was* old (circa early 1930s) and I had noticed Jill's tendency for keeling over sometimes coincided with the building having been closed for more than overnight, as in for a long weekend. On one occasion, I asked the janitor if any cleaning out of the ordinary had been done during the three-day weekend. His said no and assured me the cleaning materials used throughout the district were "all natural," "green," and approved by the EPA. Nonetheless, Maria advised me that she had ordered an internal air quality (IAQ) environmental evaluation of the Benton building. "Thank goodness," I thought, "at least someone's trying to help." I sure hoped the evaluation would reveal *something*. In the meantime, Jill was found not to have Lyme Disease which was prevalent in our geographic area and I asked Dr. Wade if we should check for lead in Jill's blood. She did. The result was three out of a reference level of zero to nine, nothing to worry about. We could move on.

CHAPTER 9

Mixed Precipitation

People treat me different.
— LILO, DISNEY CHARACTER FROM "LILO & STICH"

Principal Anne, newly appointed director of student services Bart,* special education teacher Mrs. Morrell,* school psychologist Debbie, one of Jill's regular teachers, school nurse Mrs. Williams and I were in attendance for the 504 meeting. I still did not fully grasp the difference between special education (SE) and Section 504 categories. Jill had been considered an SE student since she had started preschool but she had been switched to the Section 504 category, and I did not know why. Something was drastically amiss with Jill—I just knew it. It was not possible, when she was routinely passing out and being carted off to doctors that she would be able to keep up with her academics. The teachers reported that Jill's academic standing was relatively stable in math, reading and writing. I brought up the fainting and behavioral episodes and said doctors could not understand any of it. Mrs. Williams provided an update regarding Jill's health issues including, of course, the fainting spells and added "…not that I think she's faking it."

No sooner had she uttered that when Debbie chortled, "Well, I am!" I was stunned—and momentarily speechless. When I recovered, I said I did not think Jill actually had bipolar disorder because the psychiatrist had not addressed specifics with me as to why she felt Jill fit the symptoms associated with that disorder.

Debbie said, "Psychiatrists are not therapists" and asked me if I knew what a psychiatrist's job really was. I bit my tongue and said nothing at the time but vowed to myself that someday, somehow I would prove that Jill's health issues had a medical base. I did not know how I was going to do that, but I would.

The next week I received a "Notice of Planning and Placement Team Meeting" (PPT) and was confused again. Was Jill or was she not considered to be a special ed student? The purpose of the meeting said, "Request for homebound instruction," and I realized that was what Maria had meant when she said Jill would have to leave the school and not return "until she can get herself together." During Jill's next therapy appointment, I told Iris what had happened at the school meeting. She was furious that a school psychologist would say a student was faking *anything*. "That was completely out of line and ridiculous for her to have said! She's not an MD. Ask her what job she's licensed for at that school. She really should be stopped from staying such stupid things!" Iris groused. The same school group assembled the next week; six educational professionals and me. Bart asked for an update of Jill's medical status. I said Jill had been weaned off the bipolar medications then turned to Debbie and asked, "What exactly are you licensed to do at this school?" "I'm a school psychologist" she stammered, not nearly as confident as she had been the week before. "Are you an MD?" I asked.

"No," she replied. "Then what gives you the right to say Jill is faking *anything*? Because even the MDs don't know what's going on!"

I grabbed my tote bag from under the meeting table and said, "Last week you asked if I knew what a psychiatrist's job was." I pulled out a large Ziploc bag filled with dozens of medication bottles prescribed to Jill and Kevin over the past several months and plopped it on the table. "Well, I *do* know what psychiatrists do. They're script writers and pill pushers." Then I began to cry. I appealed to Bart, "For what it's worth, I think Jill needs to remain in the special education category." He informed me there were fifteen special education categories and told me to come up with the one I felt was most suitable for Jill, put it in writing and send the letter to him, and the committee would meet to discuss it further. In a gesture of support, Mrs. Morrell pushed a paper in my direction and circled the list of SE categories. The group then went on to discuss whether special education or Section 504 status was more appropriate for Jill. None of them seemed to know.

When I asked about special needs students, Bart sneered, "What exactly do you mean by *special needs* students?" I knew my next call would be to the State Department of Education. I had had enough of this particular school group and told them it would be interesting to see if Jill stopped fainting now that she was off the bipolar meds. Bart, in turn, advised me that Jill was to immediately start homebound tutoring at the public library ten hours a week. It would serve as her education until her behavior improved, at which point she could return to Benton School.

The State's Department of Education representative said that Bart, along with every other administrator and special education person in that room, should have been able to clearly articulate eligibility for the Individuals with Disabilities Education Act (IDEA) and the 504 Rehabilitation Act. As far as having been told to "review the special education categories and put it in writing" which one(s) *I* thought Jill qualified for, he said flatly, "What a jerk."

For the next few months, Jill was schooled at the local library. Ten hours a week wasn't much, but the reprieve from Benton and all its negativity was what she needed. She did not faint once and the tutor had no complaints or concerns about her health, behavior, attention span or academic abilities. She resumed playing basketball for Littleton's Parks and Rec league at the Main Street Elementary School gymnasium where she enjoyed seeing several classmates. She was delighted when the coach designated her one of the team's center positions. It gave her a much needed purpose. Even so, her irritability quotient during practice sometimes seemed heightened, which we attributed to having been out of the social loop and to her age in general. Ed and I counseled her to curb her temper even though some of the other players clearly did not. We returned to life—sort of.

I turned my attention to researching school building internal environmental concerns. Most of what I found discussed mold, radon, carbon monoxide, carbon dioxide and pesticides. I soon learned that a Connecticut consortium piloted by former teachers who had dubbed themselves "the canary committee" because they had sustained debilitating illnesses due to internal toxin exposure in schools, had pushed until the State enacted laws directed at school districts which required them to establish health and safety commitments. I read the book, *What's Toxic, What's Not*, the authors of which happened to be employees of Connecticut's Department of Public Health. I called one of them to ask about chemicals used in the Littleton schools. He was stymied as to why Jill's odd symptoms occurred only when she was in school, offered regret he could not help further and wished us luck.

Finished with Dr. Bludonowitz, it was time to find another pediatric psychiatrist, primarily to help Kevin who continued to struggle with depression due to his brittle or hard to stabilize diabetes. I found Dr. Nyeer,* an old school doctor. I was glad to see he took his time getting to know his patients before jumping on the medication bandwagon. As my comfort level with him grew and Kevin began to show improvement, I shared with him what was happening with Jill at school and asked if he would evaluate her, too. Fortunately, he agreed and after doing so reported, "Jill is a happy kid, other than the scary health issues she has, she's happy at school where she likes the teachers, the work and the routine." His recommendation? "Just get her a good therapist." He did not feel she needed medication or to see a psychiatrist on a regular basis. Just like that, it was 180° from Dr. Bludonowitz's bipolar diagnosis.

Since plans were being made for the Benton building to be thoroughly inspected I thought we should at least see if Jill had specific, identifiable allergies. I took her to the allergist who has treated both Ed since the late1970s and Kevin for much of his life. After submitting to a series of vile skin scratch tests, Jill was found to have low-level environmental allergies to grasses and trees. Subsequent food allergy testing indicated she was allergic only to cashews. Jill immediately decided she would never knowingly eat them. We did not pursue the chemical reactivity testing and, given what I eventually learned about her reactivity to certain chemicals, it proved to be a good decision.

About this time, Jill and I revisited the "running-through-the-Benton-School-halls" scenario that had caused me and the police to have been called to the school. Her recollection sent me reeling. After having fallen backward "straight as a board" Jill said she was left lying on the floor, unresponsive and unable to move, but somehow still able to hear what was going on around her. She said Anne called Debbie from an adjoining office. Then she heard both women step over her. She recounted a discussion in which the administrators said she was faking everything for attention and that there was nothing wrong with her. Unable to move or talk,

Jill was livid. When she was able to get up off the floor, she did not tell the women what she had heard, *"They wouldn't have believed me anyway,"* but became confrontational and that was when she attempted to run out of the office. She said Mrs. Brody grabbed her by the arm to stop her. Anne had said she merely thrust her arm out across Jill for the same purpose. Obviously, it did not matter because it was not enough to stop Jill. She had heard with her own ears the mocking accusation she was faking that the principal and school psychologist said. Incensed, she ran to a stairwell. I came. Then the police came. I was dumbfounded, "You could *hear* but you couldn't *move?*"

"Yeah. It was really weird. Then when I could move, I got out of there as fast as I could," Jill replied.

"Oh dear God—how much weirder would things get?" I worried.

Meanwhile, the school nurse had determined that Jill needed an eye exam so I arranged an appointment. The optometrist said while Jill's vision had always had an asymmetrical deficit, it had become much more pronounced since her last exam and her vision had developed a weird (my word, not his) way of processing near and far, prompting him to mention it to me. He asked whether Jill had been ill or taken any medications since her last exam. I explained about the bipolar diagnosis and the medication regimen. He said psychotropic drugs are known to have that type of neurological impact and prescribed bifocal lenses. I envisioned eyestrain and headaches as her brain made accommodations for that, too. What else would she have to contend with because she had taken those hateful drugs?

The results of the Benton School IAQ evaluation came back. It reported everything was in accordance with state and federal guidelines. I read through the report and highlighted a few things, but without knowledge to challenge anything specific, filed it away. Within a few months, Jill's tutoring at the public library ended and she was headed back to Benton School to finish sixth grade. No doubt, all involved were apprehensive.

CHAPTER 10

Worm Moon

*Be your weird, courageous, brilliant self
every single day. No matter what.*
— **ANONYMOUS**

Jill was okay for a couple of weeks following her return to Benton School. But then the fainting spells returned. When the call came this time, I arrived at the school and went directly to the nurse's office where I found Jill, unresponsive, on a stretcher. As she was wheeled to the ambulance, I noticed her jaw working as though she was chewing something. I thought, "Could this be the seizure activity they've told me about?" and focused on her face and body positioning. It was unusual for me to see her at this early stage. I usually did not see her until I arrived at the hospital—and by then she was generally alert and on the way to being released. MedCity ED's discharge papers usually noted hyperventilation as the reason for her appearance in the ED. Suddenly, a memory light bulb lit. Years before, a woman I worked with was prone to hyperventilating and periodically passed out. The EMTs would arrive, look at her and say, "She's hyperventilating." Then they would administer oxygen until she revived. One time the EMTs explained how, because oxygen is diverted from nonessential places in the body to the heart and brain when hyperventilating, the patient's hands often form into claw positions. I looked at Jill's hands. No claw. "Hmmm," I thought, "maybe instead of hyperventilation, was it possible for the opposite to occur? The opposite of hyper is hypo, right? I wonder, is there such a condition as *hypo*ventilation?" and added another topic to my "to-be-Googled" list.

After tutoring, Jill's role as bully target was cemented upon her return to Benton school. Each morning I dropped her off at school and watched the exclusion game long familiar to 'tween girls being played. One day she said a boy had spit in her face and it had not been the first time he had done so. She tried her best not to tattle and to ignore such behavior. But the spitting incident was too much. She did not complain but I put the grievance in writing because calls to the principal had not accomplished anything. Dr. Nyeer's opinion was that while of strong character, Jill did not have a bully mentality. Instead, he said, she had a sense of vulnerability and lack of malice about her that some kids were able to sniff out in order to feed their own need for control or power. It made sense to me. Vulnerability does not mean one does not have a backbone. Jill had the confidence and courage to speak out, and I was glad she refused to be pegged in a hole that others put and expected her to stay in. As the school year wound down, Jill tried her best to work her way back into the routine of school, but the bullying ramped up. A classmate whose locker was adjacent to Jill's slammed her—hard—into her open locker door. Apparently, the gym teacher heard the commotion as well as the expletive hurled at her because he ordered the boy to the principal's office. Jill was left with an angry red welt down her back. When I called Anne to complain about the incident, she said the boy would be spoken to and that his locker would be moved but, by the end of the school year several weeks later nothing had changed.

Another 504 meeting was set to plan for Jill's advancement to middle school. For the first time, I chose not to attend a school meeting for one of my children because I refused to subject myself to that unprofessional group again.

Along with the uptick in bullying, the fainting episodes returned and escalated. Once again, Jill would black out for twenty minutes or more at a time. The last episode for that school year happened on a beautiful early summer day outside on the athletic field. I was called to stand vigil with the nurse. "Just like Dorothy in the field of poppies outside the Emerald City," I thought when I saw her lying so still on the ground. We sat with Jill for the better part of an hour before she came to and slowly sat up. I helped her into the car and as we drove off, the school bell signaled the end of the school day as a single tear rolled down Jill's face.

Jill received her final report card for sixth grade; two Bs and the core classes of reading, writing, arithmetic, science and social studies hovered around C-D grades. She was not thrilled with the results, but I thought it was pretty good considering she had spent so much energy on just surviving the school year.

The DCF's Voluntary Services social worker assigned to support Jill and us proved to be one our best allies to date. Bridget* had no idea what was going on with Jill medically but recommended Vanessa* as a potential therapist to help Jill deal with the strange occurrences. Vanessa and Jill clicked from the start. Soon, Bridget called to say that because other families required the department's immediate assistance, she had to close our file. Vanessa signed on as Jill's LCSW (Licensed Clinical Social Worker) and tolerated my research predilection. She stuck with us while I investigated and reported on every possibility, no matter how ambiguous for Jill's varied symptoms. One of the first conditions I bounced off her was the hypoventilation theory. The thought of hypoventilation kept coming back to me: "…caused by medical conditions, holding one's breath or by drugs typically taken in overdose,"[20] according to Wikipedia. The phrase "medical conditions" was not

---

20 Wikipedia. Hypoventilation. https://en.wikipedia.org/wiki/Hypoventilation.

lost on me and neither was the reference to drugs and the fact that the condition could be life threatening. "Could Jill's fainting episodes somehow be related to her not being able to get an adequate amount of oxygen to her brain?" The idea seemed plausible to me and I could not shake it.

I came across a condition called obesity hypoventilation. Jill *was* overweight and frequently complained about having blurry vision, one of the symptoms. But I did not know if she snored or had sleep apnea because I did not sleep in the same room with her so that drifted to the back burner. Next, I came across Congenital Central Hypoventilation Syndrome, a rare neurological disorder characterized by inadequate breathing *and* impaired bowel function known as Hirschsprung's Disease, or Haddad Syndrome. "Were these also possibilities?" I wondered. Some symptoms matched, but a lot did not. There was also vasovagal syncope, fainting when one stands for long periods of time. This was also not likely because Jill had fainted while sitting on bleachers, on a chair in the lunch room and seated at a desk.

As I continued to research, Jill looked forward to summer. She had signed up for the Slamma Jamma Basketball Summer Camp to be held in the relatively newly constructed and much ballyhooed middle school building about a week after the school year ended. The first three days of the camp went fine. Jill reveled in the entire basketball team-bonding experience and was thrilled to get to know players from the high school team. One of the taller teammates, she often played center position and loved it. She practiced doggedly in our driveway and began dream talking about playing for the highly acclaimed University of Connecticut's women's basketball team in the future. Then on only the third day of camp, while sitting with the other players during snack time, Jill fainted. Once again, she was on her way to MedCity ED. The discharge paper cited: "Fainting (syncope)…occurs when you lose consciousness for a short time and are alert when you wake up…caused by a sudden decrease of blood flow to the brain."[21] It listed nearly a dozen potential reasons for that blood flow decrease and recommended contacting Jill's doctor if she had confusion, increased light-headedness, increased fainting episodes or any new or severe symptoms.[22]

Jill received a certificate for successfully completing the basketball camp; it was the first and last recognition she would get for participating in the game she had come to love. Summer vacation had only begun, but her fun was over. With frightening fervor, the devil had come to dance. We did not know it then, but the clue that would ultimately break the code about her bizarre illness was about to make a grand entrance. Emergency department visits and calls to her pediatrician's office were about to escalate with horrifying intensity.

---

21 MedCity* ED. Discharge summary. June 16, 2008
22 Ibid.

CHAPTER 11

Sunspots

You never know how strong you are until being strong is the only choice you have.
— ANONYMOUS

I ended up getting off the bipolar meds. Next thing you know I was fine. No attacks. My behavior even was great. So we thought, 'okay it was the bipolar meds.' I had tutoring for a couple of months then went back to regular school around December. I was fine from January until about June, except for when I fainted that time on the baseball field. I signed up for a week of basketball camp and couldn't wait to get away from Benton School and all the drama there. I needed a break. So I went to the camp and got to meet a lot of the older basketball players who were really nice to me. But on Thursday I ended up being rushed back to the ER because once again I fainted. After that attack I was fine for a month. Then all of a sudden a new but weird symptom occurred. In July I was so active, practicing my basketball, walking, swimming and jogging. I was doing this until I got the most horrible stomachache ever."[23]

One evening Jill fearfully asked where her appendix was located. Ed's appendix had burst several years earlier so when he pointed to where hers would be, it became obvious that a trip to the emergency department at Nutmeg Hospital for Children was necessary. An abdominal CT scan was ordered and Jill was admitted for observation. On continuous IV fluids and morphine, she improved. Other than inflamed abdominal lymph nodes, nothing out of the ordinary had been found and Jill was discharged the next day. A couple of days later, we attended a family picnic. Shortly after swimming and trying her hand at a few games, Jill complained of bad pain in her lower abdomen and curled up on a lawn chair. We went home where her

---

23 Jill's journal. August 2008.

pain continued. A day later, it spread to include severe back and shoulder pain—and diarrhea. She tried desperately to hold on but evening found us back at NHC'S ED. Several medical staff members came and went as we watched the clock march on: 9:00, 10:00, midnight, 1:00 a.m. Jill was wide awake and unable to sleep because of the relentless pain. To help take our minds off things, I tried various ways to amuse her. I picked up what looked like a fuzzy caterpillar from the floor; it turned out to be a fluff off someone's hairweave. Overtired and silly, Jill and I dissolved into hysterical laughter. The clock ticked on. 2:00 a.m. She turned the television on and off. I read whatever I could find. Finally, she was released. Discharge instructions noted: "Please follow-up with your therapist to discuss coping strategies for stress and illness."[24] They may just as well have written, "NUT CASE" across the paper. I had a sickening feeling that we would be back before too long.

The abdominal pain and diarrhea continued for the next several days and within the week had ramped up. Jill showed me a reddish ring, about ¼ inch in width encircling her entire abdomen. It resembled a mark left by a pant drawstring, but without the indentation. She said it did not hurt. Dr. Wade did not know what it was. She ordered a stool culture and recommended I get Culturelle for Jill "to help with the diarrhea." That night, Jill's unrelenting symptoms landed us back at NHC'S ED. The attending physician asked me to step out of the room with her. "Here it comes," I thought. Sure enough. Ever so gently she asked if Jill was a kid who liked attention. I replied "Sometimes—like most kids, but this is different. I don't know what's happening, but I know something is very wrong." I said Dr. Wade had recommended a product called Culturelle for Jill to try. The ED doctor handed me a prescription slip for it and suggested I pick it up at a pharmacy in the morning. Jill and I drove home well after midnight; she was still in toe-curdling pain.

Dr. Wade referred Jill to a pediatric gastroenterologist. Dr. Haynes* gently manipulated Jill's abdomen. She still had pain though it ebbed and flowed in severity. He recommended endoscopy and colonoscopy tests be done to see what was going on inside. Coincidentally, it was time for Jill's annual von Willebrand check up with Dr. O'Connor. He reviewed the CT scan taken when it was thought she had appendicitis and noted that her ovaries appeared to be polycystic and she was slightly anemic. He recommended we switch her to a vitamin with iron. Then he mentioned that Jill's red blood cells were "oddly" misshapen but did not know why. For a hematologist to say someone's red blood cells were distorted and did not know why unnerved me.

It was becoming more and more evident that no medical professional we had seen had any clue about what was going on with Jill, so I continued to research anything and everything remotely related to abdominal problems. I knew I was turning into a physician's nightmare, but I also knew that Jill was not a hypochondriac so I persevered. During a therapy session, Vanessa mentioned being a fan of the television show "Medical Mysteries." We tuned in and within a few segments, Jill had focused on gallbladder issues and began to worry she was having gallbladder attacks. Of the fifteen gallbladder attack symptoms she found on websites, she was

24 NCH* ED. Discharge instructions. July 28, 2008

experiencing thirteen of them; only "previous/frequent use of laxatives," and "pain between the shoulder blades" remained unchecked on the list. She had never had access to laxatives, and certainly did not need them with the ongoing diarrhea, and though she had had shoulder pain, it was not between the shoulder blades. A different "Medical Mysteries" episode featured Hunter Chiari Type 1 Malformation with several symptoms reminiscent of Jill's infant and toddler stages. But since the MRI that Dr. Bludonowitz had ordered months earlier showed no abnormalities related to that disorder, it was scratched off the list. A family friend suffered from fibromyalgia. I wondered if children could develop fibromyalgia, too. A colleague of Dr. Wade's happened to call to check on Jill, so I asked her about it. "No. She doesn't present with the symptoms associated with fibromyalgia," was her answer.

"Then, what could it be?" I asked.

"We're still not sure," was the reply.

The 2008-2009 school year was rapidly approaching. Jill was excited about attending the new middle school building, but she was apprehensive because of what had happened throughout sixth grade and the fainting episode she had had during the basketball camp held in that school. Dr. Wade gave us a letter for the school nurse and administration that said, "Jill has fainting spells of undetermined etiology. An extensive workup has been inconclusive. Precautions at this time [include] a modified gym program; i.e. no climbing, no swimming and allowing her to stop activities if she becomes dizzy, or her arms shake (symptoms that sometimes precede her fainting)."[25] Given the recent spate of symptoms, she also recommended yet another neurology consultation.

My academic goal is to stay in school as long as I can and not get sick. 20 years from now I hope to be known as a retired popular teen singer w/good money to be able to buy a good space where I could live. After my singing career I hope to go to medical school and help people out with even the hardest medical mysteries. I have already in a way helped begin my singing career by going to singing lessons and writing my own songs. But I still need to start a band, get an agent, get a manager, and my grades need to improve.[26]

In keeping with my annual custom, I emailed Littleton Middle School's principal on the first day of seventh grade to request a meeting. Mr. Tony Dithers* replied that a 504 meeting should be arranged so we "could all be on the same page." Jill euphorically sailed through her first day of seventh grade. But on only the second day, she fainted. Over the next seven school days, she fainted three times. She wore the cardio loop monitor Dr. Wade had ordered, and the school nurse faxed information following each fainting episode to the doctor's office. Then she missed a day for the endoscopy and colonoscopy procedures. That done, Jill was certain she would feel better. Instead, after spending only nine days in seventh grade, the punishing abdominal pain and nausea were back and on the tenth day she fainted again. Later that night she complained about having blood in her stool, but Dr. Haynes had warned of that possibility after a colonoscopy so we were not overly concerned. She also complained of reflux and said it tasted of blood. The gastroenterologist

---

25 Dr. Wade.* Letter to LMS* administration. August 28, 2008.
26 Jill. School writing assignment about life goals. August 31, 2008.

returned my call and suggested we "give it a few more days" regarding the resolution of the blood in her stool and prescribed Nexium for the reflux. Not only had the fainting and convulsing episodes returned within days of being in the middle school building, but also extreme abdominal pain, constant nausea and bouts of vomiting made Jill feel so bad that I called her in sick most days

Our search for the source of Jill's medical problems continued. A "Medical Mysteries" segment featured a disorder known as Sphincter of Oddi Dysfunction (SOD). Jill identified several symptoms that matched hers and became convinced SOD was her problem. "Why can't I get exploratory surgery?" she whined. I explained that exploratory surgery had been replaced by modern diagnostic equipment and/or tests and was rarely used nowadays. She remained adamant, "Unless they go inside, they're *never* going to find out what I have!"

To appease Jill, I called Dr. Haynes to ask specifically about SOD. He responded, "That's not part of a colonoscopy and no inflammation was noted, making it unlikely the sphincter was a problem. Besides, SOD can be very painful to diagnose," and did not recommend we pursue it. The doctor who had been featured in the "Medical Mysteries" segment was affiliated with Haven City Hospital within reasonable driving distance from our home. I recorded that information in my ever-present notebook for future reference.

Getting to and staying in school for an entire day became a real problem for Jill. I made an appointment with the school district's physician for a consultation to not only make him aware of Jill's odd symptoms, but to also see if maybe *he* had any idea what might be causing them. Ed, Jill and I met with Dr. Reid* to review Jill's symptoms, medical appointment schedule and checkered school attendance record of the past year and to discuss her inability to stay upright in school. Nothing registered for the doctor whose final response was, "Keep pursuing avenues with Dr. Wade. Do your best to stay in school. Good luck."

Two days later, the horrific abdominal pain was back. Jill could not be quieted and I finally drove her to Haven City Hospital's ED. The charge nurse took one look at her, felt her extremely cold hands and immediately admitted her to a room. The attending doctor could offer nothing more than what had been said by so many others. I mentioned the SOD possibility, told him about the recent endoscopy and colonoscopy and once again filled a doctor in on the many symptoms, doctors' and specialists' comments and test results. Though very kind, in the end he said the same as all the others, "Keep looking. Best of luck." Jill was no better off after we left than when we had arrived. The drive home was quiet; it was so hard not to be devastatingly discouraged. Thoroughly exhausted, after trudging slowly up the stairs to her bedroom, Jill finally slept. Sleep offered a temporary escape from the pain. The weekend was difficult. Jill had given up complaining about the pain— there was nothing we could do to offer relief. The medical community could not help. Tylenol had no effect. Jill mentioned several times that the morphine given to her when it was thought she might have appendicitis was the only thing that had helped even though she hated the weird, disorienting feeling associated with it. But it sure seemed as though morphine might be what Jill needed for the pain.

Then, one Monday morning, I realized that Jill was not up and getting ready for school as usual. By 7 a.m. I went to her room and found her still sleeping, which I found odd because the radio was on. I shook her and turned the radio up louder, then louder still; she slept on. I shouted to her and became frantic. She would not wake up. I ran to the phone and called Dr. Wade's office. The covering doctor said, "Well, if she won't wake up, call 911." "Again? *Not again?*" I was distraught. He replied, "At this point, that's all you can do." Ed arrived home after delivering Kevin to school. He, too, tried to wake Jill by pulling her up into a sitting position. She flopped down. He yelled to her. We both yelled at her. Nothing. I called 911. The EMTs came, administered oxygen and took her to MedCity's ED. By the time I arrived there she was awake. I asked if she remembered anything from that morning. She remembered waking to her alarm then nothing until she had awakened in the hospital. It was now about 8:45 a.m. and she had "come to" just before I had arrived. That meant she had been out for over two hours—the longest stretch of unresponsiveness she had had so far. And what was so terrifying was that the symptoms had happened *at home.* "What in God's name was going on?"

As I agonized aloud in the hospital room about what was causing Jill's weird attacks the attending ED doctor cautioned, "When you hear hoof beats, look for horses—don't look for zebras." I was so discouraged. The bizarre episodes were making our family crazy. Swirling questions seemed always to be on my mind: "Was it possible the ever-present abdominal pains were somehow connected to the fainting episodes Jill was experiencing? And if so, how?" My mind raced back to toddler Jill's head and abdominal problems and I wondered, "Had a connection between the brain and the gut been figured out over the past ten years or so? What about narcolepsy? Was it even possible for a kid to have that sleeping disorder?" I went back to Google and Bing. Up popped various articles but nothing really seemed to leap out at me, but I figured I would ask the doctor about narcolepsy, too. And still another possibility came up: hypersomnia in bipolar depression. Here we went again with the bipolar business. Besides, Jill still did not appear to be depressed though it certainly would have been understandable if she were. We were scheduled to meet with the second- (actually third-) opinion neurologist the next day. That night I prayed *something* would come out of the appointment.

CHAPTER 12

Thunder Clouds

The eye sees only what the mind can comprehend.
— HENRI BERGSTON

Ever since I got sick, my mom talks a lot about time. She says there's our time, there's school time, there's hospital time and there's God's time. When it's my time I try to get one step closer to making my dream of being a singer come true, when it's hospital time you never know when you'll get out but they give you the help you need; the school time well, we all know what that's about whether we like it or not it's what helps us to reach our goals in life and finally there is God's time, the one who in the end calls all the shots.[27]

In spite of persistent abdominal pain, Jill was cordial and responsive during the neurology examination. I explained to the doctor about the endoscopy she had had as a toddler and said the neurologist at the time had mentioned that a connection between the gut and the brain had been acknowledged but was not well-established. I wondered aloud, "There's *must* be more known about it by now." Dr. Tourtellotte* responded, "The only thing I can think of that connects neurological problems with the abdomen is something called porphyria—but it's very rare." She waved a hand dismissively, "Don't worry, she couldn't have it. Like I said, it's extremely rare—and she's too young."

I stashed the info in my head and asked, "Is there a test to determine whether or not she has this rare disease?" Dr. Tourtellotte left the room and came back with a completed lab slip. She had gone to look up the spelling of the enzyme porphobilinogen deaminase (PBG-D), the blood level of which she said could diagnose porphyria. And to rule out the question of narcolepsy, she suggested another EEG, one that would require a controlled setting with lots of stimulation so that Jill's brain

---

27 Jill's journal. October 2008.

waves could be monitored in the event she had another fainting or sleeping episode, which they would be attempting to provoke. The neurologist handed over the test orders for blood, twenty-four hour urine and the EEG tests. She also suggested I take a couple of weeks to check with other doctors we had seen to ask if there were any other conditions to look for so Jill would only have to have one blood draw. She appeared not too concerned about the diagnosis so I made a light comment but the doctor's solemn response, "It might be something insidious," really scared me.

Nonetheless, I left elated because I had been given a *clue*. God *had* answered my prayers, "Thank you, thank you, thank you Lord," I praised. My hope was beyond measure for the first time in so long. I could not wait to start researching. While Jill had the word pegged the first time she heard it, I had trouble pronouncing it. "Mom, it's *not* pro-fear-ee-ya, it's *poor*-FEAR-ee-ya!" she corrected over and over until I got it. As it happened, the next day we had an appointment with Dr. Rice's associate, Dr. Weiderman.* "Porphyria," he said when I told him, "tough. Rare. But an absolute possibility which means *don't* wait two weeks—get the tests done ASAP." Within a couple of days, Jill's blood had been drawn and a completed twenty-four hour urine jug had been left at NHC's lab. I had already begun researching and soon learned that porphyria is actually a group of metabolic genetic disorders that affect the liver and are separated into two distinct categories, the acute porphyrias and the cutaneous porphyrias. My mind raced, "A *genetic* disorder! Jill's adopted. *If* she had a type of porphyria, had it come from her birth mother or birth father?" Did it really matter? I was riveted and took notes from many sources about the blood-building process that takes place in the liver's home biosynthetic pathway that involves eight sequential enzymes, one for each of the eight porphyrias, how porphyrin precursors and intermediates known as aminolevulinic acid (ALAs) convert to porphobilinogen (PBGs), and that iron is converted into protoporphyrin by the enzyme ferrochelatase to form heme, which enables the cells to use oxygen.

I found the reference to oxygen interesting because it had intrigued me since early on in Jill's ordeal. Then, "A common feature in the porphyrias is the accumulation in the body of porphyrins or porphryin precursors, [which are natural body chemicals but normally do not accumulate]."[28] I was hooked on learning more about these strange disorders and set about making lists of symptoms for each type of porphyria. I soon discounted the cutaneous porphyrias which are characterized by skin reactions to bright light. Jill had spent many hours outside, at the beach or swimming in our pool and never had a problem being in the sun. She had never developed lesions or blisters or complained of painful skin of any type; in fact, she had never even been sunburned. Reading about the cutaneous porphyrias, I remembered seeing a television news program years before about children who could play outdoors only after the sun went down. No, that did not fit Jill at all. But some of the symptoms associated with the acute porphryias definitely matched. Described as neurovisceral in nature, I cobbled together a list of symptoms from various websites and scrutinized each to consider how or if it related to Jill's complaints:

---

28 *Porphyria, Acute Intermittent.* WebMD. http://www.webmd.com/a-to-z-guides/porphyria-acute-intermittent.

- pain in abdomen, progressing to back and/or thighs (*yes—**very** bad stomachaches*)

- darkened urine (tea- or wine-colored) (*no.* I hadn't seen that and Jill had never mentioned it)

- severe gastrointestinal/liver/kidney/uterine pain (*yes*)

- lymphocytic inflammation (*yes*)

- nausea (*yes*)

- vomiting (*yes*)

- constipation or diarrhea (*yes—diarrhea*)

- numbness and/or tingling (*yes*)

- acute neuropathy (*yes*)

- central nerve paralysis (*yes*)

- cardiac arrhythmias and tachycardia (*yes*)

- respiratory distress (*yes*); can move quickly to respiratory insufficiency

- depression and personality changes (*yes*)

- disorientation (*yes*)

- agitation (*yes*)

- confusion during attack; difficulty remembering details (*yes*)

- bizarre, even disruptive behavior (*yes*) (super)

- mental disturbances, including mania, anxiety, paranoia and hallucinations (*yes*)

- seizures/convulsions (*yes*)

- muscular weakness (*yes*)

- paralysis (*yes*)

- coma (*no*—but those weird, lengthy "sleeping periods" *were* worrisome).

Having to look up the majority of the medical terms made the research all the more tedious but, even so, something was beginning to come together. Of the twenty-two symptoms I had identified, Jill had "presented," as is said in medical vernacular, at one time or another with twenty of them so I forged ahead. I read member stories posted on the American Porphyria Foundation (APF) website and searched for other stories on the Internet. Though hard not to jump to conclusions, the bulk of Jill's symptoms (nervous system involvement often with severe abdominal pain, vomiting, peripheral neuropathy and mental disturbances) sat squarely in the acute porphyria category: Acute Intermittent Porphyria (AIP), Variegate Porphyria (VP), Hereditary Coproporphyria (HCP) or ŏ-Aminolevulinic Acid Dehydratase (ALAD or ADP) Porphyria. Attempting to narrow the field, I learned that AIP attacks could be precipitated [triggered] by "the four M's: medication, menstruation, malnutrition, maladies." [29] I considered each as it related to Jill:

1) *Medication:* She had been taking bipolar medications when all this started and over the ensuing months had been given various medications for one problem or another. Perhaps some or all of them had contributed to her problems?

2) *Menstruation:* She had started her menses at age ten, but I had not noticed if the weird "attacks" coordinated with her menstrual cycle.

3) *Malnutrition:* At the beginning of sixth grade Jill had not only begun to skip meals in an effort to lose weight, but she had also inexplicably sometimes lost her appetite and had no interest in eating. Would simply missing a few meals now and then be considered "malnutrition"?

4) *Maladies:* She often complained of various aches or pains, from earaches and sore throat to achy leg, arm and body muscles, or that the flu was threatening; oddly, her body temperature sometimes fluctuated during those times.

I focused on AIP and uncovered information about the phenomenal level of pain its attacks can provoke: "[abdominal] pain could be extremely severe, frequently out of proportion to physical signs and almost always requires opioids to reduce it to tolerable levels. Pain should be treated as early as medically possible due to its severity. Nausea can be severe [and] may respond to medications but is sometimes intractable." [30] Jill's abdominal pain appeared to be extraordinary, and only morphine, an opioid, had brought her relief the time it was thought she might have appendicitis. My head bells were clanging as a memory of baby Jill howling in pain, her legs pulled up to her abdomen, came to mind. Then the dime dropped, the light bulb lit and I got it. My own gut and head were in sync. Based on the symptoms that had dogged her for the past several months, the four M's, the similarity between Jill's symptoms, the many AIP member stories I had read on the Internet, and intuition, I *knew* Jill had Acute Intermittent Porphyria. Now, how was I ever going to prove *that*?

The blood test results came back with a PBG-D level of 6.9. The comments section of the report stated the expected value for porphyria was 7 and 6.0-6.9 was deemed "indeterminate." The accompanying interpretation stated, "In this sample, the erythrocyte porphobilinogen deaminase (PBG-D) activity is minimally decreased. Enzymatic activity levels in this range have been described both in affected and healthy individuals...." [31] The twenty-four-hour urine test interpretation

29 *Acute Intermittent Porphyria.* Wikipedia. http://en.wikipedia.org/wiki/Acute_intermittent_porphryia
30 *Porphyria.*Wikipedia. http://house.wikia.com/wiki/Porphyria
31 Jill's Porphyria Profile. Mayo Clinic, received by NCH. October 7, 2008

was that no acute intermittent porphyria was detected. "Could the 6.9 out of an expected value of 7.0 be considered 'borderline,' if there is such a thing where porphyria is concerned?" I asked Dr. Wade. She emphatically answered, "No. The urine test was conclusive. But," she continued, "the sample might not have been handled according to clinical expectations, contributing to the outcome." To my "Mom Doctor" way of thinking, 6.9 out of 7 was a pretty good indication we were on the right track. So she ordered another test. My head was swirling. "How many times was Jill going to have to submit to tests and evaluations before this frightening ride would be over? *Would* it ever be over?" As it turned out, it would, but not before many more challenges and a lot more knowledge came our way. I wondered what actually defined an attack? When Jill fainted? When her body was "shaking"? When her heart was racing? When she was nauseous and vomiting? When her abdomen hurt so badly? All of the above?

I set about collecting every medical and academic paper, invoice or report we had acquired since Jill had first seen Dr. Bludonowitz. Then I developed a computerized log of episodes, appointments, tests and evaluations. I compared and scrutinized months of data but could not identify patterns. "Dear Lord, what, what, WHAT in the world was going on?" Every day and night, my thoughts and prayers revolved around Jill's condition. It seemed I knew nothing more than I did a year ago, but at least my "event log" better prepared me to answer professionals' questions, not that it made a difference. Most doctors still looked at us as though we were speaking Martian.

In spite of everything going on and the exhausting, debilitating pain Jill lived with, she had a new passion. She wanted to take singing lessons. Truly motivated, she identified a singing teacher not far from us. It was obvious she was willing to work at this new interest. Before long I had agreed to let her start singing lessons with Lora.* As it turned out, Lora was recovering from a long-term illness herself and readily agreed to my request for schedule flexibility. She also told of her success with alternative diagnostic techniques and homeopathic treatments, which appealed to my predilection for alternative treatments.

Lora tried from the start to dissuade Jill from the professional music industry, but it did not work. Jill wanted to sing professionally and was completely infatuated with the Jonas Brothers and with the fact that the Jonases were devout Christians. She was particularly smitten with Nick, the youngest of the three singing siblings who, like her brother Kevin, had Type 1 diabetes. Hospitalized during the appendicitis scare, she had missed the chance to attend a Jonas Brothers concert but attacked her ancient piano with gusto, belting out JoBro songs. Jill was happiest when singing, but frankly, her singing and piano playing combinations at times assaulted the eardrums. Kevin complained nonstop about it, but I shushed him. If nothing else, I knew singing would take Jill's mind off the health problems that plagued her. She suffered every day with crushing abdominal pain and endured frequent, humiliating fainting episodes at school. "The least we can do is put up with her singing," I told him and prayed for the time when her voice would mature.

CHAPTER 13

Blustery Winds

Some people just suck the nice right out of me.
— ANONYMOUS

The subject of Jill continuing to miss school raised its head. A 504 meeting had been scheduled, but Jill was not one iota better. In fact, she was worse. Intending to be more prepared than I had been for the Benton School meetings, I had researched federal guidelines for the Special Education (SE) Other Health Impairment (OHI) classification and Section 504 of the Rehabilitation Act of 1973 laws. Jill had started preschool with the SE, speech and language (S&L) designation. In order to release her from Special Education, by federal law a planning and placement team (PPT) meeting should have been arranged and the district would have had to make its case and request Ed's and my approval to make that change. At that point, there was no doubt we would have approved the change; as taxpayers, we knew special education services cost the school district taxpayers over and above "typical" student's needs. However nothing had ever been broached with us, so I was unaware that Littleton had switched Jill's educational status to 504.

Vanessa was slated to accompany me to the meeting to recommend that Jill receive homebound tutoring at least until a medical diagnosis was determined. A bleak, rainy day arrived. Jill was home nursing her daily bout of debilitating abdominal pain. Vanessa's car was not in the parking lot; it looked like she was not going to make it after all. The meeting started with principal Tony,* the school nurse, the school psychologist, Jill's math teacher and me in attendance. So they could better understand Jill's questionable health status, I began by telling the group about her fainting episode at the summer basketball camp held in that school; the new and worsening symptoms; the fairly recent neurologist appointment and the porphyria question that I hoped would be answered soon. I said Jill was sick at home and though her therapist was not able to make the meeting, she was in favor of resuming tutoring. Going with my experience with the give and take format of past school meetings, I said my research into the porphyrias made me believe we were moving in the right direction regarding Jill's health problem. "I don't how I know, I just know she has an acute porphyria," I said. "Now, I have to prove it." They all stared at me. Guidance counselor Yvette* breezed into the room and asked for an update. School psychologist Karen* told her I had just asked about resuming homebound tutoring for Jill.

Yvette asked, "Oh, you're going to home school Jill?" I replied, "No, I'm asking the district to resume tutoring until her medical condition stabilizes or until we get a diagnosis. Her therapist, who can't be here today, strongly recommends that." At that, Tony derided me about "coming in here with all of this paperwork" and mockingly repeated my statement, "I don't know how I know, I just know" that Jill had porphyria.

Then he got nasty. "Jill needs to be in school," he snarled, pounding the table with each syllable. Continuing with a scornful tone and motioning a quick, brushing action beneath his nose, he said, "If she gets a little nosebleed, she can go to the nurse." He had obviously never seen a von Willebrand nosebleed and by saying that, confirmed that Littleton must have reclassified Jill when she had been diagnosed with von Willebrand—without having involved us. As the conversation progressed from bad to worse Tony roared, "Jill needs to be in school!"

I leapt to my feet, "*You want her in school? You got her--*and you better provide a wheelchair because if she faints and hurts herself or grabs onto another student while attempting to steady herself and causes that student to fall YOU'VE got problems!" I snatched my belongings and headed for the door, "*I'll be back with Jill—and you better have that damn chair ready when we get here.*" As I reached for the door handle, Tony held out a paper for my signature. I recoiled, "Are you *serious*? There is *no way* I will sign *anything*. I totally disagree with everything that has happened here. You want something checked off? *Do it yourself.*" I stormed out through the pouring rain to the car and drove home where I informed Jill she had to get dressed because she *had to go to school*. She was terrified, horribly pale and in extreme pain. During the drive to school I told her for her own and other students' safety, she had to use a wheelchair while in school. She was so demoralized. It was all I could do to hold back my tears. As we walked into the building, Tony came with the wheelchair and Jill sank into it. She had not showered that day, her clothes were a mess, she looked like she had seen a ghost but, by God, she was *in school*. I went back through the lobby seething. The "WHACK-A-Jill!" game had begun.

Jill lasted only a few hours in class before ending up in the nurse's office. Over the next few days we tried again, and again. Vanessa advised me to call Jill in sick whenever she felt she could not make it to school—every day, if need be. She was in favor of continuing the tutoring and not forcing a child in medical distress to attend school. I did my best to get Jill into school because she *had* to be there. She really tried to make it through her classes but the unbearable pains forced her to tears—and the nurse's office—time and again. The other students were clearly curious and wary. Some stared, others looked away, unable to meet her gaze, except one boy who made a point of sneering at her whenever he caught her eye which added to her humiliation. To make everything worse, Jill was barely getting any sleep. As I continued to learn more and more about the porphyrias, I made more connections between Jill's suffering and acute intermittent porphyria. I knew I was on the right path. But I still had to prove it—to *everyone*.

A couple of weeks later I received the 504 meeting notes. Tony had handwritten on them that I wanted homebound instruction "but the team did not see any reason for that." Other than my request for it, there had been no discussion whatsoever about homebound tutoring during that meeting. Dr. Wade's letter had not been brought up for discussion, either. I had requested tutoring and Tony had gone off on his rant which in turn sparked my anger. For academic accommodations his report read: "Jill may leave class immediately for medical attention if she is ever having a bleeding episode. There will be no school or work penalty. May opt out of PE class." We were most definitely not on the "same page." After all these years, within a matter of months I had experienced what so many parents of special needs students had complained about—the insensitivity and *hostility* of Littleton's school representatives toward them and their children. For years, we had been protected, probably because largely through insurance companies' coverage and out-of-pocket payments, Ed and I had financed a plethora of tests and evaluations aimed at helping our children navigate school life which saved the school district a whole lot of money.

Just days after the 504 debacle Jill's health deteriorated severely, plunging both of us into deep despair. In addition to the daily complaint about severe pains riddling her body, especially her lower right abdominal area, the bloody tasting reflux was back and she had started an extraordinarily heavy menses. The pain became even worse, if that was possible—a twelve on a zero to ten pain scale. And, oddly, she was complaining about unbearable pain in her *ankle* (as she had in sixth grade). Once again, we trekked to Dr. Wade's office. This time, her medical partners came in to inspect Jill, too. They prodded her abdomen, made her lift each leg and bend it out to the side while lying on her back. Then Dr. Wade handed me orders for an ultrasound and told me to immediately get to NHC's radiology department. To Jill's horror, the ultrasound technician pressed the scan firmly all over her abdominal area. Somehow, she held her screams in. We returned home only to find ourselves returning to NCH's ED in a few hours. Jill was hemorrhaging and the abdominal pain was at screeching levels not helped, I was sure, by the pressure associated with the ultrasound. Driving back and forth to the hospital was an ordeal in and of itself. The highway was undergoing repairs and every bump in the road, no matter how slight, caused excruciating leaps in Jill's pain register. Notes from that ED visit stated:

> 12 yo female with heavy menses and ab pain. Seen by PMD today, s/p ultrasound for re-eval for appx--negative…abdominal pain began at 4 am; diffuse, but most intense in RLQ [right lower quadrant]. Also feeling pain in lower back and between shoulders. Pain is constant byt [sic] has waves of more intensity.

Diarrhea x6, 'watery' ... Menses heavier than usual; using 1 pad/hour... Cramping in groin area started today; pt doesn't usually get cramps... Also complains of sore throat, decreased appetite, no vomiting, no fever, no known sick contacts; has missed school for approx. 3 weeks."[32] The report also noted the onset of abdominal pain as being two months ago and the "Complaint is intermittent." The physical exam indicated "Increased respiratory rate, intermittently tremulous at rest."[33]

Jill was insulted about having been asked if she was sexually active and if it was possible she might be pregnant. "Who would ask a 12-year-old-kid something like that?" she demanded once we were alone. I explained to her that indeed, some 12-year-old-girls were sexually active, either by choice or otherwise. She snapped, "What are you talking about?" It was time for the incest and peer and date rape situations talk. "Ugh, that is so gross!" she said after I explained to her why hospital personnel sometimes saw sexually active 12-year-old- (or younger) girls.

Once again, blood was drawn and a urine sample taken. But since no one would listen to me about AIP, no one checked for that. She was given 650 milligrams of Tylenol every 4 hours and put on a drip with 5 milligrams of oxycodone hydrochloride. When asked what level her pain was on a scale of zero to ten, ten being the worst she'd ever felt, she readily rated it a ten. Hours later, "...pain still a 10 out of 10, post oxycodone. Pain is still constant"[34] the report said. Still, through everything, Jill was politely responsive to the medical personnel's questions and submitted to their prodding and pushing tests.

The report indicated, "Child laying on bed, conversive [sic] and interactive"[35] so the ED doctor decided to discharge her. Upon hearing that, Jill began sobbing and begged to stay in the hospital. I could not stand the thought of bringing her home only to writhe in pain so I took up the plea, too. "Please, let her stay overnight to get some relief from this horrible pain," I begged on her behalf. She was admitted to the hospital, received an IV drip through the night then was discharged the next day with a prescription for Amicar Syrup for the heavy menses. The pain was held at bay only for a couple of days, just enough time to see Dr. Wade again for a follow-up visit and for her to give us an order for another porphyria blood test and a request for a thoracic/lumbosacral (spine) X-ray. She prescribed Neurontin for the pain.

Jill returned intermittently to school. About one and half hours at a time was all she could achieve before retreating to the nurse's office. Vanessa continued to lobby for tutoring and school administrators continued to ignore the subject. I connected the severe pains, diarrhea and other symptoms Jill was having to AIP attack activity and became more desperate than ever to get a doctor to verify that.

32 NCH* ED. Medical report. October 5, 2008
33 Ibid.
34 Ibid.
35 Ibid.

CHAPTER 14

Purple Storms

Be sure to put your feet in the
right place, then stand firm.
— **ABRAHAM LINCOLN**

I was beyond excited to learn that a member of the APF Scientific Advisory Board, Dr. Brownell*, practiced at a university health center in our region but then was disappointed to learn that he had recently relocated to a medical facility in a southern state.

Meanwhile, Jill remained convinced that she either had gallbladder problems or SOD. I contacted Dr. Jasson,* the SOD doctor featured on "Medical Mysteries" to see if he would consult with us. We were able to schedule an appointment with his associate, Dr. Hummel.* He did not think Jill presented with SOD or gallbladder impairment, but said a hepatobilliary (HIDA) scan would answer the question. He also urged me to continue to pursue the porphyria trail. Jill was despondent. She had been certain Dr. Hummel would have answers and begged me again to ask "somebody" for exploratory surgery. Jill needed somebody to do *something*! But things were about to get even more wacky. For months, I had relentlessly tapped the encyclopedic Internet for answers to questions medical personnel did not have answers for, thus improving my familiarity with AIP. I relied mostly on porphyria support organizations' websites in America, Australia, Canada, England, South Africa, Sweden, United Kingdom (UK) and Wales. From these sources I identified hospitals, individual experts, insurance companies, medical higher education venues and other avenues for further investigation. I double- and cross-checked information as much as possible and became more and more convinced that Jill had AIP and that it was *active*.

Less than two weeks after the appointment with Dr. Hummel, Jill had another attack. This time, her chest began to hurt terribly. I was in my home office one evening when she handed me a note that said, "I just can't breathe." I told her to go lie on my bed and put the ceiling fan on high. I called Dr. Wade to say Jill was in distress with chest pain and respiratory difficulty. The covering doctor asked if she was able to talk so I asked her a question. Her reply was weak but the doctor was able to hear her. "OK, that's good. Are her lips blue?" I looked at Jill's lips. Actually, they were gray, I said. I explained that I was convinced Jill had a rare liver disorder known as acute intermittent porphyria and that Dr. Wade knew I felt this way. Furthermore, I said, in order to confirm AIP activity, everything I had read said that blood, stool or urine samples should be taken while an attack was happening— and an attack was clearly underway. I asked the doctor to call NHC's ED to see if it would it possible for them to take samples to be refrigerated until they could be sent out with the PCP's orders to test for AIP again. The doctor told me to pose that question to the hospital staff and urged us to go there. It was about 10 p.m. By then, Jill could barely stand up. I helped her down the stairs, out to the garage and into the car. Once again, every bump, swerve and stop on the drive to the hospital brought her waves of agony.

I zoomed onto the hospital's emergency entrance ramp, jumped out of the car and raced for a wheelchair. I got Jill into the lobby and told a nurse about the possibility that Jill might have AIP, her lips were gray and she needed oxygen *immediately.* Then I went to park the car. I returned to find Jill with her head between her knees, holding a small paper bag to her mouth. I grabbed the bag out of Jill's hands and cried, "Please help her! She can't *breathe!* She needs oxygen, not a paper bag!" She was immediately moved into a room and transferred to a bed. As the attending physician approached the room, I started to tell him about the porphyria possibility. Surprisingly, he had heard of it. He asked if I'd seen the movie about Mad King George potentially having had the disease. "No, but I sure am glad that *somebody* around here has at least heard of it," I said anxiously.

"Really!? She might have porphyria?" he continued. "Wild!"

Before I could say, "Wild is right!" Jill went into the hardest convulsive activity and rapidly declining SAT (oxygen saturation) numbers I had seen yet. The ED report noted:

> She had shaking of her extremities, rapid eye movement. It was to be noted that she had no incontinence during this time. She was administered Ativan intravenously and given oxygen and the episode resolved, but it was questionable by the observers if it was a true seizure. Due to the episode of shaking and questionable seizure and the severity of her abdominal pain according to Jill, it was decided to admit Jill for further evaluation."[36] The ED records continued, "Initial studies were obtained in the emergency room where Jill presented. She had a normal sugar at that

---

36 NCH* ED, medical report. October 16, 2008.

time, normal electrolytes, normal magnesium. Calcium as [sic] slightly low at 8.9. White blood count was 10.3. Hemoglobin was 11.9, hematrocrit sedimentation rate was 13. A prolactin which was obtained to help differentiate whether the episode in the emergency room was a seizure: Prolactin level was 23, which is in the normal range. Phosphorus was normal.[37]

According to the report, hyperventilation was listed as the reason she had been brought to the ED. Questions and possibilities exploded and ran roughshod over my thinking. I wondered what was happening to Jill's body and brain during these attacks and desperately wanted to know more about porphyria-related breathing problems. That topic would have to wait because Jill had to stay in the hospital for a week. It was the worst week of her life. As sure as I was that she was not consciously or unconsciously manifesting the symptomatic episodes, I soon found out medical professionals were just as convinced that was exactly what was going on. Nonetheless, her urine sample taken during that ED encounter was recorded as "Brown" and a nursing note "Pt being tested for acute intermittent porphyria" had been made. Unfortunately that particular sample was never sent for ALA/PBG analysis. I would not find out until years later that her blood level PBG-D at that time had registered at the lowest level yet—5.3.

After a stress-filled night, Jill received IV fluids and rested somewhat comfortably during the next day. I decided to stay overnight with her and slept on a hospital sofa bed. I went home the next morning to shower, gather more reading material and, as usual, access the Internet to continue researching AIP. I also took the opportunity to fax a message to the chair of the APF scientific advisory board about the latest circumstance:

> Went to [hospital] with continued severe abdominal, flank, back pain and breathing difficulty. Observed plunging SAT numbers and seizure type activity. Still in severe abdominal pain which migrated to include chest pain just before breathing problems escalated. They gave her oxygen and after 10-15 mins she came to. The IV glucose/fluid helps ease the pain somewhat. PLEASE HELP.

I then cancelled the HIDA scan appointment and after considerable research to find the number, placed a desperate call to Dr. Brownell's office to say I needed to know how to go about getting DNA testing for AIP. His assistant, Clarice* said his clinic used only two labs for porphyria testing: one was in Texas and the other in New York. She was unsure if Dr. Brownell would see Jill. I faxed him a letter, concentrating on the recent health issues and potential porphyria connection:

> Perhaps it would make sense for me to bring Jill directly to you for testing, or should I get her to the New York lab for the test

---

under your orders?" I continued, "The doctors here are unfamiliar with porphyria. None of the blood tests were drawn during an actual attack. A high carb diet, glucose tabs, fluid infusion and morphine are the only (minimal and intermittent) relief she has found. I would very much appreciate hearing your thoughts as quickly as possible. I am truly scared for Jill's safety.

There was nothing left to do but go back to the hospital and wait. I would not give up.

When I returned to her hospital room, Jill was still complaining of stomach and side pains and in short order began seizing and exhibiting signs of breathing difficulty. The nurse seemed hesitant, but I begged her to give Jill oxygen through a mask not just through a cannula. Reluctantly, she put the mask over Jill's mouth then gave her a shot of Ativan. Shortly after the oxygen began to flow, Jill revived. Dr. Wade's dictation from that morning read:

> The abdominal pain continued. Jill rated it approximately an 8 on a scale of 1 to 10. She again had a shaking episode with some random eye movement. Again it was questioned whether this was a seizure. She was given Ativan intravenously, administered oxygen. The episode resolved within a few minutes and again it was questioned by the observer if this was a true seizure.[38]

The next day brought the worst series of medical occurrences we had experienced so far—in a hospital, no less. Jill's pain level had been marching steadily up the scale when all of a sudden she sneezed and her nose started bleeding—heavily. I reached for the call button and requested immediate help. Two residents arrived. "She needs Stimate right away," I said. The hospital pharmacy was contacted. Fifteen minutes went by with no medication. I said, "Look, I will call my husband, he can bring our bottle of Stimate."

No, they said, it would come from the hospital pharmacy. A river of blood flowed from Jill's nose. It took forty-five minutes for the medicine to arrive; one spray and the blood flow lightened. Then Jill began seizing again. Ativan was administered but this time she mouthed "*help*" and "*can't breathe*," and I knew she was really in trouble. Trying desperately to stay calm, I urgently asked for someone to get oxygen on her again—NOW. The two residents simply stood there. I said, "For God's sake, *why are you just standing there*? Can't you see she needs help?" I could not take seeing Jill like that, with no one willing to help and ran sobbing into the hallway. Several nurses immediately surrounded me, attempting to calm me. I knew we were in the hematology/oncology department where plenty of parents before me had sought the hallway or other areas to collect themselves but could not stop the screaming in my head, "My kid *doesn't have cancer* like you are all familiar with; she has a treatable condition—and she's going to die if you *don't do something*!" But

---

38 NCH. Dr. Wade hospital report. October 18, 2008.

of course, no one but me believed that. The logical side of my brain took over. I had done a lot of research and had increased my AIP knowledge and awareness. But the doctors, nurses and other medical personnel did not have confirmation about *what* Jill was suffering from so they could only do what they knew, what they had been trained to do. As much as I hated it, I realized medical ignorance could result in Jill's death. But I also knew that administering oxygen was a reasonable request, so I went back into the room.

Looking at the monitor, one of the residents, Dr. Green,* said Jill didn't need oxygen because her stats were "within range."

Pushed to the edge, I snapped, "I don't <u>care</u> what your *stats* indicate! If you value that M.D. you've worked so long and hard and paid so much money for, then you had better get that oxygen on her <u>NOW!</u>" Dr. Green abruptly left the room. Her partner attempted to placate me, but I was too worked up, "<u>Don't</u> patronize me! You guys obviously know nothing about this *porphyria*. But eventually you will know that Jill has acute intermittent porphyria!" By this time, the oxygen mask was sitting squarely over Jill's mouth and she had settled into sleep mode. My gut, my soul and my heart hurt like hell. But we were only in the middle of the trial that had begun the afternoon Jill had handed me the "I just can't breathe" note.

CHAPTER 15

Atmospheric Instability

...for all the times we cried I always felt that
God was on our side...
— SUNG BY HELEN REDDY

As I slept fitfully on the sofa bed in Jill's room, her monitor's alarm began to sound during the early morning hours. "What now?" I muttered. Nobody responded. "Bomp. Bomp. Bomp." Still no one came. "Bomp. Bomp. Bomp." So I started counting. On the forty-second "bomp" I got up, went over to the monitor and read, "Sleep apnea >64 seconds." The bomping continued. I looked at the oxygen mouthpiece over Jill's mouth. There was no vapor and no mist. She did not seem to be breathing. "What the...?" I jostled her, she started breathing and the bomping stopped. I went back to the sofa bed. After a while, the alarm sounded again, but this time, only for a couple of bomps.

When Dr. Wade came by the next morning, I asked if she knew what had happened to make the alarm sound off for so long during the night and why the screen had said "Sleep apnea>64 seconds." She, replied, "Oxygen is a medicine. Too much can be bad. She doesn't need it," and left. Shortly thereafter a nurse removed the monitor and attachments. Things were not looking good. Jill was given scrambled eggs for breakfast that made her sick. I felt sick, too—and angry that Dr. Wade was not taking Jill's condition seriously. As the primary care physician, she had not once asked why I thought Jill had AIP. I did not have time to find another PCP for Jill but determined that a change *would* be made.

Jill told me that while I had been home showering, "some other doctor" had come to talk with her about what had been going on during the past year. I had begun to suspect the NHC medical professionals were of the opinion that, like Benton Middle School cohorts Debbie and Anne, Jill was in some way manifesting her symptoms, which was confirmed the next day when Ed, Vanessa and I attended a meeting with NHC's medical and psych teams. Ed, Vanessa and I joined three psychiatric doctors; Dr. Wade; Dr. Tourtellotte, the neurologist who had first mentioned porphyria to us; a resident who had been attending Jill and the hospital's insurance coordinator. Jill was supposed to attend the meeting, but nobody remembered to get her. Dr. O'Connor was conspicuously absent. From Dr. Wade's dictation:

> A team meeting was held to discuss the complex issues that Jill has...her abdominal pain which is a chronic issue and her episodes of syncope have been intermittent and also the newer question of seizures being present...One differential diagnosis entertained was acute intermittent porphyria. A workup for this has been started and is being continued and will be continued until a definitive diagnosis is made. Discussion on how to manage the episodes of syncope and the episodes of dizziness and shaking of the extremities and fast breathing were discussed, and it was felt by all the physicians present that a calm, supportive approach would be the best, medication should not be given on an acute basis...It was stressed that care should try and not be in the emergency room for Jill but through her primary physician pediatrician's office and ongoing outpatient psychological counseling was recommended to be continued for Jill, twice weekly on an outpatient basis...This would be through [Vanessa]...

> [Dr. Marlone*] spoke...about conversion disorder. She felt that this diagnosis should be entertained with Jill...Treatment at this point was supportive and included psychological outpatient counseling. A school reentry plan was also discussed and highly recommended that Jill reenter school as soon as possible. Jill did well throughout her hospitalization and extensive work up again was undertaken to try to delineate the etiology for her complex symptoms. She was stable and it was felt by all physicians involved that she should be discharged home."[39]

Someone finally remembered that Jill was supposed to be in the meeting, too, and sent for her. Upon her arrival, one of the doctors informed her she would be discharged the next day and that Vanessa would see her twice a week. Jill would resume going to school (which scared me) and that other supports such as the Pain Relief Clinic were being planned to help her. Jill was angry. "You're supposed to be helping me but you're not doing anything for me," she said, turned around and walked out. Back in her room, another gushing nosebleed developed. The calm,

---

39 NCH.* Dr. Wade's* medical record of October 22, 2008 meeting.

supportive approach the psychiatrists had recommended was shown to be a facade when Dr. Smart* angrily snapped, "She's got to learn to deal with life."

The next day was discharge day and though apprehensive, Jill was packed and ready to go when a nurse came in to say that more blood work would be required. "I'm just waiting for the lab to identify the right 'tube top' colors," she said. To me, that meant they had not tested for porphyria even though Jill had entered the hospital a week before and endured numerous attacks. I thought, "Once again, she isn't in attack mode so it'll be a waste of time and insurance money." In a short while, the nurse came back and handed me a completed lab slip for porphyria testing. Then Dr. O'Connor appeared in Jill's room. He said he had asked to attend the meeting but had not been paged. I was dismayed that his request had not worked out; he could have been a voice of reason. When I asked about the blood work that the nurse said was still required, he seemed surprised. About the last test Jill had had, he said there was no evidence of cancer, but there was a "low red blood cell count," and the latest twenty-four hour urine test results showed no 'porphyria' in the urine, so Jill "doesn't have acute intermittent porphyria," he finished confidently. "We'll just see about that," I thought to myself and knew that soon there would be no more doubt about it. I could just feel it. I just had to figure out how and where to get it done. Clarice had mentioned labs in Texas and New York City as the ones Dr. Brownell relied on. I prayed Jill would be able to hang on until the DNA testing happened.

A few weeks later I ordered complete hospital records from that week and read, "… consultations were requested with the psychiatry division of NHC, also Hematology, and also a pain management clinic evaluation was requested…The patient was seen in a psychiatric evaluation by Dr. Marlone*…The impression of the consultant at that time was chronic abdominal pain and probable conversion disorder."[40] I could see they were intent on proving Jill was a mental case and now understood why the monitors in Jill's hospital room had been removed; they weren't going to "coddle" her anymore and were convinced she could stop the symptoms on her own "if she really wanted to." I was angry that a "psych consultation" had taken place without my prior approval and that I had not known about it. If I had, I would have then confronted them about it during the "team" meeting. But they had made up their minds. Nothing was said or documented about the times of respiratory distress, the lengthy nosebleeds or sleep apnea of more than 64 seconds. To them there *was* no physical medical diagnosis to speak of; their psych diagnosis would stand. "Entertained until a definitive diagnosis is made" [about porphyria] was also in the records. I had brought up the possibility of AIP multiple times during the meeting and was never assured that it would be pursued at all. Apparently, they weren't interested in looking beyond their psychiatric diagnosis. I was disgusted and knew they would all be surprised when the AIP diagnosis was finally made.

Next, Jill and I met with the Pain Relief Program professionals. Their plan recommended that school tutoring be maintained during gradual school reentry, beginning with one-half hour per day, and indicated Jill showed evidence of a

---

40 NCH.* Dr. Wade's* medical record dictation. October 21-22, 2008

condition called postural orthostatic tachycardia (POTS). They provided a transcutaneous electrical nerve stimulation (TENS) unit to reduce the pain level "…if only she would let it" and "Physical Therapy–the more you do the better you feel" and finally, biofeedback to "help teach relaxation skills…."[41] Obviously, they were taking cues from the NHC psychiatric and medical reports. "And why wouldn't they," I thought, "Who would they take their direction from—the medical experts they worked with or a *mom* who knew her daughter had something other than what all of these medical experts could identify?" My despair grew—it was all so agonizing!

---

41 NCH's* Pain clinic report. October, 2008.

CHAPTER 16

Sun Peeps

*For whatever is hidden is meant to be disclosed, and whatever
is concealed is meant to be brought out into the open.*

— MARK 4:22

*"I was in and out of tutoring. I was in the hospital, on my death bed every other day, it
seemed. The seizures, body aches, horrific stomach pains, even the small symptoms like
nausea, vomiting, dizziness, fevers, fatigue was too much for my body to handle, yet NO
ONE BELIEVED ME!!!"* [42]

I finally got the opportunity to speak with APF's head of the scientific advisory
board. Shortly into the conversation he said, "[The numbers] just don't appear
to support that Jill has porphyria." I called Dr. Brownell's office again and spoke
with Clarice who said the most marvelous thing, "Call Tri-State Laboratories* in
New York and speak with Andrea Davis.* She will tell you what to do to for genetic
testing." I thanked her, had a brief relief cry and then called Andrea who advised
me to get a prescription for a phlebotomy draw with a note from Dr. Wade saying
it was okay to release the sample to the patient. She said to retrieve the online
genetic testing requisition form, print and complete it and send a check and insurance information in case the insurance would cover the cost, which it did not. She
instructed me to find a sturdy box, get the blood drawn at a lab and send the sample
to her attention at Tri-State Labs via overnight carrier. Surprisingly, she said it did
not need to be kept cold. The previous blood and urine tests had had so many strict
parameters about stabilizing the sample that I wondered if it would really work
out. I coordinated the necessary steps and spent considerable time filling out the
forms—I did not want to make a mistake. The porphyria tests included the acute
porphyrias: acute intermittent porphyria (AIP), hereditary coproporphyria (HCP),
or variegate porphyria (VP) and the cutaneous porphyrias. For $1,750.00, the
option of testing for all three acute porphyrias was available. As sure as I was that Jill

---

42 Jill's journal. November 2008.

had AIP, I opted for the "package deal" and mused about how much our insurance company had paid for tests and evaluations for over a *year* that had found absolutely nothing. I put the completed paperwork, the check and a St. Jude prayer card into the container, collected Jill and went to the lab. As soon as the sample was completed, I put it into the container and taped the mailing label onto it. Then I drove to the UPS store, said a prayer and off it went. Andrea called the next day to say the sample had arrived intact. She suggested I "settle in" as results would take three to six weeks.

In keeping with the Pain Relief Program's recommendations, Jill met with a biofeedback therapist and started physical therapy. The recommendation was to attend the program once or twice a week for eight to twelve weeks. She also continued to see Vanessa twice a week as we had agreed at the NHC "team meeting."

For weeks, my mind was distracted by wondering about the DNA results. Then, two days before Thanksgiving, Andrea called to say, "I'm sorry to tell you that Jill has the mutant gene associated with Acute Intermittent Porphyria." I cried with relief.

"Thank you, thank you, *thank you*, Andrea. I *knew* it. I only did what I thought doctors are supposed to do—especially once the possibility of porphyria surfaced. I researched the symptoms and connected them to Jill. *No one* took me seriously. Not one medical person sat down with me to review the porphyria symptom list I'd compiled and compare them to Jill's complaints. Not one.

I *knew* from the beginning that Jill wasn't making anything up," I blathered on.

Andrea replied, "Well, you've been able to do something that some of the best doctors were not able to do." Fourteen months after her symptoms had surfaced we had proof that Jill indeed had a *medical* condition.

Andrea recommended we bring Jill to Tri-State's Porphyria Center as soon as possible, so I made an appointment. Then I called Dr. Wade's and Dr. O'Connor's offices to tell them the news. Then I faxed the results to them. Dr. Wade's skepticism was evident. She said, "Well, it says under Interpretation: 'Identification of the splice-site mutation, IVS10-31A>G in one of Jill Gould's HMBS alleles [variants of a particular gene] is consistent with the diagnosis that Jill Gould has Acute Intermittent Porphyria (AIP).' It doesn't actually say that she has it. That word 'consistent' is the one I'm concerned about."

On the other hand, Dr. O'Connor said, "I'm so sorry. I really *didn't* think she had it." Because he had been treating her for von Willebrand, I asked if he would be willing to take on AIP through Jill Gould. My relief was palpable when he agreed to do so. Finally, it was time for a brief "happy dance." I told him of the APF's website, the upcoming Tri-State Lab's Porphyria Center appointment and of finding Dr. Brownell. I said we would get answers about treating AIP and I would continue to research and share what I learned with him.

But, of course, AIP was in charge and all too soon Jill was back in the ED with yet another bout of the gripping abdominal pain. This time, I brought the Tri-State Lab's DNA results with us. The resident who had been teamed with Dr. Green a few months ago came into the room. "Oh, it's you guys again," she said nonchalantly.

I said, "Yes, it's us again and here's proof that Jill has Acute Intermittent Porphyria. We have a meeting coming up at Tri-State Lab's Porphyria Center in

New York City in a couple of weeks and depending on how that goes we've located a porphyria specialist in Georgia who has agreed to see us." The resident stared at the DNA paper so intently it was almost as though she was willing it to talk like something out of a Harry Potter scene. Jill lapsed into seizures. Ativan, oxygen, a few hours of rest and we left—again.

Our appointment with the Porphyria Center clinicians was scheduled on Kevin's birthday. We decided to take the train to New York City, get settled in the hotel and then celebrate Kevin's birthday with dinner. The next day the Porphyria Center team took an extensive health history from Jill. In addition to the porphyria experts, a gastroenterologist joined the group, explaining he was there to learn more about porphyria. Andrea was there, too, saying, "It's always good to put a face to the voice on the other end of the phone." Ed and I were given a research form and asked if we would consider filling it out and signing it on Jill's behalf. Their intent was to compile a national database of information about porphyria patients. Happy to help others, Ed and I signed on.

Jill was examined, her vital signs recorded and blood and urine samples collected to be analyzed. But the conversation became vague when the subject turned to treatment. Apparently, proving AIPorphyria was one thing but treating it was another, especially because Jill was a juvenile. I knew Panhematin was the drug of choice for treating AIP. But no one seemed to be aware of how much to use or could even recommend its use. I persisted, "She's got the mutant gene; frequent and strong *active* symptoms—seems to me she needs to be treated for acute intermittent porphyria." Andrea nodded in assent. I began to think no one there had actually treated a case of porphyria in so young a patient.

Ed and I realized we had gotten all we were going to get from the group of assembled experts so we left and collected Kevin, then our family spent time in the city before catching the train back to Hartford. Once on the train, I called Clarice at Dr. Brownell's office. "We just met with the Porphyria Center team." I told her, "Truly wonderful people, but quite honestly, Ed and I both felt they got more out of us than we got out them. Could Jill please see Dr. Brownell as soon as possible?" Clarice said the next available opening was in January. "We'll be there," I said gratefully.

I signed Jill up as a member of the American Porphyria Foundation and soon a three-ring binder filled with information about AIP arrived in the mail—with my name on the cover. Jill was ticked. "I have porphyria—not you," she said. I did not think it was a big deal and explained that as her parent, medical people would look to me for help in treating her and that is probably why my name had been inserted. Jill would not buy my explanation; the binder was for and about her so Jill wanted *her* name on it. I called the APF office to ask for a replacement insert. Fortunately, they sent it right away. Jill was so pleased and proud of her new possession. For her, the binder was tangible proof that she had AIP and had not been faking *anything*. We immediately put the Tri-State Lab's DNA diagnosis paper into the binder. I added the running log of Jill's health-related experiences and appointments so that we could easily and quickly tell what had happened when. Every medical discharge paper went into the binder. The lengthy yet comprehensive Canadian and Swedish

Porphyria Foundations' *Patient's and Doctor's Guide to Medication in Acute Porphyria* was added for reference. I had begun the building of an information binder aimed at supporting Jill.

I re-read APF member stories, focusing on AIP narratives this time that mentioned health concerns during childhood. A full 60 percent made mention of symptoms they felt were attributed to AIP. Many told of living with hellish symptoms that no one could figure out. Not surprisingly, the signs had been ignored or dismissed. Still, it seemed the extent that symptoms had manifested in Jill as an eleven-year-old was extraordinary. I contacted the APF's executive director to ask if it might be possible to accumulate anecdotal information from AIP members about their childhood health. We emailed back and forth but my attention and energy was increasingly pulled into Jill's fight with porphyria. Talking to Dr. O'Connor about my hope of gathering the information, I vowed, "I know it won't be a 'structured, scientific' study but if I have to, I'll survey AIPorphyrics myself." Dr. O'Connor smiled.

PART III

Batten Down the Hatches

*I know that God won't give me anything I can't handle.
I just wish He didn't trust me so much.*

— **MOTHER THERESA**

CHAPTER 17

Partly

These are times that try men's souls.
— THOMAS PAINE

A few days before we were to leave for Georgia,* Clarice called to ask us to bring twenty-four hour urine and stool samples to the appointment for testing. Since we planned to fly down the afternoon before the appointment it meant we would have to carry the samples with us. I packed each with plastic frozen packs into thick, Styrofoam containers and duct taped them closed. It was by far the nastiest thing I had ever had to travel with. Jill and I arrived at the airport with our bags and her samples. The next morning, a nurse took the noxious samples away, showed Jill and me to an examination room and introduced us to a pediatric nurse who, because the practice did not typically see children, said she was required to be in the room during the consultation. I asked if they had ever had a juvenile patient with AIP before. The nurse said she remembered only one child having been tested for the disorder, but the result had been negative.

It was a relief to be in Dr. Brownell's presence. Compared to all the doctors we had seen, he oozed AIP knowledge. Though he questioned whether Jill's AIP was active, he advised us about Panhematin, also known as heme, and cautioned us about its side effects. He said Dr. O'Connor should use the APF's guideline for using Panhematin and said they would talk. As our time with him came to a close, he said he would await lab results from Jill's blood, urine and stool samples before making his final diagnosis. I knew he'd be looking for those PBGs and ALAs. Before I could attempt to stop them, the words shot out of my mouth, "Doctor, *what if kids don't always* produce these markers you're looking for? What if children are not little adults in that respect as far as AIP is concerned?"

Dr. Brownell's look seemed to say, "Sigh, another parent wishing and hoping what she is saying will be true." Jill and I flew back to Connecticut. I realized I had forgotten to ask Dr. Brownell if he himself had ever treated a juvenile with AIP or if he was aware of any other cases of childhood manifest AIP that required heme treatments. Within two days of returning from Dr. Brownell's consultation, Jill received her first heme infusion. She tolerated it well and over the next eleven days, received four heme/dextrose (D10) treatments. The foreseeable future started to look good for the first time in a long time. Jill continued to work with Vanessa and went to physical therapy sessions. Another school meeting had been scheduled in hopes of returning her to school because she was once again in tutoring.

This time the school meeting went more smoothly. The school nurse had been appointed Jill's case manager and he produced a 504 meeting/report that included the AIP diagnosis and acute attack symptoms. The academic goal was to "keep Jill in class and school while assisting in the management of symptoms associated with acute exacerbations of AIP." The action plan was laid out: "If any one or more symptoms are reported or observed, contact the nurse IMMEDIATELY... Symptoms may progress rapidly to a life threatening neuromuscular weakness that may result in paralysis and/or Respiratory Failure (stop breathing)." The report indicated the degree of impairment (mental or physical) that limits major life activity (attendance at school) to be SUBSTANTIAL (#4 in the range 1-5, 5 being highest).[43] Our request that Jill be transported to NHC ED to receive heme as soon as possible was noted. However, because Littleton is in MedCity Hospital's emergency coverage area, it would continue to be problematic.

Though I had provided the DNA results report to the school administrators, they understandably wanted a definitive diagnosis from Jill's physician. Dr. Wade was intimidated by the whole AIP diagnosis, but Dr. O'Connor produced a medical protocol that helped, "If Jill has severe abdominal pain, mental status changes, seizure activity, please offer Oxygen by face mask; D10 ½ NS + 10 mEq KCL/l at150 ml/hr; May use small doses of Ativan 0.5-1.0 mg IV; Pls check sodium and blood pressure and treat hypertension and correct hyponatremia [low blood sodium] as indicated."[44]

Though the Pain Relief Program team had recommended a gradual return to school, Littleton decided she would start back full-time and Jill was anxious to return, so back she went.

A letter from Dr. Brownell arrived about two weeks after our meeting with him, informing us that the test results from Jill's samples were "entirely normal... with no evidence of any biochemically active acute intermittent porphyria...similar to the results obtained at [Tri-State Labs]."[45] He concluded Jill was a genetic carrier of AIP but remained uncertain "as to whether or to what the extent the symptoms you have been having are due to Acute Intermittent Porphyria." He went on to say that Panhematin therapy could be considered but might not lead to significant

---

43 LMS* school nurse. Medical Management Plan. February 9, 2009.
44 Dr. O'Connor.* Letter To Whom It May Concern. April 10, 2009.
45 Dr. Brownell.* Letter to author. January 27, 2009.
45 Ibid.

improvement in Jill's symptoms..."which may...not be arising from the underlying genetic defect...Most patients with the genetic defect are latent or 'silent' carriers of the genetic abnormality, and clinical features are usually thought to be unlikely if urinary excretions of ALA and PBG are normal."[46]

According to Webster's dictionary, latent means "present and capable of becoming but not now visible or active" and silent means "not exhibiting the usual signs or symptoms and presence."[47] I was thinking more like Dr. Wade's dubious reaction to the DNA report and so "unlikely" was the word I focused on. Unlikely meant doubtful. Doubtful meant "open to question...uncertain in outcome...undecided... lack of conviction."[48] Unlikely and doubtful were not convincing enough for me, an MD, mom doctor, who'd watched my child's slight symptoms explode into life-threatening signs of real medical peril, especially when none of the clinical samples had been taken during an actual attack.

I had come across mention of Isabel Allende's book "Paula," written in memory of her daughter who died agonizingly of porphyria. The fact that AIP was a known, potentially life-threatening condition was not lost on me, and the reality that another mother's daughter had lost her battle with porphyria horrified me. I wasn't yet ready to read the book but stubbornly thought to myself, "Jill's AIP is *active!*" But, really, who was I, a mom with a business degree and marketing background to challenge a doctor who had made AIP his life's work? I responded to Dr. Brownell's letter and thanked him for the time he had taken to detail the heme and dextrose treatments during our meeting. I said that I recognized his typical porphyria patient demographic was adults, but noted this "adult onset" disorder, said to show itself in the second through fourth decade of life, had appeared to such a degree that it required treatment with an orphan drug in now-twelve-year old Jill. I closed by telling him that Jill was responding well to the heme/glucose infusions and decided it was time for me to survey AIPorphyrics about their childhood recollections.

I had a feeling that Jill was not done with her attacks and after seeing the monitor's "Sleep apnea >64 seconds" notice, became fixated on the AIP oxygen-binding problem. I found information supporting my feeling that Jill's breathing difficulty was not, as the NHC residents insisted, just her brain thinking it could not breathe, "[n]euromuscular weakness can progress rapidly to paralysis and respiratory failure,"[49] and emailed a question to the website about porphyrins and how or if they might interfere with tissue oxygen-binding. Dr. Frederick Plapp of St. Luke's in Kansas City Hospital replied, "While the exact mechanism underlying the neurovisceral complaints is not well understood, various hypotheses have been put forth:

- Direct neurotoxity caused by PBG or ALA;

- ALA promotes the generation of reactive oxygen species (ROS) in vitro

---

46 Dr. Brownell.* Letter to author. January 27, 2009
47 *Latent.* Webster's Ninth New Collegiate Dictionary. Merriam-Webster. 1985; *Silent.* Webster's Ninth New Collegiate Dictionary. Merriam-Webster. 1985.
48 *Unlikely.* Webster's Ninth New Collegiate Dictionary. Merriam-Webster. 1985; *Doubtful.* Webster's Ninth New Collegiate Dictionary. Merriam-Webster. 1985.
49 *Porphyria.* ClinLabNavigator. http://www.clinlabnavigator.com/porphyria.html.

which may result in oxidative damage to membrane structures within the central nervous system. ALA-induced lipid peroxidation in the cerebellum and hippocampus was reduced by melatonin in a rate model, suggesting that it may reduce neural damage in humans with AIP;

- Inhibition by ALA of gamma-aminobutyric acid (GABA) release at central synapses;

- Loss of heme in the central nervous system, which may be deleterious for the synthesis of important heme proteins such as Cytochrome P450 (involved in the metabolism of chemicals, vitamins, fatty acids, and hormones… very important in transforming toxic substances into excretable materials);

- Decreased activity of hepatic tryptophan pyrrolase, a heme-dependent enzyme, leading to increased levels of brain tryptophan and increased turnover of 5-hydroxytryptamine, a neurotransmitter;

- Decreased plasma melatonin levels, with enhanced ALA-mediated lipid peroxidation."[50]

Dr. Plapp's explanations re-ignited my interest in the condition known as hypoxia or oxygen deprivation which means the body does not have sufficient oxygen to function properly. Knowing that oxygen is carried by the blood and AIP is a disorder where the binding of heme and oxygen is problematic, I searched for more information about the connection between AIP and hypoxia. Several sites told how pilots are trained to recognize the causes, types and stages of hypoxia. I found the symptoms of hypoxia to be particularly interesting: "dizzy" feeling, inappropriate actions, vision problems, forgetfulness, headache, nausea and the most critical—loss of consciousness.[51] Another resource cited "lack of appetite, vomiting, headache, distorted vision, fatigue and difficulty with memorizing and thinking clearly." [52] I thought, "Hmm, the same symptoms Jill exhibited in school—*with* and *without* the bipolar meds" and immediately began wondering if there was a possibility of reduced oxygen (fresh air) in Littleton schools' IAQ. More research produced an article that spoke about AIP attacks having been precipitated by international air travel. Apparently, the combination of dehydration, missed meals, alcohol use, infection, chronic hypoxia, premenstrual syndrome and stress that may occur during international air travel is considered a risk factor and AIP should be suspected in individuals presenting with these symptoms, particularly unexplained abdominal pain, following international air travel.[53] Further research on that would have to wait because AIP was again attacking Jill's liver.

---

50 Plapp, F. Saint Luke's Regional Laboratories. Email to author, January 28, 2009
51 Frushour, Dr. S. *Hypoxia and Flying*. Published online at "International Bird Dog Association." http://www.ibdaweb.com/surgeon_pages/hypoxia.htm. 2000
52 O'Neil, D. *Adapting to High Altitudes*. http://anthro.palomar.edu/adapt/adapt_3.htm. 1998-2012
53 Peters, TJ and Deacon, AC. *International Air Travel: a risk factor for attacks in acute intermittent porphyria*. Published online by "International Journal of Clinical Chemistry" via EuropePMC. http://europepmc.org/abstract/MED/12927685. 2003

CHAPTER 18

Wind Confluence

Patience often gets the credit that belongs to fatigue.
— FRANKLIN JONES

Jill was back at LMS* and though she missed time for heme treatments, was doing relatively okay. Then Kevin began complaining of rapid heartbeat, feverishness and bouts of diarrhea and the genetic aspect of AIP began to gnaw at me—was it possible that he, too, had inherited the gene? I contacted Andrea who sent testing swabs for Kevin. A few weeks later, she called to say he did not have the AIP gene. However, I knew that he and Jill had multiple biological half-siblings that had been adopted by other families. Knowing what we were going through, I felt if there was a chance that any of the other siblings might have inherited the AIP gene, they and their families should know. So I called DCF and was connected with social worker Karli.* Within a week, she had made contact with Kathy who agreed to be tested for the AIP gene. A few days later Karli and I met with Kathy, and I explained Jill's diagnosis to her. Gesturing to her abdominal area, she offered that Jill's biological father had been sick "a lot but no one could figure out what was wrong" and said the two had lost contact long ago. She followed the directions for the mouth swabs and then slipped them into the envelope for mailing. A few weeks later, Andrea called to say Kathy was not a genetic carrier for AIP. That meant Jill's birth father, whereabouts unknown, had bestowed the AIP legacy.

Near the end of February 2009, lethargy dogged Jill. One morning she could not make it to school. "Oh no! Here we go *again*," I moaned and reached for the phone to call NHC's Hem/Onc department. Since this did not constitute a full attack, Dr. O'Connor said to bring her in for a D10 (dextrose) infusion. I had hoped that would fortify Jill, but two days later she collapsed at school. Though we had asked for her to be sent directly to NHC and her 504 plan clearly stated this, when

I arrived at the school, the EMTs said to meet them at MedCity ED. I hurried there and asked if Jill had arrived. "No, not yet," said the receptionist and motioned me to the waiting area. I took a seat, and I sat, and sat. I checked frequently to see if Jill had arrived. About an hour later, the receptionist beckoned me her desk and said, "Call your husband."

Puzzled, I asked, "Call my husband? Why?" She shrugged. I called Ed who said someone from the ambulance company had just called to say Jill was at NHC. I asked, "Why hadn't the ED receptionist been told this so she could have told me instead of letting me sit here for all of this time, worrying about Jill and let Jill wonder what was going on, especially after I'd asked that she be brought to NHC to begin with?" I rhetorically grumbled and hit the road.

As it turned out, MedCity's ED had been full, so the ambulance crew was told to bring Jill to NHC. During the trip, once again, Jill was unresponsive but able to hear what was going on. She heard one of the EMTs laugh about ending up at "the same place the mom had asked for to begin with." Though it was nothing more than a quip about an ironic twist, Jill was insulted.

When I arrived at NHC's ED, she said "Jerry* laughed at you," and told me once again, when thought to be "out of it," she had heard what was going on. This was the second time it had happened. It would not be the last.

One day, notice of a new online forum, www.rareshare.org appeared in my email. Intrigued, I checked it out and noted "acute hepatic porphyria" was among the roster of rare diseases. I joined the forum and posted a message. I received a response within a week. My excitement heightened as I read, "It took almost 3 years to diagnose my daughter. We all know the story. There is a pediatric hematologist in the D.C. area with a solid background in treating porphyria. I highly recommend her. We now have a treatment regimen and plan." She said the porphyria expert was Swedish-born, bred and medically trained. I thought, "Washington, D.C.—drivable distance—YES!" I felt we had just caught a lucky break.

Within a week, Brenda Wilhemina,* mother of twenty-three year old AIP patient Jordin* and I were communicating via email regularly. Jordin was older than Jill by ten years and had gone through terrifying medical experiences, "During one hospitalization, she coded during a seizure. A urine sample that had been forgotten on a shelf turned color. A hospitalist brought up the possibility of porphyria. She not only has the abdominal pain, [she has] psychiatric issues, skin lesions and a sunburn-like rash." Brenda described her daughter's abdomen during AIP attacks as turning the "color of a ripe plum." That Jordin had marked skin coloration interested me—perhaps Jill's mysterious red "abdominal ring" *was* connected to AIP after all. Brenda brought up the matter of a port, "[Jordin] now has a port to relieve the horrors of trying to get an IV going or to take blood and will get regular heme treatments in an attempt to avoid future attacks." Though I had read that Panhematin should be infused through a central line, Jill was still undergoing regular IV sticks and often, multiple sticks to find a suitable vein. As a result, her arms were bruised and battered. Still uneasy with Jill's breathing difficulty and medical personnel's sometime hesitancy to administer oxygen during her attacks, I asked Brenda if Jordin was similarly affected and if so, what was done about it. She replied: "I insist they put oxygen on her even though SAT (blood oxygen saturation) levels say she is fine." With the subject of oxygen came the fear of losing Jill simply because someone could not or would not understand that sometimes she really *couldn't* breathe when AIP was in control. Brenda shared, "Christ's example and presence gives me great comfort. No matter what happens, my daughter will be loved wherever she is. That, I know." My heart grew lighter than it had been in a long time. Brenda was right—if God decided to take Jill, she most certainly would be loved and her earth troubles would be over. Nonetheless, I would of course continue to do everything in my power to keep her on this side.

I continued to consume and digest everything I could find about AIP. I finally felt strong enough to read the story woven by Ms. Allende for her daughter Paula who for months lay in a porphyric coma before succumbing to the disease. As I did so, I was on alert for anything that might correlate to Jill's symptoms, and I did find similarities to Jill's circumstances. One was that Paula had inherited porphyria from her father as Jill had, who was prone to depression. Ms. Allende wrote that one day "...he fainted."[54] In fact, "Michael fainted so frequently that we all became accustomed to it."[55] Just like Jill! "We had never heard the word porphyria, and no one connected his symptoms to that rare metabolic disorder...."[56] Just like us! The story was spellbinding but I was morbidly drawn to the straightforward account of porphyria's control of and ultimate defeat of Paula's life. I *needed* to know all that porphyria was capable of. The heartbreaking story of Paula's deteriorating condition interwoven with the unwavering hope of loved ones standing vigil steeled me. Now able to understand the horrendous force of porphyria, I knew I would remain Jill's sentinel and, from one mother to another, I thanked Isabel Allende from my heart's depths.

Inspired by what I'd read, I immediately changed my tack on researching AIP and searched "childhood onset acute intermittent porphyria." A report, "Acute intermittent porphyria in childhood: a population-based study" appeared. Published by a Swedish team of doctors, the article discussed urine samples in children affected by AIP: "...to establish age-adjusted reference intervals of urinary delta-aminolevulinic acid (U-ALA) and porphobilinogen (U-PBG) in children, and to analyse [sic] the frequency and type of clinical manifestations of acute intermittent porphyria (AIP) in childhood."[57] The pivotal conclusion was what I had been wondering about: "AIP symptoms in children maybe [sic] vague and of short duration and U-ALA and U-PBG levels are often elevated only slightly or not atall [sic]; thus, symptoms and signs may differ from those in adults."[58]

As I read I thought: "Oh Lord, thank you! This means that Jill *isn't* the only one to not produce the 'hallmark' urine!"

---

54 Allende, I. *Paula.* (New York: Harper Perennial), 280.
55 Ibid.
56 Ibid.
57 Hultdin, J et al, *Acute intermittent porphyria in childhood: a population-based study.* Published online at "Acta Paediatrica" via Wiley Online Library. http://www3.interscience.wiley.com/journal/119924471/abstract?. 2003.
58 Ibid.

Jill often complained about being barely able to catch her breath when navigating the school stairs. Once again, head bells jangled; could something in the school building be interfering with the heme/oxygen binding problem already going on in Jill's liver? Could the physical exertion of walking up and downstairs carrying a backpack make it difficult for her to breathe? I convinced the school administration to give her an elevator pass, but it was another thing to try to persuade Jill to use it; doing so was yet another reminder of her weirdness.

Another article that excited me was a PowerPoint presentation detailing the case of a teenage girl diagnosed with AIP. I could barely contain myself when I read through "Behavioural Aspects of Acute Intermittent Porphyria" presented by specialists at the University of Tel-Aviv and noted many of the symptoms listed that I'd seen in Jill. But the clincher appeared in the *Neurotic symptoms* category: "Anxiety (26%), restlessness, agitation, depression (13%), hysteria, phobias, conversion disorder, chronic fatigue syndrome and somatization disorder."[59] To me, this meant conversion disorder was a *symptom* of AIP—not the other way around! I shared the report with Vanessa who said, "Can you imagine how many people have been carted off to mental hospitals, halfway houses or other places away from the mainstream or written off completely because nobody had a clue they could have porphyria?"

"Yes," I said, "I can." And, having parented a kid who had had so many potential conditions bandied about, the realization that it could happen to Jill scared me. While I could not prove that the symptoms she had exhibited from birth could be attributed to porphyria, neither could the multitude of doctors, specialists and professionals who had labeled her with disorder after disorder *disprove* it either.

The initial heme/glucose treatments seemed to have worn off and Jill finished March with continuous complaints about feeling sick, many bouts of diarrhea and headaches that persisted for weeks.

---

59 Luder, A and Schoenfeld, N. *Behavioral Aspects of Acute Intermittent Porphyria.* www.pigur.co.il/bio/porphyria.ppt (Note: url has apparently been changed since original access.)

CHAPTER 19

Relentless, Pounding Rain

*With the Lord a day is like a thousand years, and a
thousand years are like a day.*
— PETER 3-8

Attempting to regain the relief that heme/D10 treatments regimen had offered Jill, another round was scheduled over the next several days, each requiring a new IV insertion. Accessing her veins was getting harder and harder so a nurse suggested leaving the IV setup in overnight since we had to come back the next day for another treatment. We agreed. The nurse put Heparin in the IV lock to keep it from clogging, covered it and instructed Jill about how to keep it dry. During the drive home, she mentioned that her hand was tingling.

The next day Jill said she was tired, sat on the living room couch and slipped into seizure mode. This time the ambulance took her directly to NHC's ED; I followed in the car. By the time she arrived at the hospital her convulsions were stronger and she was given Ativan. She recovered from the convulsive attack but was paralyzed from the waist down. At about that time, we were scheduled for the heme treatment so she was transported on a stretcher to the Hem/Onc clinic where she promptly became argumentative. This was the first time Jill had aimed negativity at NHC staff and it unnerved me. Thankfully, I had read about central nervous system (CNS) involvement including agitation, possible paralysis and hallucinations. While concerned, I was not as terrified as I would have been if she had been so affected when this all started. As the Panhematin flowed into her liver Jill calmed down considerably and regained movement in her lower body. When the infusion was done, she was able to walk on her own and we left the clinic.

The IV setup was left in again the next day in order to reduce needle sticks. This time, though, Jill's hand became so swollen it resembled a cartoon character's. Once home she took the IV out herself. Head bells began jangling. I realized Jill had not been exposed to Heparin before yesterday so I Googled "Heparin" and read "…a highly sulfated glycosaminoglycan."[60] Knowing that porphyria and sulfa drugs aren't compatible, I wondered, "Could Jill be supersensitive to sulfa/sulfur? And if so, how much was in Heparin?

The next day Jill was at the Littleton Public Library with her tutor Lizabeth* who called to say that Jill had become very lethargic, could not stay focused and needed to be picked up. I arrived to find an ambulance parked in front and quickly made my way to the room that served as Jill's classroom. She was non-responsive and convulsing. I was shocked that she had reacted in the library. I asked that she be brought to NHC. The EMTs insisted because she was non-responsive she would be taken to the nearest hospital, which was MedCity. There, they said, she would be stabilized and if need be, sent via another ambulance ride to NHC. The whole idea was ludicrous to me—after eighteen months of dealing with Jill's fainting/seizure episodes and multiple trips to different emergency rooms, it seemed only logical that she should be taken directly to NHC to get much-needed heme into her liver as soon as possible. But all the professionals we talked to about the issue said it was a "state law" that an unresponsive patient had to be brought to the nearest local hospital though no one could cite the actual law.

I made my way to Jill's ED room and was relieved to see, though she was still seizing, that an oxygen mask had been put over her nose and mouth. The nurses turned to acknowledge me and I thanked them for administering the oxygen. Since this was the time when information regarding what was happening when she collapsed was collected, I told them that Jill had been getting daily treatments of Panhematin at NHC and, to help reduce the number of IV needle sticks, the nurses had put Heparin in the IV lock and sent her home. Shaking her head from side to side one of the nurses declared, "No one uses Heparin anymore."

I replied, "Well, NHC did yesterday and the day before, too. Her hand swelled up both times. She had seizures yesterday and was sent to NHC where she got a heme treatment. They left the IV in again and put more Heparin in it. But last night, her hand swelled so badly that she took the IV out herself. The swelling went down, but as you can see, now she's seizing again. I really think Heparin might have something to do with this." One of the nurses grumbled that she had been "told in our training not to use Heparin." Then they both abruptly left the room. I sat with Jill. I went into the hallway every ten minutes to see if anyone was around who could administer Ativan, as Dr. O'Connor's protocol required and as had happened the previous times she had arrived in seizure at MedCity. Finally, as the time approached 2:00 p.m. (I had received Lizabeth's call from the library before noon) and after I'd been back and forth between the hallway and Jill's bedside multiple times, I recognized Mario,* a former Benton School nurse. I asked him if he would please get someone to give Jill Ativan to stop the seizures.

About fifteen minutes later Dr. Berkov* came in, stood at the foot of Jill's bed and announced, "She is *not* having seizures."

---

60 *Heparin*. Wikipedia. http://en.wikipedia.org/wiki/Heparin

I tried to remain calm and replied, "I know she's not having actual seizures. She has acute intermittent porphyria and one of her symptoms is convulsions—but "seizures" is on the list of AIP symptoms. Ativan generally relieves them. Can't you please give her some to make them stop? The doctor who treated her last time she was here did that and she recovered fine." The fiasco that followed was something I hope never to experience again. Jill continued to convulse and my calmness went out the window. I was about to lose my temper. I could feel it coming and other than the doctor administering Ativan to Jill right away, there was no way to stop it. I asked Dr. Berkov how many porphyria patients he'd cared for. "Two or three," he said nonchalantly.

I truly doubted him. Trying so hard to steady my voice, I said, "Look, when she was brought unresponsive to this hospital some time ago, the attending doctor told me not to look for zebras. Well guess what? I found a damn zebra." I felt a surge of panic and my voice became urgent and strained, "And her problem is *not* in her head—*it's in her liver*! She has acute intermittent porphyria! PLEASE! All she needs from you right now is a shot of Ativan. Why won't you just DO that?" I asked to talk with the nurse coordinator with whom I had been speaking on the phone for a week or more regarding the "state law" about the ambulance's inability to transport Jill directly to NHC where she could get the treatment she needed. Berkov said she was out for the day.

"Then I want to talk with the head of the ER," I said.

He replied, "I *am* the head of the ER." Jill was still convulsing. I hurried through my theory about the IV lock/Heparin situation, said I had found out that Heparin is a "highly sulfated" drug and that I suspected it somehow might have played a role in Jill's current convulsive state. I did not know what exactly caused the sulfa/porphyria problem, I said, nor did I know if sulfur/sulfa/whatever contributed to what was happening. "Look," I said, "two incidents of Jill ending up in the hospital following Heparin use in as many days just can't be coincidental."

Dr. Berkov said, "*Highly sulfated* does *not* mean it's got sulfur in it—or, it might have a trace—but not enough to create this type of reaction." So he was conceding Jill *was* having a reaction! I was trying so hard to get back to some semblance of calm.

In my head, I yelled, "*So DO something about it!* But aloud I said deliberately, "Then at least *look* at her records from the last time we were here and follow that treatment—it works." Dr. Berkov and I were standing on opposite sides of Jill's bed. She was still convulsing. I lost my composure which prompted him to admonish, "*Why* are you giving me such a hard time?" I snapped, "*Me* giving *you* a hard time? *Really*? My kid is flopping around like a fish out of water, YOU'RE not doing a *damn* thing to help her though you claim to have treated 'three or four' porphryics and I'M giving YOU a hard time? What about *you* giving *a patient* who needs medical attention a *hard time*! He raised his voice, "*You* need to calm down. Would you like me to step out of the room?"

I turned from the bed and yelled, "*I'M THE ONE LEAVING THIS ROOM! YOU NEED TO STAY RIGHT HERE AND HELP MY DAUGHTER!*" I ran into the hallway and looked back through the window in the door that I had shut behind me. Jill was still convulsing. As I stood with my hand on the doorknob, my head was reeling and I began rambling, "Hippocratic Oath be damned, this doctor is not making any effort to help Jill. No one seems to know, or care to know, anything about this hateful disease! What in God's name is going to happen to her now? He probably doesn't even know about Panhematin!" I still had my hand on the doorknob when Berkov grabbed it from the inside, attempting to come out into the hall. I pulled it back and reminded him, "You need to help Jill!" He roughly yanked the door open, stormed by me and yelled for security. Then he addressed Mario, "Is she always like this?" Mario answered no. I tried again to calm myself and succeeded— a little bit that is—until I returned to Jill's bedside. She was still convulsing. Two security guards entered the room. One stood at the foot of the bed, the other across from me on the opposite side of the bed and asked what the problem was. Jill was still convulsing.

I yelled, "What's the problem? Really? Look at her!" I hooked my thumb at the doctor and continued, "He's the problem! He's a doctor who's refusing to help his patient. He's not doing anything to stop her seizures even though he easily could. OK, I'm not an M.D. I am a M.O.M. and my daughter needs help and"—stabbing my finger in Berkov's direction with tears running down my cheeks—"HE WON'T HELP HER! What would you do if a doctor refused to help YOUR sick kid even though he could? Just stand around wringing your hands? I doubt it. THAT, sir, is my problem."

The security guards and Dr. Berkov took off, leaving me alone with convulsing Jill. I grabbed my cell phone to call Ed. I was so distraught I could barely concentrate on what I was doing and could hardly talk when he answered. Not knowing I had left the house to begin with, he attempted to get me to calm down and tell him what was going on. I said, "I got a call from Lizabeth. She said Jill wasn't doing well and asked me to come get her. By the time I got there, the ambulance was there, too, because Jill went into seizures—at the library! They wouldn't bring her to NHC and brought her to MedCity again. And the doctor won't even give her Ativan! He says she's not having seizures! It's been over TWO HOURS and she's still convulsing! I want her to go to NHC now!" Ed said he was on his way. By this time, ED Chair Dr. Maxim* arrived in the room; Jill was still convulsing. I demanded that since Berkov would not treat her, she immediately be transferred to NHC to get the Panhematin she needed. Ed arrived and began talking to Dr. Maxim about the NHC/MedCity ambulance debacle. He asked if MedCity Hospital was going to accept Jill as a patient in the future, would they be willing to keep Panhematin on hand to treat her? Dr. Maxim said that would be unlikely as there were few if any known porphyrics in the entire state, never mind the hospital's service area. When asked if Jill could be sent directly to NHC as had happened numerous times already, he said he would "try to get that to happen" and would get back to us with an answer. Then, because he said he would transfer her to NHC, I left to get there before Jill did. Ed stayed until she left in the ambulance. By the time she left MedCity via ambulance transport, Jill was in the same condition as when she had first entered that ED—convulsing. In spite of having been finally given Ativan during the ambulance ride, when she arrived at NHC, her torso, hands, limbs, head and jaw continued to sporadically spasm. She was utterly exhausted, as was I.

CHAPTER 20

Unstable

Couldn't Stand the Weather
— STEVIE RAY VAUGHAN ALBUM TITLE

Following that ordeal, Jill had a conveyor belt of attacks. She ended up at NHC again the next day with seizures that started at *home*. Over the next week, she had three more. Because so many people, medical and otherwise, found calling Jill's convulsive activity "seizures" to be problematic, I took to calling them "convulsive attacks." I feared that time was running out; Jill was collapsing nearly every day. Her packed hospital bag was always at the ready, and I was constantly running between NHC and MedCity hospitals. It was a routine I dreaded. Jill would lapse into convulsions, I'd call 911 and she would be transported to a hospital. Regardless of where she was headed, I would pray she would survive the attack and wondered how much more her body and brain could take. I spent lots of time by her bedside as she lay either convulsing, receiving heme/dextrose or recovering. I kept a small notepad in my purse with questions I had written to hold up for her to read after an episode calmed. On one page I wrote, "Can you hear?" On another, "Can you talk?" She would reply by either nodding "yes" or shaking her head "no." Sometimes there was no response—no recognition she even knew who I was or what was happening.

The trips to NHC ED had become so frequent that a couple of the nurses commented about how calm and collected I appeared. "You're obviously familiar with what's going on," a nurse said to me one day when Jill had been put into the trauma room because of a lack of beds. Jill had the "lights are on, but nobody's home" look about her and could neither speak nor hear. Suddenly, she pointed at something on the ceiling and motioned that whatever she saw was moving down. I was eerily intrigued. The heme/D10 treatment had been ordered from the hospital pharmacy and the infusion was to take place in the trauma room. I supposed that meant the usual hours-long timeframe so, not having been able to cancel a brief appointment on such short notice, I told the nurses I would be back before the heme arrived. I made it back to the hospital in relatively short order only to find the room in chaos. Jill was yelling at the nurses and I thought, "Well at least she regained her speech!" To make matters worse, a little boy was in the next bed. His father was with him and it was clear Jill was disturbing everyone. It was one of those times when I wished the floor would open up and swallow me whole. I tried enticing Jill with lunch, a drink, anything. Finally, the heme began to reach Jill's liver and she calmed down, made it through the post-hydration infusion without further incident and regained her personality. She and I left the ED not knowing when the next attack would come.

During one of Jill's regular treatments, I told Dr. O'Connor that I had made a connection with the mother of an AIP patient who was older than Jill. She had given me the name of a pediatric hematologist who was of Swedish descent, had been medically trained in Sweden and was very familiar with AIP. "I'm going to contact this doctor and see if she would be willing to consult with us about Jill's case," I said. I had told Ed a week earlier that Jill was not getting enough heme to keep the attacks at bay. "In my "mom opinion," I'd said, "she needs heme until."

"Until what?" Ed asked.

"Until the symptoms stop," I replied, "and I have no idea how much heme that is." So to Dr. O'Connor, I asked, "How long should a heme treatment last anyway?" He said he didn't know. "Okay," I said wearily, "then I will make an appointment with this Dr. Piersen,* bring Jill to her office, get the information and bring it back to you." Dr. O'Connor asked if having an oxygen tank at home would make Jill feel better. It occurred to me he was still in sync with NHC's psychiatric team about Jill having conversion order. "Well, maybe she does have conversion disorder, I conceded to myself, but the fact that she had AIP was incontrovertible and in my mind, that needed to be figured out first. To that end, having oxygen available at home would make *me* feel better. So I said, "yes," and he signed us up for the program. We soon had the opportunity to try the apparatus out when Jill collapsed on the couch and began convulsing just five days after the Berkov/MedCity ED debacle. I raced for the face mask, put it on her and started the oxygen flowing. Then I called 911. The ambulance arrived with strict instructions to take Jill to MedCity Hospital—Dr. Maxim's orders, the EMTs said. Upset, I said, "Are they going to put Jill through hell again?" I begged, "*Please* bring her to NHC. *Please.*" I was furious. So much for Dr. Maxim saying he would see what he could do about sending Jill to NHC. "*How* can they continue to do this?" I yelled at God. "*Why* are you doing this to Jill? Why?" The ambulance pulled out of the driveway. Jill was on her way to MedCity Hospital, and there was nothing I or anyone could do about it.

We went through the same drill the next day. Jill said she was tired, reclined on the couch and went into convulsions. I put oxygen on her and called 911. This time the police chief and an officer from the Littleton Police Department arrived along with the first response medical team. It was a relief to have the officers there; others would witness what was happening. Jill was unresponsive and convulsing. The first response team members moved her to the floor and replaced "our" oxygen supply with theirs. As usual, I asked the EMT team to take her to NHC. One of the EMTs, a woman named Vivian* said no, they would follow the protocol established by Dr. Maxim, which was to take her to MedCity. Jill was transported to MedCity Hospital and transferred to NHC later that night. When she had recovered enough to be able to talk again, she was perturbed about something she had heard in the ambulance. Vivian had apparently been one of the EMTs present in the early stages of Jill's fainting episodes at the Benton School when she was being treated for bipolar disorder. Evidently, Vivian had not heard about the porphyria diagnosis. This time when the EMT crew arrived she had heard me say Jill had AIP, but apparently like Debbie and Anne before her, Vivian knew more about Jill's "problem" than anyone else did. And it was obvious that rather than being unable to hear like the attack she had suffered just five days prior, this time her hearing was working fine. Filled with indignation, Jill said, "Mom, Vivian said you have *Munchkin by Peroxide!* She mimicked, 'Poor Jill. Her mother thinks she has a disease that she doesn't have. She has bipolar and she goes off easy and gets mean and nasty.'"

Stifling a laugh, I said, "Do you mean Vivian said I have *Munchhausen by Proxy?*" Jill was annoyed because she hated that Dr. Bludonowitz had labeled her bipolar to begin with. "That was a misdiagnosis," she says in all seriousness. This was Jill's third bout of hearing while she suffered convulsive seizures and was considered non-responsive. Even though Lizabeth and I had a good laugh over Jill's *"Munchkin by Peroxide"* interpretation, I registered a written complaint to the ambulance company, the hospital, and the State department of public health about Vivian's indiscretion.

Though Jill adored Lizabeth and was doing well in tutoring, Ed and I were concerned about the isolation and ten short hours a week that served as Jill's "schooling." But what could we do? It was the State's minimal requirement. And it was clear to us that Jill's health was very precarious. I so hoped this Dr. Piersen would help us figure out AIP.

CHAPTER 21

Mix of Clouds and Sun

Ask and it will be given to you; seek and you will find;
knock and the door will be opened to you.
— MATTHEW 7:7

Dr. Wade continued to prescribe medications for Jill with no regard about whether or not they were on the APF or Swedish/Canadian (S/C) safe drug lists. The Hysocyamine she had prescribed for menstrual cramps was noted "probably safe" on APF's list but "probably porphryinogenic" and "prescribe only on strong or urgent indication" on the S/C list. The Klonopin she had said would help was rated unsafe on both lists. She had not even asked how or if the Panhematin was working for Jill. Before meeting Dr. Piersen I wanted to find a replacement primary care physician (PCP) who was not intimidated by AIP's challenges. I called a doctor friend who provided names of possible pediatricians for Jill. I settled on Dr. Alaimo* because she had affiliations with both NHC and Haven City hospitals and made an appointment for Jill and me to meet her.

Amidst the drama of fainting episodes, hospital visits, heme/D10 infusions, physical therapy appointments, tutoring and therapy sessions with Vanessa, Jill kept up with her weekly singing lessons. Her voice teacher Lora was patient, kind and encouraging—a good soul for Jill to have connected with. Singing was Jill's stress outlet and she continued to regularly give the antique piano, and with it, Kevin's nerves, a workout. In the meantime, Vanessa said she had to miss the next appointment because she was having some health issues and a colonoscopy was planned. Jill gamely told her not to worry—she had recently had one herself and it had been no a problem at all. We wished her good luck and said we would see her again in a couple of weeks.

Brenda and Jordin continued to provide email support to us. Brenda said she had already told Dr. Piersen about us. She extended an invitation to stay in her home when we came to Washington, D.C. I'd already looked into flights and had printed door-to-door driving directions from our house to the doctor's office. I was excited about getting ready to be on our way. Brenda's emails sustained me. She wrote, "I know how you feel… do you want to just stand in the middle of the road and scream in frustration because your child is very ill and no one is listening?" At the time Jordin was getting weekly heme infusions which were wearing for Brenda, too. In addition to being the first person I could talk to who understood the highs and lows we were dealing with, Brenda offered pragmatic advice. She told me of Jordin's port and offered, "You might want to talk with Dr. Piersen about getting Jill a port, too. There's an anesthesiologist at the medical center who is very familiar with porphyria because he worked in Africa with porphyria patients. He did Jordin's anesthesia and the surgery went off without a hitch."

Jordin, herself in and out of the hospital with recurrent AIP symptoms, emailed Jill and shared some of her own before and after port insertion experiences. She explained to Jill that she received her first treatment through a vein in her leg as that was the only vein they could access. Unfortunately, the vein was damaged and took over a month to heal. Because of the ordeal, Jordin decided to have a port surgically implanted. She admitted to being nervous prior to getting the procedure, "Because it made the fact that I was sick all that more real and that my AIP wasn't going to disappear. I got over that though. It's been a Godsend." Jordin included a photo to show the exact location where the port had been surgically implanted so Jill could see where hers would be located. Soon, she was looking forward to getting a port.

Before long, Dr. Piersen's assistant called to schedule an appointment. Ed preferred not to fly so we began planning a road trip. Meanwhile, the meeting date with Dr. Alaimo arrived. She admitted she knew little about porphyria but was willing to work with us and Dr. O'Connor, based on the input we received from Dr. Piersen. I shared Jill's AIP binder with her, emphasizing the S/C "drug list." She handed me a note to give to Dr. Piersen asking if it was all right to administer immunization shots Jill was due for. We talked about the ambulance company's "unbendable" rule about bringing Jill directly from home or school to NHC anytime she was unresponsive and explained they had done exactly that on several occasions. When in attack mode, Jill needed to get heme ASAP, I said, and the delay in bringing her to MedCity to be "stabilized" when oxygen and Ativan could be administered in the ambulance on the way to NHC made no sense to me. I told her what had happened with Dr. Berkov and explained MedCity's decision not to carry a supply of Panhematin for the single AIPorphyric identified in their coverage area. She pulled out a prescription pad and wrote "To whom it may concern. Please take Jill directly to NHC's ER if she is having seizures or unresponsiveness." With that, Dr. Alaimo became Jill's new primary care physician.

I faxed documents including the Tri-State Lab's DNA report, the lab report from eight months prior with her PBG-D values, observations I had made regarding Jill's symptoms and a series of questions I was hoping to get answers for to Dr. Piersen's attention. She called prior to our making the trip to ask how Jill had been responding to the Panhematin treatments. I said, "You know, it *is* helping, but no one seems to know how many treatments to give her."

Dr. Pierson responded, "Clearly, DNA proves Jill has AIP. I recommend she be given a heme bolus of four treatments—that means one treatment of a bottle of Panhematin per day before our appointment." She said she would talk with Dr. O'Connor about it. Once again, I felt that things were beginning to look up.

Soon, Jill was scheduled for the four heme treatments. When we arrived for the first one, the nurses had trouble finding a suitable vein for IV access. My stomach churned as nurse after nurse tried. Jill was doing her best, even trying to joke as vein after vein "blew," until Natalia* arrived and took care of business. She selected her spot carefully, fastened the rubber tie and plunged the IV needle into Jill's left wrist. Jill burst into tears. Five nurses had made separate attempts of up to three sticks apiece until a vein had been accessed. They all agreed it was time for a port. Although this was true, it would not help Jill for the immediate future—she still needed three more heme treatments before we met with Dr. Piersen. Like the trooper Jill is, she went back each time with anxiety in her heart and a smile on her face and endured three more series of dreaded IV sticks.

With time moving quickly toward our D.C. trip, Jill contacted Brenda herself to let her know we were coming, "My mom told me that you've invited [us] to stay with you, and I would love that if it's ok with you. But," she warned, "I would have to see how I'm feeling when I get there. If I'm good, I would like to take the offer up and stay with you guys. On the other hand if I don't feel that great I wouldn't wanna have you taking care of me or possibly rushing me to the ER or having to call 911 for me. Sometimes when I'm not feeling well my attitude is really moody." She signed off, "I LOVE going around to other places. I'll let you go because I have to go watch the Jonas brothers TV show. Until next time, tell Jordin I said hello and to stay healthy."

Brenda welcomed Jill for a visit, "I was thinking you could share Jordin's room with her. That would give you the chance to get to know each other and share porphyria stories that only those who have the disorder can understand."

When we arrived, Brenda hugged us all around, introduced us to her son Lenny* and the delightful felines that shared their home and made us feel comfortable. As it turned out, Jordin was recuperating from her most recent AIP go-round so Brenda led Jill upstairs. She then returned to visit with Ed and me to share AIP stories. She told us of the time Jordin had had one of her worst attacks and her urine sample had been put aside and left for a while. It had darkened in color and that was how it was decided she had porphyria. It was getting late and having met Brenda, Ed and I decided if Jill asked to stay the night that would be allowed. We exchanged cell phone numbers and returned to the hotel but shortly after retiring, Jill needed to be picked up. The long trip and the excitement of meeting Brenda and Jordin had taken a toll; Jill was exhausted and her abdomen hurt. We got her settled into bed where she slept fitfully until it was time to go to Dr. Piersen's office. Ed filled out the requisite paperwork and we were ushered into an examination room. The doctor arrived and proceeded to examine Jill. As she did, she provided answers:

- Was Jill's AIP was manifest or latent? "Indisputable. Her AIP is active. As such, her attacks require treatment/maintenance according to the Swedish Porphyria Foundation's recommendations (carbs, safe/unsafe drugs, lifestyle, eating habits)." Dr. P told us that in the area of Sweden that she called home, AIP prevalence was approximately 1:1000 people (and in one particular village 1:50).

- Could AIP be considered to be the cause of Jill's varied and odd symptoms? "Yes. Attacks can be considered mild, moderate, severe or critical in nature and should never be dismissed, no matter the level."

- Regarding the psychiatric/psychological symptoms Jill sometimes exhibited, she said, "If Jill has them, they are secondary to the AIP" and continued, "when anyone back home is exhibiting psychotic symptoms and taken to hospital, tests are done to check for porphyria before any medication is administered and other diagnoses considered."

- What about the Swedish article I had found regarding the darkened urine symptom not always seen in children with AIP? "Recordable urine porphyrin elevations are sometimes not seen until the late teens/early adulthood and possibly later," she said.

- She called the "seizures" pseudo seizures, yet when pressed about respiratory rates and low finger pulse-oximeter stats, she said, "Leave the oxygen on. It won't hurt and since it helps Jill to recover, that's what is important."

- What about the bout of paralysis that Jill experienced? "Not to be taken lightly. As attacks continue and/or worsen, paralysis can become permanent. Nip attacks as early as possible; it is best to avoid them altogether."

- Should Jill have a port? "Panhematin should be administered via a central vein," she said and recommended Jill get a port as soon as possible, claiming not to do so was "cruel and unusual punishment."

The examination and parent question session essentially over, Dr. P turned her attention to Jill with advice:

- Stay well hydrated to avoid kidney stones, a common occurrence in AIP patients.

- Avoid contraceptives; they are a *huge* risk for AIP attacks.

- The doctor asked Jill if she'd ever noticed a change in "how things taste—particularly orange juice?" Jill said yes. Ed and I confirmed that Jill sometimes complained about the taste of it. Dr. Pierson said a little thing like that can be an early sign of impending AIP activity.

- Jill was troubled by weight gain yet Dr. P. underscored a mandate: NO fasting. In fact, she recommended, "You need 250 g of carbs per day—go with whole/multi grain choices vs. sugar carbs." She suggested three meals and three snacks daily to achieve that carb goal and said "exercise is critical for weight loss, so start slowly and try to work up to swimming, bike riding, etc."

- Most importantly, she stressed: "Always and forever—avoid alcohol and recreational drugs."

- "Before taking any medication—over the counter (OTC) or prescription (Rx) *always* check the safe drug list—and when prescribed drug(s) are required, make sure any doctor you see in the future does the same."

- "Prior to any surgery (port included), carbo-load the day before and never fast before surgery. Be sure your doctor knows that you require glucose infusion (D10) before and during any surgery and until you are able to eat for yourself. For any necessary dental work requiring local or general anesthesia, again, check the drug list to be sure that safe ones are selected." [Note: For dental work, we have found that Jill tolerates Bupivacaine numbing agent well.]

- Finally, "To help reduce the risk of liver cancer, take vitamins and supplements." However, she said to always avoid the herbal remedy St. John's Wort as it is *very* dangerous for porphyrics.

- Dr. P then gave us a Panhematin treatment/maintenance schedule to be started immediately:

Week 1: Heme bolus (4 treatments/1x per day)

Week 2: 3 treatments/1x per day

Week 3: 2 treatments/1x per day

Week 4: 1 treatments/1x per day

Week 5: Heme bolus (4 treatments/1x per day)

Week 6: 3 treatments/1x per day

Week 7: 2 treatments/1x per day

Week 8: 1 treatment

Week 9: 1 treatment

She stressed that it was critically important for Jill's blood levels be checked regularly with particular focus on the iron level in order to avoid iron overload. If her iron count crept up, she recommended the treatment be reduced until a stabilized iron count had been achieved. Once this regimen had been completed, Dr. Pierson recommended paying attention to Jill's body's signs and symptoms and modify the protocol as seemed medically appropriate. At that point, Dr. Piersen said, she might be ready for one treatment per week—or she might require the heme bolus again. Ideally, the goal was to get down to one heme treatment per month. However, because female hormones are in charge, if needed, she said to add a treatment just prior to menses. "Follow this program," she said, "and Jill should be ready to go to school with her classmates in September."

CHAPTER 22

Moon Shadows

In youth, we learn; in age we understand.
— MARIE VON EBNE-ESCHENBACH, AUSTRIAN WRITER

Clearly, Dr. P was familiar with and not afraid to use heme "until." We left her office uplifted and relieved and ready to spend the afternoon in Washington, D.C. In spite of being worried she might have an attack, Jill got into the tourist spirit and we all enjoyed an abbreviated visit to our nation's capital. During the drive home, I called Dr. O'Connor's office and learned the port surgery was set for the end of the week. Jill looked forward to it and, thanks to Dr. P's guidelines, the surgery went fine. But when Jill woke in the recovery room she *hurt* and confided, "I'm *so* glad I didn't get exploratory surgery!" That afternoon Jill received her heme/D10 treatment through the new port.

Jill was eager to tell Vanessa about the horrible multiple IV stick ordeal; meeting Brenda and Jordin; the appointment with Dr. P; visiting Washington, D.C.; the heme treatment protocol plan and her port surgery, so I called to arrange a therapy session. Vanessa's voice mail picked up and I left a message. Her husband returned my call to say surgical difficulties had been encountered and it might be some time before Vanessa was able to get back to us. Jill and I were worried; no one likes to hear of problems associated with surgery. It was a few weeks before we saw Vanessa again. When we did, she told us about what had happened during the colonoscopy. As she recounted the story, she said though she had felt miserable, she had gotten a chuckle remembering the door-pulling escapade with Dr. Berkov I'd told her about. I said I was glad at least I had been able to bring a smile to her face during such a harrowing time, but more than anything, Jill and I were thankful Vanessa was on the way to better health.

Having received Dr. P's letter confirming Jill's diagnosis of active AIP, I sent a copy to Bart and wondered what, if anything, would come of it. Meanwhile, a notice about the International Conference on Porphyrins and Porphyrias to be held in Stockholm appeared in the APF newsletter and nudged my Internet research impulse with another search focus. First it had been simply "porphyria," then "acute intermittent porphyria," then "childhood and/or juvenile onset acute intermittent porphyria." Now I Googled and Binged with new gusto: "Swedish Porphyria Foundation," "International Conference on Porphyrins and Porphyrias," "AIP in Sweden," "AIP in Europe," "AIP in Australia," "AIP in Canada," "AIP in Spain," "AIP in France" and other countries.

As I read through the multitude of articles, I learned AIP is said to be the most common and the most severe of the acute porphyrias. It is found in all races and on every continent and is known across the globe by many different names: acute intermittent porphyria, acute neurologic porphyria; acute neuropsychiatric porphyria; chronic porphyria; hepatic porphyria; intermittent acute porphyria; neurovisceral porphyria; neuroporphyria; porphyric hemophilia; porphyrunuria; pyrroloporphyria; Swedish porphyria and probably others. AIP has confounded USA and other countries' doctors for generations. It may be referred to as a liver, blood, enzyme, metabolic or neuropsychiatric disorder. However, from a medical standpoint because AIP patients' problems result from a faulty blood-making process, U.S. cases are most often managed by hematologists.

The word *porphyria* is derived from the Greek word for purple and is so named because purplish-red pigmented porphyrins can be excreted in the urine of AIPorphyrics. It is said that AIP has its roots in the Northern Scandinavian indigenous people known as the Sami. Sweden's Dr. Einar Wallquist "was able to construct a family tree displaying eight generations [with acute intermittent porphyria] back to 1701."[61] The first reported case of acute porphyria was in 1889 when a female patient died after taking sulphonol.[62] At the time, her physician, a Dr. Stokvis observed and "described 'two peculiar urinary pigments' but did not believe they were connected to the drug. [Then] two years later he showed that the drug was indeed the cause of the urinary pigments."[63] It is reported that Swedish physician Dr. "Waldonström and his coworker Arthur Engel [skied] through the vast countryside [and identified] farmsteads of interest by aid of the red urine spots in the snow beside houses."[64] At the time, the illness was known as the "family" disease or the "red" disease. Then, in 1937, Dr. Waldonström published a thesis based on 106 AIP patients in that country. Because the condition typically manifests quickly in acute or sharp, severe, excruciatingly painful episodes at varying intervals,[65] he named the illness "acute *intermittent* [because the symptoms can come and go with

---

61 Bylesjö, I. *Epidemiological, Clinical and Studies of Acute Intermittent Porphyria*. Medical dissertation, Umea University. www.diva-portal.org/smash/get/ diva2:141227; FULLTEXT01.pdf. 2008, 3.
62 Ibid.
63 Ibid.
64 Thunell, S. et al. *Porphyria in Sweden*. www.biomed.cas.cz/physiolres/pdf/55%20Suppl%202/55_S109. pdf. Porphyria Centre Sweden. 2005.
65 Socialstyrelen. *Acute Intermittent Porphyria*. http://www.socialstyrelen.se/rarediseases/acuteintermittentporphyria

maddening unpredictability] porphyria." The condition then became known as "Swedish Porphyria."

The exact worldwide AIP prevalence is unknown but what is known is that Sweden's AIP prevalence is generally estimated to be 1:50 to 1:1000 with two Northern Sweden municipalities having the highest prevalence of AIP patients in the world. U.S. AIP prevalence is estimated to range from five to ten per100,000.

The name of a Swedish doctor who had collaborated on numerous porphyria articles and studies frequently came up in my online searches. I saw that he was scheduled to present at the porphyria conference. I decided that since I could not go to the convention in Sweden, maybe I could get his attention, so I emailed him. There was so much I needed to know—most importantly, how typical Jill's case of juvenile AIP was. He replied via email that her AIP diagnosis had been well established, she had entered puberty, had ingested a porphyrinogenic agent (risperidone) and said she could well be expected to move into an acute attack of porphyria. I then asked if there was a possibility that juvenile-onset AIP might be addressed at future porphyria conferences. He said he could take the issue up with the doctor responsible for planning the next porphyria conference and also one of his colleagues.

Dr. Piersen's recommended heme schedule worked wonderfully; Jill was attack-free for seventy eight days. But then on June 30th she spent the entire treatment time not feeling well. Upon returning home I detected a faint odor throughout the house. When I asked Ed about it, he said he had applied a small amount of ant killer in the basement the day before. The smell was weak and I did not think too much about it. The next day Jill was not feeling well again and asked for a bed for the treatment. As the pre-hydration D10 was administered, her body began trembling. An hour later it was time for Panhematin to be infused when she fell into sleep-mode. Then she abruptly started convulsing. The nurse, the nurse-practitioner and the on-call physician, Dr. Goddin* were with us. This was the first AIP attack of Jill's that this particular medical team had witnessed. Oxygen, Ativan and Panhematin were administered and the convulsions ceased. After the heme supply had been fully infused, Jill regained consciousness, but was unable to speak and mimed that she needed to use the bathroom but could not walk. Elena* helped her with a bedpan. When her speech returned, she asked what had happened. I told her she had just had an attack and everyone had done the right things to help her through it. She was groggy, but still had an hour of post-hydration D10 to complete. Thankfully, when that infusion was finished, she was able to walk and talk again, and we went home.

By this time, I had deduced that Jill must have had reacted to the pesticide in the basement so when I got home I opened doors and windows to ventilate the house. It worked because Jill was okay for the rest of July and August. However, the issue of toxins remained on my mind. Jill's reaction to the chemical in our basement was very much like what she had experienced in the Littleton schools and the Heparin problem: shivering, tremors, falling asleep, convulsions, sensory impairment, paralysis. Knowing she would be returning to school in a few weeks, I called Littleton's school facilities director to ask about specific products used in the schools. "Would it be possible for me to get specifications for all cleaning products used as well as a list of where and when pesticides are applied on school property?"

Mr. Bell* said, "We use a 'green' hydrogen peroxide-based cleaning product. Completely safe. A super sanitizer. Healthy for people and the environment." I reminded him what was safe for most might not be safe for AIPorphyric Jill and maybe others who might be unusually susceptible to the substances. He said he would collect the necessary product specifications and to call him in September to arrange a time to meet.

CHAPTER 23

Sun Behind the Clouds

Tou saw we, se pa sa.
(Nothing you see is what it seems.)
— CREOLE ADAGE

Vanessa referred Krista Williamson,* an MSW with a state initiative for children with special health care needs, to us. Krista came to Jill's next infusion session to learn more about AIP and its effects on her. During the meeting, Jill expressed anxiety about returning to school; she was afraid that the fainting spells would resume. She was also worried about potential upcoming inevitable absences due to the heme infusion maintenance schedule. Many adults can attest that middle school is challenging for most children and students with perceivable differences know firsthand how tough peers can be. Jill knew that, too. She had hobbled through sixth grade and much of seventh grade. While the other students had spent seven hours a day sitting in classes, passing through hallways and interacting with each other during lunch period and/or on buses, traveling on field trips, watching and/or playing intramural sports, she had been sitting in the local library or at a small table in our living room with a single teacher for ten hours a week. She felt like damaged goods—out of sight and out of mind. I asked the NCH APRN for a supply of Ativan tablets to be given to the school nurse if or when Jill's anxiety increased at school. She readily agreed, and provided me with a prescription slip.

Dr. O'Connor arrived in the infusion center and we discussed the treatment protocol. He shared that he was more concerned about the CNS involvement during the attacks than liver damage. "The liver can regenerate itself," he said, "but the damage done from CNS depression might not be an easy cure." I was relieved he had voiced a concern about another thing that had been on my mind; this CNS stuff made me nervous—no pun intended.

A friend who taught in a city school system told me of a student with a chronic illness in her class. She said a group of medical specialists, along with the school nurse and the child's parent, had conducted an informational session about the student's illness, its treatment and how the student might be affected such as absence from school, treatment at the hospital, late arrival, early dismissal, and lethargy. She said, among other things, the discussion helped to build peer empathy and support for the student. Having heard similar stories that schools allowed information about various conditions such as allergy to peanut butter and other allergies, diabetes and leukemia to be disseminated or discussed, I suggested arranging for a similar discussion with Jill's peers, perhaps in a health class setting. As an employee of a state public health department funded entity, Krista readily agreed it was a good idea. I added that to my to-do list and thought the principal or student services director would be the person to start with.

One day, knowing beforehand that Krista would be visiting her at NHC, Jill brought her CD player and the CD she had made with the help of NHC's "Mike the Music Man." She played the song for Krista. As discussed, singing was Jill's coping mechanism. Each week, she presented the latest song she had written to Lora who would play piano as Jill sang. Being the 'tween that she was, Jill occasionally missed a lesson because of something she'd said or done. So Lora asked if she could talk with Jill about respecting parents and if she could give Jill some literature geared toward young people. I said that would be fine. When Jill brought the information home, they were easily identifiable as being of the Jehovah's Witness faith. Our family is Roman Catholic; I'd been either a CCD (Catholic religion school) teacher or assistant teacher since Jill was in first grade. That alone would have been enough for some people to have summarily dismissed the information. But after reviewing them I decided that to ignore the books would not be fair to Jill's budding interest in religion, nor to Lora who was offering genuine assistance. Jill would soon be confirmed as an adult Catholic. No, I wouldn't simply banish the books. God had given Jill a heavy cross to bear. If there was even one point in those books that could help her when she needed it, I felt they were meant to be in her possession.

The stars must have aligned because Jill, who had been trolling the Internet to keep up with the Jonas Brothers' concert tour schedule, discovered they were to be in Boston before the start of the school year. A couple of weeks after meeting Krista, Jill and Ed were off to Bean Town to see the Jo Bros live and in concert. She was ecstatic—a dream fulfilled. The next weekend found us at the annual family cookout. Jill was relieved when this time she was able to swim, play games, spend time with her cousins and be a regular kid. Things were beginning to look promising.

About two weeks later, our family attended a summer awards ceremony for a college-prep program Kevin attended. Jill was happy to see that a former classmate whose older brothers Kevin knew, was there, too. Yearning for updates about school life, Jill cautiously approached Beatrice* and before long the girls were reconnecting. Jill filled Beatrice in as to why she had been absent from school for the year—and to tell her she had attended the Jonas Brothers' concert in Boston. Beatrice herself had reentered Littleton schools only the year before after being homeschooled by her mother, Sherilyn.* During the limited amount of time Jill spent in seventh grade, she had noticed that Beatrice hovered in the periphery of the clique of tough girls of which Cameron was the leader. This bothered Jill immensely and, during her homebound tutoring term would periodically express concern for Beatrice. "She's not as strong as I am," Jill would say. "I hope they're not doing the same thing to her they did to me." I had noticed police reports in the local newspaper about a domestic situation at Cam's residence months before and counseled Jill to be particularly careful about school social issues when she returned to LMS, "You've missed a lot. Be yourself but try to keep your distance, especially from the kids who weren't very nice to you back then." I was pleased to see Jill had done just that with Beatrice. I had always told her, "All you need to get through school is one good friend." Maybe Beatrice would wind up being that friend; the potential certainly was there.

The girls got together soon after the awards ceremony. Jill was excited about Beatrice being from a bible-based Christian family, "Just like the Jonas Brothers," she said.

Sherilyn dropped Beatrice off at our house and before leaving to run errands informed me that she and her husband Mickey* were "going through a contentious divorce." Surprised, I conveyed my sympathies or otherwise, depending on her feelings and said to let me know if there was any way we could help. When Sherilyn returned for Beatrice, Ed and I invited her in to visit. The topic of public school social problems came up as we chatted. I mentioned that we were concerned that a trio of boys who had bothered Jill at the local fair might give her a hard time when she returned to school. Though I had spoken to the boys myself that time, Ed and I expected school problems to be handled by the administrators, we said. Sherilyn readily agreed. Throughout this time Beatrice and Jill were playfully running around. I was tempted to tell them to tone it down; after all they were not little children anymore. In the end I decided to let it go—Jill had had such difficult times, it was good to see her having fun again. When Sherilyn was ready to leave, the girls appeared with several items Jill had apparently given to Beatrice. Then Jill asked if she could give a rather pricey bedroom item to Beatrice because "I don't want it anymore." Beatrice and Sherilyn looked at me.

I shook my head, "I'm sorry, but no. Jill might want to pass it onto her own child in the future." My head bells rang. The last time Colton,* Beatrice's oldest brother, had visited Kevin he'd tried to wangle a piece of electronic equipment by telling him, "I'll invite to you my party—you can give it to me for a birthday gift." Kevin had said sorry, but no.

Then Jill asked, "Beatrice invited me to go to church on Sunday with them. Can I go? Please?" "Put any misgivings aside," I told myself. "There's a divorce happening in the Martin home—lots of things up in the air."

Sherilyn interjected brightly, "It's okay with me. We can pick her up and bring her home after." Jill's eyes were pleading.

How could I say no a church/friend visit? "Besides," I thought, "Jill is interested in Bible-based Christianity like the Jonas Brothers religion. It is an opportunity to let her see how other people worship God." I bet to myself that doing so would eventually turn her firmly in the direction of continuing to follow Jesus as a Catholic. "Okay, you can go," I said. The girls had already rummaged through Jill's closet to select suitable church wear. Over the next couple of days Jill prattled on about how Beatrice did this, Beatrice said that.

I wondered if she knew Beatrice's parents were getting divorced. That was answered when she said, "Beatrice is kind of mad at her dad; her parents are getting divorced."

"Well, divorce can be hard on kids, just be careful with what you say and how you say it to her. She might get moody sometimes and need space," I said.

Then Jill said, "You know what? When we were in my room, Beatrice said 'Catholics are fake!' I was so shocked, my jaw just dropped!" I was taken aback too. We have always taught our children to respect others' religious choices so I was uncomfortable that Beatrice would spew anti-Catholic rhetoric even if she was just a child.

I asked Jill if she had responded; she said no, she'd been too surprised. "But I know I would never say anything like that to her or anyone about their religion," she said.

I drove Jill to the Martin home in time for them to make it to the church service. When they returned, Sherilyn raved, "Jill has turned into a lovely young lady. She's grown up so much!" I honestly could not say the same about Beatrice; my jury was still out on her. The girls had seated themselves at the old piano and Beatrice was playing a tune. Impressed, I asked her if she took lessons. Sherilyn immediately answered. Imitating a violinist, she said yes that while Beatrice took piano lessons, she, Sherilyn, took violin lessons. Not having any musical ability, I expressed admiration for such talent. Sherilyn went on to say she was resuming an interest in the violin she'd had as a child. As the conversation went back and forth, Sherilyn offered that she had been an only child. I mused to myself, "An only child who married and mothered four children in short order could find circumstances a bit overwhelming." To me, taking on the additional burden of homeschooling seemed to be tempting burnout. I was aware that her father had passed away a few years' earlier; missing her father and the comments she tossed out about her soon-to-be ex-husband gave me a glimpse into the depths of Sherilyn's discontent.

CHAPTER 24

Cold Front Approaching

Their mouths are filled with…deceit and oppression;
under their tongues are mischief and iniquity.
— PSALM 10:7

Invitations for Jill to join Beatrice for church services came frequently. Jill was like a bug drawn to a lighted bulb on a summer's night. I sincerely doubted Sherilyn and her husband Mickey would have allowed any of their offspring to have a vice-versa experience. One time Jill came home ruffled about a conversation Sherilyn and her aunt, who had accompanied them to church, had engaged in during the car ride home in which Sherilyn repeatedly referred to one of her sons as the "problem" child." She had said that to me years earlier so I wasn't surprised to hear it. I was concerned, though, the two women had had the discussion in Jill's and Beatrice's presence. Jill, fancying herself our family's 'difficult' one, was really bothered by Sherilyn's portrayal of Josh.*

As visits to our home became more frequent, Ed and I soon realized that Beatrice was definitely *not* bashful. In fact, she was precocious, sometimes rudely so. As Colton had done with Kevin, Beatrice introduced Jill to Facebook where it became obvious that Jill had not needed to be so concerned about Beatrice's social positioning after all. Though she voiced strong, negative opinions about members of the "tough girl" clique, they were all her "Facebook friends." Beatrice had introduced Jill to a few girls on Facebook and she began spending quite a bit of time on it. "Mom!" she said reverently one day, "Kaitlin* says she'll have my back when we get back to school!"

Jill's thirteenth birthday was approaching. She asked to have her hair styled in a salon and to go to the Red Lobster restaurant. She asked if Beatrice could come. Ed and I said yes. We planned for Beatrice to accompany Jill to the hairdresser's.

Then we would all go to the restaurant after which the girls could take a quick swim in our pool. Beatrice expressed disappointment in our time choice and said her mother wanted her home at a different time than we had planned, so we changed the timing. The day arrived. At the hair salon, Beatrice settled into the chair next to Jill's, happily chatting away. I left them to their girl talk and went to run errands. When I returned, Jill proudly displayed her reddish highlights. We went to collect Kevin and Ed for the next phase of the birthday celebration. On the way, Jill commented about how she'd "almost" gotten her hair cut "in spikes" in addition to the highlights. I told her I would not have been happy to have seen her hair cut that way without my permission.

Beatrice piped up, "Well, it's her hair, right?"

"Yeah, but *I'm* paying for it," I retorted. "And when she's old enough to take care of herself *and* pay for it, she can do what she wants with her hair—including spiking it!" I sensed a rebel lurking beneath Beatrice's outwardly complacent Christian girl persona.

With our tight budget, sit-down restaurants were a luxury, so we were all looking forward to a sumptuous lunch. Walking into the restaurant lobby, Beatrice spied the lobster tank and loudly demanded, "I want a whole Maine lobster!"

Jill picked up the notion, too, "Yeah, can I have a whole lobster, too?"

I eyed the empty lobster pot in the restaurant lobby and said, "Weird, but I don't think they have lobsters today." Ed looked doubtful. Kevin looked annoyed.

"Whaddya mean they don't have whole lobsters? This is Red *Lobster*, right?" Beatrice chirped.

A more subdued Jill said, "Well, if they have whole lobsters I'd really like one." A look at the menu told us whole lobsters were not available that day. Ed and I informed the girls and suggested they make a different selection. As we waited for our meal, Beatrice attempted to engage us all in a memory game. I said, "Sorry hon, my head just won't cooperate. I'm going to have to pass." Kevin said he wasn't interested.

"Boy, you guys are boring!" Beatrice said flatly. My teeth went on edge. Our meals arrived and everyone began to eat. Everyone, that is, except Beatrice who had a running log of complaints. It was turning out to be a long day. Finished eating, Ed, Kevin and Jill went to the restrooms. A waitress came to ask if there was anything else we needed. Beatrice told her it was Jill's birthday and asked if "something" could be done for her. I said Jill would not like the attention and suggested merely putting a small lighted candle in whatever dessert Jill ordered. Shortly after the others returned to the table, a group of servers appeared loudly singing "HAPPY BIRTHDAY TO JEN!" and set the dessert decorated with an overly tall lighted candle in front of Jill. Even though they had sung "Happy Birthday" using the wrong name and she despised that kind of display, Jill good-naturedly went along with it.

When we arrived at our house, the girls and Kevin went for a swim. A short time later, Beatrice declared, "I was supposed to be home an hour ago. Can you bring me home right now?" When we arrived, Beatrice went directly into her house and Sherilyn came out to the car. She proceeded to discuss among other issues, the factions her family had split into because of the divorce. She said she wanted to move to the same town as her sister, but because it was out of state, she did not know if the court would allow it. I excused myself and Jill and I went home. On the way, we talked about Beatrice moving. Jill had already lost a couple of friends to moves so was resigned to the fact it was going to happen again. Then it occurred to me that Sherilyn had told me she was an only child. I wondered what was this about wanting to be near her sister?

Chinks appeared in the Beatrice and Jill friendship the next day. Jill was worried because Beatrice said she needed to "take a break" in the friendship.

"This is just the typical middle school girl friendship up and down thing," I supposed. "Best friends one day, haters the next," and told Jill to just ride it out.

It had been two weeks since Jill's last heme treatment and we were about to start the pattern that Dr. Piersen had recommended of getting her down to two then ultimately, one treatment a month. She had had only one attack during the entire summer and that had been connected to the ant pesticide. She had kept up with her weekly singing lessons with Lora and therapy sessions with Vanessa. Jill desperately wanted to return to school; she longed for a semblance of normalcy. But that was not going to happen. The devilish AIP was on its way back to challenge Jill in the educational arena yet again. Just when the medical root of Jill's illness and finding a treatment program had settled, real problems with the Littleton school system were about to occur. My record-keeping and documentation skills were about to replace much of the time I had spent researching AIP. Jill would come to know her true inner strength—and to see that being a strong, confident, female youth would invite a social backlash aimed at breaking her spirit. It would not be easy or pleasant to witness.

CHAPTER 25

Cool Downdraft

*Courage doesn't always roar. Sometimes courage is the
quiet voice at the end of the day saying,
"I will try again tomorrow."*
— ANONYMOUS

*20 years from now, I hope to be known as a popular/retired teen singer with good money to
be able to buy a good space where I could live. After my singing career I hope to go to med
school and help people out with even the hardest medical mysteries. My academic goal is to
stay in school as long as I can and not get sick.*[66]

Jill had been delighted when school Principal Tony Dithers* announced during
the first day school assembly that bullying would not be tolerated at LMS. She
recounted to me the unacceptable conduct he had listed: name-calling, harassment,
intimidation, excluding others. Respect and responsibility were the LMS themes,
he vowed. Jill's first week of eighth grade went so well that superintendent Maria
even called to say everything was going smoothly. We had no idea things were about
to deteriorate.

While Jill was happy to be back at school, some of her peers seemed downright
aggravated about her return. Beatrice seemed to be trying to avoid her. Jill was confused and worried about possibly losing the first friend she had had in more than a
year. Her Facebook account was registered through my work computer and I had
her password, my prerequisite to be allowed onto Facebook, so I could spot-check
her online activity. By the middle of the second week of school, I sensed something
was off, so I checked Facebook. I wasn't too surprised when I saw messages from

---

66 Jill's first 8th grade writing assignment. August 31, 2009.

Beatrice berating Jill for being "annoying." She replied to Jill's messages with slap-down responses. I knew middle school could be tough and was worried about Jill's psyche, but intent on not interfering.

A few days later, Jill, Beatrice and MaryAnn* were involved in a gym class scuffle, which I was really surprised to hear about considering school had been in session for such a short time and Jill had been so eager to return. Jill said in the heat of a game the class had been playing, MaryAnn had fallen and Jill had accidentally stepped on her hair, causing MaryAnn and then Beatrice to rear up against her. After the dustup, Yvette,* the guidance counselor, had called a meeting of the girls to iron things out. But the end-of-school bell interrupted it and the meeting was to be continued the next day. Before the next day's end, I got a call from Yvette saying Jill needed to picked up because she had "acted out."

"What the heck?" I thought as I drove off to collect Jill. My mind whirred. "Acting out? What's that all about? Let's see, it's been fifteen days since the last heme treatment and she's scheduled for another tomorrow. She *should* be doing okay," I thought. As it turned out, Yvette had reconvened the meeting with the girls and allowed Mary Ann to read a list of complaints that Beatrice had compiled against Jill, things that had occurred out of school. To make things worse, *Sherilyn* had contributed to the list—after speaking to *MaryAnn's mother* about it. Jill was outraged and let her displeasure be known or "acted out," so I had been called to retrieve her. I could scarcely believe it. For what had started as a gym flare-up, the guidance counselor had allowed what amounted to four complainants, Beatrice, MaryAnn, *Sherilyn* and *MaryAnn's mother*, to gang up on Jill. Jill barely knew MaryAnn, had not really spent a substantial amount of time with Beatrice and had never met MaryAnn's mother. Why, I wondered, hadn't we, Jill's parents, been called about this? I was as outraged as Jill. The school year was less than two weeks old. How could an administrator subject Jill to this level of stress? I could not believe three adults had behaved so irresponsibly. My intentions of not getting involved in middle school drama withered. I called Yvette to ask her to explain why Beatrice had been allowed to present a list of complaints prepared by *her mother* in the school setting about things that allegedly had happened outside of school—and that it had been presented by *MaryAnn*. Yvette replied, "Oh, but it really *was* Beatrice's list—her mother just wanted to help her because she gets nervous speaking in front of others." I told her I disagreed with allowing two middle school students to square up against a single one in such a format—*and* that she, Yvette, had de facto allowed the other girls' mothers into the room. I asked that the "list" of grievances be sent to Ed and me so we could address them directly with Jill. She responded she had told the girls to "stay away from each other from this point forward." Fair enough. But what she really meant was that *Jill* was to stay away from Beatrice and MaryAnn. We never got the list.

Meanwhile, Kevin was involved in his own Martin family-related drama that day. His friend, Pete,* had handed him a small pocketknife at school and said, "Colton said to give this back to you, he doesn't want it anymore."

Confused, Kevin said, "Where did he get it?"

Pete said, "He said he stole it from you."

Kevin took the knife home and checked his room where he found another, almost identical knife. Standing in front of me, he held out his hand with two knives in it. He said, "*This* one is mine. It's been in my room for a couple of years." He pointed out a slight difference between the knives, "I don't know where he got this other one." He then said he was going to return the one that was not his to Colton the next day.

"Kevin, you can't take that knife back to school," I said, "If you get caught with it, you'll be expelled. Really, you shouldn't have kept it on you all day. I'll drive you to his house so you can give it back to him in person—outside of school." Not being one for confrontations, Kevin kept both knives and never addressed the situation with Colton.

Monday dawned. Jill went off to school. The phone rang mid-morning. The caller ID registered LMS. Jill was convulsing and I was asked to come right away. When I arrived, Jill was being loaded into the ambulance to be taken to MedCity ED. I thought, "Only two days after a heme treatment and she ends up in a convulsive condition at school again?" She had been in school for *two weeks*, had behavioral issues and she was nonresponsive *again*? And this time there was no fainting—she'd gone straight into convulsions. "*Please, please Lord, what is it? What is causing Jill to keep doing this?*" My mind was reeling as I made my way to the math class where Jill had collapsed. The math teacher was in the now empty classroom. "Mrs. Menard,* by chance, was Kaitlin in this class?" I asked. Kaitlin, who had promised via Facebook to "have Jill's back," had instead been apparently trying to make her mark as one of the tough girls and let Jill know frequently she was "on Beatrice's side" for whatever transgression Beatrice had complained to her about Jill. Kaitlin had been "talking junk" to Jill whenever the opportunity occurred, out of adults' hearing range.

"Why, no, she wasn't," Mrs. Menard said.

I was uneasy and knew the hospital staff would be asking questions: "What class was she in when she fainted? Had she eaten breakfast? What time was lunch? Does she have math anxiety? Was anyone bothering her?" I had this experience before and was arming myself with information.

By the time I arrived at MedCity, thankfully the staff had already contacted Dr. O'Connor and received the go-ahead to infuse D10. Once that was going, I asked the ED doctor if he could think of anything in a school building that might have such a noticeable effect on the human neurological system. Though he sympathized with me, he said no, he couldn't offer any suggestions. I was desperate and pressed, "How does one go about testing for toxins?" He did not have an answer for that, either. I mulled it all over and could not get past the notion that besides bullying peers, *something* in the school was triggering Jill's reactions. Several hours later, fortified by D10, Jill perked up. They brought dinner, and as she ate, she told me she had been in math class when all of a sudden, she had fainted. She was discharged from MedCity ED later that evening with the diagnosis of pseudo-seizure. She seemed revived by the D10 infusion, but I had already called Dr. O'Connor's office to arrange another heme treatment. I had read that Panhematin is a preventative medication for AIP attacks and found myself wondering, once again, how much heme was needed to counter whatever was making Jill sick in school? How full of heme did her liver have to be to not react to the triggers she was encountering there every day? Could heme levels be measured? If so, how? And *what were* the triggers that set her off?

Jill went back to school the next morning. Shortly afterwards, a call came in from the guidance secretary. She had been told to arrange a 504 meeting for Jill. I wrote down the dates and said I would get back to her. Because Jill's medical/educational dance was getting too complicated for Ed and me to deal with alone, I decided to call Krista Williamson before agreeing to a meeting. Krista expressed concern about what had happened with the Beatrice/Mary Ann/Sherilyn/Mary Ann's mother situation and suggested I contact an attorney before agreeing to any school meeting. Based on her recommendation, I called Attorney Troiano,* a special education lawyer. It was obvious she was familiar, and not favorably impressed with, the Littleton school district. Nonetheless, she said I had a good handle on the medical aspects and recommended I present all the info I had about Jill's medical condition to the school administrators. She explained her retainer was fairly substantial, and it seemed to her we were on the right track and did not need her services at that time. "Remember, as the parents, you have the law on your side," she said. After talking with her, I read her blog and decided to forge ahead.

Unexpectedly, Mickey Martin* called to say he had some items Jill had "loaned" to Beatrice and wanted to return them. "Sure," I said, wondering what had prompted this. He arrived at our house with the items Beatrice had asked Jill for and been given along with the unused nail manicure kit from Jill's birthday goody bag.

As he was leaving, I remembered Kevin's dilemma with the knife and Colton's role in that. I asked him if he knew anything about it. "What kind of knife is it?" he asked.

"I don't know exactly but it's small, about so big," I indicated, moving my fingers apart.

"Does it have wood on it?" he asked. "Yes," I said.

"Oh, it's one of those Scout knives; they earn them once they've proven they're responsible enough to use it properly," Mickey replied.

I said, "Well, it's not too cool that Colton brought a knife to school–*and* claimed he stole it from Kevin. Kevin earned his own years ago, so now he has two." Mickey said he would look into the matter. "One more thing," I said, "do you monitor your kids' Facebook accounts?"

He answered, "As a matter of fact, I do. And my sisters are also on my kids' "friends" list, so we have it covered."

"Okay," I said, knowing that unless he knew his children's passwords and checked both their sent and received messages, he did not have "it covered."

CHAPTER 26

Bad Moon Rising

As far as physical and mental health are concerned, a child's plight is a parent's fight.
— JOYCE GOULD

Ed dropped Jill off at school the next morning. What happened after that could not be corroborated. Beatrice had one story, Jill another and there were no security cameras, or witnesses to step forward. But just after having been told by Yvette to "stay away from each other," they had ended up face-to-face on the sidewalk in front of the building. Beatrice said Jill had threatened her and "put hands" on her before she, Beatrice, ran to the principal's office to report her version of the scene. Jill's story was that Beatrice approached her and asked, "What's up with the knife?" evidently referring to the incident between Colton and Kevin.

Knowing only the barest information she had heard me talking to Kevin about, Jill replied "What are you talking about?" At that point Jill said Beatrice dismissively pushed her aside. This prompted Jill to begin pursuing her asking, "Why'd you push me?" which caused the teacher on duty to see what was going on, and Beatrice bolted to the principal's office.

I told Jill it was too bad that she had not gone to the principal's office herself immediately after Beatrice pushed her and explained to him what Beatrice had said and done. Then covering principal Mr. Boyle* would have heard about the knife episode and Beatrice would have had to explain why she was asking about it, breaching the "stay away from each other" mandate. Instead, Mr. Boyle told Jill Beatrice's version of what happened was that Jill had "gotten in her face" and that is why Beatrice pushed her. Thankfully for Beatrice, at that point, Jill was badgering her, so she had run to the principal first in tears. But Mr. Boyle did not pursue what had prompted the incident. To him, it was clear. If former homeschooled, good girl Beatrice had cried, Jill was the agitator.

Matters got worse—a lot worse. Though we did not know it at the time, the next day Sherilyn called or went to school and demanded Jill be removed from classes that she and Beatrice shared. So Yvette concluded that because *Jill* had not obeyed the "stay away from the other girl" mandate, her schedule was changed. Jill became distraught, and I was called to pick her up again.

When Jill told Ed and me that Yvette had changed her schedule, we were angry. For the second time, she had not contacted us about a problem involving Jill. I called Yvette to find out why she had changed Jill's schedule without even talking to us and cluing us in on the "problem." I was unprepared for the story she told me. She said on the evening of the morning sidewalk incident Jill had telephoned Beatrice. Ed and I knew nothing of this. Sherilyn had answered the call and words ensued that prompted Sherilyn to go to the school and request that the classes Jill and Beatrice had together be changed. Flummoxed, I immediately called the Martin household. Sherilyn said Jill had indeed called their house that day and asked to speak to Beatrice. Sherilyn was not articulating clearly what had been said between Jill and herself, other than "Jill called me a bitch!" I was startled—something must have been terribly wrong for Jill to have spewed that out. Sherilyn went on to say Beatrice had worked so hard during seventh grade to fit in socially. I reminded her that Beatrice had missed years of public school because *she,* Sherilyn, had made the choice to remove her to homeschooling. Jill, I said, had missed nearly a year and a half because of *illness.* I said, like Beatrice, Jill would have to work her way back into the middle school social structure. Sherilyn went off on tangents. She said, "There are so many scary things happening in schools today. How about all the predators? Teachers having affairs with students?" Then abruptly she continued, "My kids are not allowed to go to dances." I had always respected parents who chose to home-school their child(ren) and was aware of many situations where homeschooled students excelled academically and were well-balanced. Sherilyn and Mickey, it seemed, had sequestered their children merely to keep them away from society's evils. I jogged Sherilyn's memory with the fact that our houses are just a few miles apart and asked why she had not just called us, or driven to our home, to complain about the phone call? She said, "I couldn't! She called right back!!"

"What do you mean *'she called right back'*?" I asked. Sherilyn began to ramble again so I changed the subject and asked why she had had a certain conversation in Jill's presence on the drive back from church. "Apparently, you discussed how Josh is your 'problem child.' Of course Jill heard that, among other personal matters, which I think is inappropriate for you to have done," I said. She said she had only called Josh her "challenging child" but she clearly did not understand, and didn't want to understand, that to Jill, that sort of talk was tantamount to "back-stabbing." After hearing Sherilyn's negative ravings about her soon-to-be ex-husband, also in Jill's presence, I was beginning to understand why Jill had called her a bitch. It was Jill's first exposure to such family hostility and negativity; the picture was coming into focus. Things were starting to make sense to me in an odd way. By then the conversation had turned into an effort in futility for me. I thanked Sherilyn for telling me her "side" and said the one thing I agreed with Yvette about was the girls should stay away from each other from now on.

Just before hanging up, she said in a lowered voice, "*I was so scared!*"

I thought, "Why was *Sherilyn* so scared? And what had she meant by 'she called right back'"? I knew I had to talk to Jill about why she had called Beatrice. I was fuming. Yvette had punished Jill by changing her schedule for something that had happened outside of school—and for the second time in a week, had not notified us. I filled Ed in on Sherilyn's story. It was evident to both of us that Sherilyn was mired in drama. When we finally found out what had really happened, the small amount of sympathy or liking I had had for the woman was gone.

The phone rang a few hours later. The caller ID unit registered LMS's number. Jill was in convulsions. "On no, here we go *again!*" I moaned. By the time I arrived at the school Jill was on her way by ambulance to MedCity ED. Thankfully, by the time I arrived the doctor on duty had administered Ativan, called Dr. O'Connor's office and D10 had been ordered from the hospital pharmacy. We were able to leave the hospital relatively early. As an added precaution, Dr. O'Connor ordered another heme infusion for the coming Wednesday. We were back on the school and hospital merry-go-round. "For heaven's sake, why isn't Panhematin *preventing* these attacks?" I worried.

I had heard Sherilyn's version of the phone call; now it was Jill's turn. She said Yvette had told her during the day to apologize to Beatrice for the morning confrontation. I wondered, if she had ordered them to stay away from each other, *why* would she send one to apologize to the other? Jill said while passing through the afternoon bus crowd that day, Beatrice mimed talking on the phone and told her to "Call me." So, Jill called her. Sherilyn answered the call and told Jill "*No, you can't talk to her. Don't call here ever again!*" and hung up. Jill impulsively redialed, and when Sherilyn told her again, "Don't ever call here again," Jill called her a bitch.

"OK, we were getting somewhere. Not smart and rude for Jill to have done, but at least things were beginning to make sense," I thought. "Jill, why in the world would you make things worse than they already were? Why would you call her a bitch?" I asked rhetorically.

"I just wanted to talk to Beatrice so we could work things out," Jill replied. Ms. Booker told me I had to apologize to her plus Beatrice put her hand up to her ear like this and said to call. So I did."

I replied, "Sorry, Jill, you're going to have to pretend Beatrice has already moved. Forget trying to have any relationship with her. And remember when Beatrice said 'Catholics are fakes?' Well, I talked with Sister Marguerite* about that. She said, 'Well, some Catholics *are* fake.' And she's right. There are fakes in every religion. That's been the root of wars all over the world for about forever. Every religion, even Bible-based Christians have fakes in their midst, too."

The saga kept going. Jill said Yvette made a comment to her alluding to police involvement. Jill did not know what she was referring to. I called Yvette to discuss Jill's version of her phone call to the Martin household. I said had she coordinated a venue for Jill to apologize to Beatrice, or for them to apologize to each other, especially since she'd just told the girls to stay away from each other, this might have all been avoided. By not doing so, I added, she had been asking for trouble. Yvette countered that perhaps a "cocktail of meds like some of our other 'impulsive' students take" would help Jill. I was shocked that a school administrator would make such an irresponsible, illegal statement and told her so. Ed called Yvette also to ask if she'd consulted with Tony or Bart before changing Jill's schedule. Her reply, "It was *my* professional opinion to change Jill's schedule." Ed was not happy with Yvette's response.

From the start, both "new" classes turned out to be problematic for Jill. Several students—girls and boys, but mostly girls—simply would not accept Jill into "their" Spanish or gym classes. Camerin and her clique were after Jill in force. She could not bear going to the "new" classes where she was neither welcomed by peers nor supported by teachers. Looking for guidance, she went to Yvette and was told, "I can't talk to you without a note from your mother or father." Jill was mystified as to why Yvette would say this; so were Ed and I.

It turned out that many of the Facebook friends Beatrice had connected Jill to had issues of their own. Mary Ann and Kaitlin were relative newcomers, having arrived during Jill's seventh grade absence. Each girl was trying to find her way in the LMS social structure in which "newbies" are thrown to the lowest rungs on the totem pole where "Camerin & Company" held court. Jill had had that gym problem with MaryAnn early on. Kaitlin had told Jill on numerous occasions that she was going to punch her in the "f#cking" face. Jill had been uneasy but she did not respond. Tammy, who had been in Camerin's clique for years, nastily informed Jill that she dressed like a whore because she wore "full black." By this time, Jill had begun favoring black pants, of which she had several identical pairs, and had abandoned her colorful tees and other shirts in favor of black.

Our family had just come off two years of challenging medical crises. It now felt like they were starting up again. Whatever her reason, Sherilyn Martin had dragged us into ridiculous middle school drama. Disgusted, I did an about-face on my position of expecting children to fight their own battles. As far as Jill was concerned. I would sit squarely in my daughter's corner because she was at a true disadvantage, and it was clearly evident that Littleton school peers and adults were after her.

CHAPTER 27

Slippery Black Ice

You're a liar, the wind and the fire,
you know don't always get along.
— FROM "WIND IN THE FIRE" BY JILL GOULD

Things had gotten so preposterous that Ed and I called a meeting with Tony and Bart. Assuming things could not get any worse, we found they already had. Tony chided me for having told him that Beatrice "held Jill's psyche in the palm of her hand and was crushing it."

I said I had mentioned Beatrice's hold on Jill's psyche because 1) I knew my daughter, 2) I'd seen evidence of Beatrice's attempts on Facebook to control Jill and 3) I remembered how middle school girls operate. I said I had spoken to Dr. Nyeer and Vanessa and both supported my statement of Beatrice holding Jill's psyche as being spot-on, and they questioned a middle school principal's claim to not understand how a seventh or eighth grade girl could wield power over other middle school girls. I reminded him that other than her tutor, no one from the Littleton school district had had direct contact with Jill for the year and a half she had been away from school. As such, I said, she was considered to be a social outcast by the students and through them, the school administration—a true tail wagging the dog situation. I added it had been unfair to drop her into regular school without orientating her. I rhetorically finished with, "After missing virtually her entire seventh grade school year, she's had an interesting welcome to eighth grade, wouldn't you say? We want a full explanation as to why the administration felt it appropriate to make such a drastic statement by switching Jill's schedule in the first two weeks of the school year."

Tony said, "Jill's schedule was changed because 1) she had violated the agreement to stay away from Beatrice (clearly, no one believed Jill's version that Beatrice approached her first that morning); 2) she'd called Beatrice's home and used pro-fanity at the mother; and finally 3) the mother had gone to the school to request that Jill be moved out of Beatrice's classes to insure there would be no interaction between the two girls." Ed asked, "If no interaction was the goal, why hadn't the girls simply been moved to different corners or sides of a classroom? Why the extreme?" And as far as Jill calling the Martin home, it happened outside of school and as her parents, Ed continued, "We would deal with it; the action shouldn't have changed her *school* schedule. As far as Sherilyn requesting Jill be moved out of Beatrice's classes—the school was wrong to not have discussed that with us." Tony went on to tell us after the phone call with Jill, Sherilyn reported she had filed a complaint with the Littleton police department about Jill's "threatening call" and her daughter's safety, so that's why they had moved Jill from Beatrice's classes. Tony said, "We couldn't move Jill to other classes of the same time frame because none was available." He also said a school security guard had been assigned to monitor Jill's activities. Ed and I were stunned—and seething. It was the first we had heard of a police complaint having been made by Sherilyn. This put a new, serious spin on things. It also explained why Yvette had made the snarky comment to Jill referenc-ing the police.

Incensed, Ed brought up Kaitlin's frequent opportunistic bullying of Jill and said emphatically, "Get that security guard off Jill—*now*. And let this serve as our formal complaint about this Kaitlin kid's threat the other day to punch Jill in the f#cking face *again*," he added. To us, it appeared that the school administrators were skating on thin ice; they had singled Jill out and were harassing her. This meant discrimina-tion. At that point Bart suggested a change in Jill's school counselor, from Yvette to school psychologist, Karen.* Ed and I readily agreed. We felt the farther Yvette was away from Jill, the better. Tony then indicated Jill would be allowed to go to the nurse's office, Karen's office or the rest room at any time during the school day if she felt she needed a calmer environment.

Following the meeting, Ed went to the police station to see if a complaint had been filed as Sherilyn had reported to the school. I told him not to be surprised if she had fabricated the whole thing. When Ed returned home he said, "Nothing. No complaint. Seems she lied about that." He then called Tony to tell him the same thing. To his credit, Tony apologized for not having verified the claim himself. Ed replied, "Yes, Tony, you *should* have verified it, but the real onus was on *Sherilyn Martin to tell the truth*."

I solicited opinions about the school's actions from Krista Williamson, Attorney Troiano, Vanessa, Dr. Nyeer and Dr. Alaimo. The professionals' responses included: "Careless, reckless, inappropriate, irresponsible, outrageous, slanderous, harass-ment; and he/she calls him/herself a (fill in the blank)?" Dr. Alaimo sent a letter to the LMS administration reminding it that undue stress was detrimental to Jill's health. Vanessa requested Jill's schedule be restored to its first of the school year status. But the school ignored all comments and refused to reinstate Jill's original schedule. Members of Camerin's "posse" were split between the classes so, to avoid stressing Jill further, Ed told her that rather than going into the classrooms at class time, to instead go to the nurse, call him and he would pick her up. When told that from now on she was to go to Karen, not Yvette, with any concerns or questions, Jill was relieved. We also told her Tony had said she could go to the nurse or to the school psychologist's office any time she felt overly stressed.

After missing more than a year and a half of regular school, Jill's academic life had been turned upside down in only twenty-one days. She had endured stress above and beyond what returning to school should have been. It was clear to us that Sherilyn had pulled her children out of public schools to be homeschooled where *she* was in charge and could change whatever, whenever she wanted. She obviously believed she had the same power over LMS—and it had worked. In a matter of weeks, she had twice insinuated herself into middle school matters, proving to me and Ed she had not meant "what happens in school should be taken care of in school." And she had made a false statement to LMS administrators about going to the police regarding the phone call incident. As Mark Twain once said, "A lie can travel halfway around the world while truth is putting on its shoes." Sherilyn Martin lied and while the Gould family was diligently putting on its shoes, the rest of LMS was enmeshed in her false claim—and punished Jill for it.

Because she had been so rude to an adult, Jill was not allowed to attend the Littleton Fair. I told her she had to write a letter of apology to Sherilyn, but was advised by Vanessa and Dr. Nyeer to not send it. They questioned Sherilyn's stability and said sending the apology could re-ignite issues. After Jill told me during the first week of the school year about Tony, "He's the weirdest principal I've ever had—but I kind of like him," now, not surprisingly, her opinion of Tony had drastically changed. Because Jill had been out of mainstream school for such a long time, she had lost daily opportunities to learn to "let things roll of her back" and similar socialization techniques.

Karen, Jill's newly appointed counselor, was nice but not effective in helping her manage dysfunctional middle school tactics. Then, it appeared she might have found an ally in Geoffrey. The two used to shoot baskets in fifth grade and that had prompted rumors Jill had a crush on him. The truth was in those days she was no more interested in crushes than she was in becoming an astronaut. He was nice and she appreciated that. Still, the boys in his clique were not happy about Geoffrey being friendly with Jill. His friend, Stan,* was the boy who had spit in her face while in Benton School. Fast forward to eighth grade and, not surprisingly, Stan was the leader of the LMS "tough boy clique."

Geoffrey and Jill ended up in the same science class and began joking and chatting between lessons. He told her she had "changed." She said he "drove her nuts" because he was always "talking during class" and had a penchant for poking her with his pencil, which she hated. But at least no one made nasty cracks to her in that class.

An extroverted personality and a hard worker in those fifth grade days and before, Jill had always had a smile on her face. Through the years, many teachers had told me they looked forward to seeing Jill's smile as she moved through the school. But the trauma of having missed so much school; being poked, prodded, transfused and infused; being embarrassed because of fainting and convulsive spells and the horrific "welcome" back to eighth grade had wiped the smile from her face.

So it was a relief when Geoffrey took a playful approach to her in science class. He seemed concerned when she missed school for treatments. He asked if her port "hurt" when he saw the sometimes visible scar at the neckline of her shirts. She took some comfort in his niceness. Later, Jill would find out there was a mean method to his madness and it would hurt.

CHAPTER 28

Cyclonic Circulations

Fall down seven times; stand up eight.
— JAPANESE PROVERB

When I went back in eighth grade, people were welcoming, but not for long. Everyone started telling me to become tougher, not show my emotions. So I did that. But people turned on me as soon as I did. The name calling came back: bitch, slut, fat, ugly, etc. Then I started getting sick again. When I went on Facebook I saw people saying stuff like every time she falls down and faints there's an earthquake or she should lay off the burger king. Everyone would laugh. At school I would try to stand up for myself but would get yelled at by the principal. He would tell me I was an antagonist and deserved what was happening to me. Every single day the name calling and harassment got worse and worse. I felt like everyone was out to get me.[67]

Another October emerged and leaves were changing. But the same old school routine held true: Tony called to say Jill was in convulsions and she was on her way to MedCity ED. I arrived at LMS just in time to see the ambulance zoom off to the hospital, but this time to NHC for a heme treatment. She had been fine all summer and after only a month in the building she had had her second attack and several incidents of irritability. Jill assured me. "It's just the stress, Mom." I was not convinced. This time she'd been in the chemistry lab working on an experiment. Jill reported, "All of a sudden I got the worst headache I ever had and I don't remember anything else."

I thought, "It's obviously not safe for her be in the chemistry lab. I'll talk with Mrs. Morrison* to ask if the room can be fully ventilated before Jill enters it—and based on what happened, she shouldn't be present anymore during chemical experiments."

---

67 Jill's journal. January 2010.

Jill also received her progress report. With the exception of PE/Health for which she had medical excuses; mathematics, "Class absence affects performance, interest in area should be encouraged;" and Conversational Spanish, one of the classes that had been changed, "Danger of failing"—after it had been made intolerable for Jill to go into the room thanks to her peers and ineffective teacher management, all other classes reflected "Average" for academic status and "Satisfactory" for effort and conduct.

Meanwhile, Jill had begun forging a friendship with Miranda,* who like Beatrice, hovered in the periphery of Camerin's clique. I remembered dropping Jill off at school in the mornings at Benton School; Miranda would usually be hanging around the sixth grade tough girl faction, but appeared friendly enough toward Jill. Jill was relieved when Miranda ended up in a couple of her classes. One day Miranda's mother, Jane*, telephoned to extend an invitation to Jill to attend a local fair with their family during the coming weekend. The invitation included a sleepover. Other than what I had seen and Jill telling me that Jane was a teacher, I knew nothing about Miranda or her family. But not letting her go would probably precipitate a conniption. I agreed to her going, and knew I would have to hope for the best. "Thank you for thinking of Jill," I said. "She will be over the moon!" I took Jill to Miranda's home as arranged and briefed Jane on the liver disorder, saying she had just had a treatment a few days before and should be okay. Jane said, "Yeah, Miranda says she passes out a lot!"

I showed Jane Jill's medical ID, told her about the list of "unsafe medications" that Jill kept in her purse, gave her our cell and home phone numbers and told her, "If she should happen to faint, please call 911, then call me. Ask the EMTs to put oxygen on her and get her to NHC asap. They'll know what to do." Jill would have had a fit if I had gone any further. I retreated and prayed she would have a good time and would not have an attack while she was with Miranda's family. I didn't want Jane and her family, or Jill, to have to deal with a possible medical problem. I also knew I could not shelter her forever.

The next day Jill mentioned the man we'd thought was Miranda's father was actually her soon to be stepfather who smoked cigarettes. Jill said she had had no breathing problems while with the family. She enjoyed the fair. Soon she and Miranda were talking regularly after school on Facebook and posting photos of their escapades. Based on what I had seen in a mishmash of middle school Facebook communications, I decided to stay tuned periodically to Jill's account. As the school year went on I would be glad I did.

Before too long Jill would tell me that Miranda and their friends sometimes hit each other "in fun." At first I did not think much of it; joshing around was a typical child thing and a friendly swat was not something to be made into a big problem. But one afternoon I noticed Jill rubbing her arm and wincing and saw she had a bruise. "What'd you do now?" I asked.

"Oh, Miranda did that. She's stronger than she thinks," Jill said. Head bells chimed. I told Jill to "punch me in the arm as hard as Miranda hit you." She did. It *hurt*. I told her that sort of punch did not constitute "playing around" and told her not to hit others. "Remember the rule: hands to yourself?" I said, "It's in place for a reason." I did not like *anyone* pushing, pinching, punching or kicking another in the name of friendship. I told her being friends should not hurt. I knew that given her luck, it was highly likely if Jill did hit someone, the chances of the other student complaining to a teacher, parent or other adult was high, and she would be the one in trouble.

Jill laughed it off, "We're only joking around; everybody does it." Vanessa told Jill that type of behavior from eighth grade girls was not appropriate and supported my contention it could lead to her accepting future possible abusive relationships. We both advised Jill to begin to steer clear of Miranda and avoid her "subtle" abuse. "Doesn't anyone see this at school?" I asked Jill, "teachers, paras, other students, janitors, librarians, *anybody*?"

"Oh, the kids in our clique see it all the time but no one else does," she said. I counseled her to not encourage them by laughing and to stick up for herself by saying "That's not funny," or "Don't."

Jill would sometimes sing softly to herself at lunch or other downtimes during the school day. Miranda criticized and ridiculed her, "You sing it too slow...don't draw it out so long."

"She doesn't understand that you don't have to sing it exactly like the artist does; you have to make it your own!" Jill, the budding singer and songwriter, said. My head bells jangled, but I assumed the exchange was definitely "middle school stuff" and Jill would have to deal with it like any other student would have to. To my way of thinking, it did not constitute the need for parental involvement.

CHAPTER 29

Gray Days

"I lift my eyes to the hills—from where will help come?"
— PSALM 121:1

Krista was alarmed by Jill's and my reports of school happenings and suggested she accompany us to the upcoming 504 meeting. She asked Jill if she wanted to attend the meeting, too. When Jill apprehensively answered, "yes," Krista recommended that she write a statement and, if she felt strong enough to do so, read it at the meeting. If she did not feel comfortable enough to read it, Krista said she would do it for her. Jill took the assignment to heart and labored over it. We assembled in the conference room with Tony, Bart, Karen, the school nurse and Mrs. Menard.* Krista opened the meeting by asking Jill if she wanted to read the letter she had prepared. Jill said yes and read it aloud. As soon as she had finished, Tony launched into a condemnation of her behavior, reminding her of every "bad" thing she had just "admitted" to (like calling Beatrice's home and calling her mother by a swear word). The WHACK–A-Jill! game was on—in front of everyone. Krista looked stricken. Jill left the room. Ed whacked back. Not one to tolerate blatant bullying and unfairness, he had heard Dr. Piersen's confirmation of Jill's AIP activity and knew the shenanigans Sherilyn, Yvette and Tony had pulled since the start of the school year. He picked up where Jill left off and backtracked to the Beatrice and Jill morning confrontation that had sparked the schedule change. He pointed out though Sherilyn had professed Beatrice was allegedly *"scared"* of Jill, he said because he was the one who drove Jill to school, he had seen Beatrice approach the group that included Jill and move into the conversation nearly every day. He brought up the Colton and Kevin knife incident and repeated Jill's version of how when Beatrice could not get information from Jill, had pushed her aside in a dismissive manner. Then when Beatrice realized what she had done, *she* was scared because she herself had just violated the

125

"stay away from each other" order. "There were no witnesses," Ed told them, "so it's one student's word against the other." He went on to say that Beatrice had been in our home on enough occasions that he was comfortable in saying she was neither quiet nor shy. He then reminded everyone that *he'd* discovered Sherilyn had made the false allegation to the police. He also pointed out because we had been told by Tony that Jill could go straight to the nurse, her counselor or the restroom any time she felt pressured or stressed, like when she was met with students making nasty comments and avoidant actions toward her in the "new" Spanish class. At this point Krista turned to Tony and expressed quite clearly, "*That's* bullying." Ed continued, "When the teacher who called Yvette to report that Jill was reluctant to go into the classroom, Yvette said, 'Either she goes in the room or she can get to the principal's office.' Why didn't that teacher call Karen, Jill's 'new' guidance counselor?" he asked. Ed then said *he* had told Jill to go to the nurse and to call him to be picked up. "*I made that decision, because we know that stress can be a trigger for Jill,*" he ended.

Bart asked if we had any more recent information or confirmation about the varied disorders Jill had been suspected of having over the years. I said, "No. Except for early speech & language; a visual processing problem; the questionable mood disorder; von Willebrand and the AIP, no one has ever put anything on paper." He then floated the possibility of Jill undergoing a psych evaluation. Both Ed and I readily agreed to that with the caveat being whoever was selected to conduct the evaluation would be willing to learn about AIP before settling on a psych diagnosis. After the bipolar misdiagnosis, the NHC conversion fiasco and the fact that AIP symptoms are known to mimic symptoms of mental disorder, we were wary about any potential attempt to label Jill with a psychiatric diagnosis.

The night of that meeting happened to be the first eighth grade dance of the school year. Jill craved social interaction and was looking forward to it. Like any middle school girl, she selected her outfit carefully. Then Ed drove her to the dance. I was worried about her being back in the building again, but everything worked out. She said she had danced with Geoffrey but he had also been texting and checking his cell phone during the entire time and talked to every boy or girl who came near him. Yet, she said, when she turned to talk with someone in her proximity, he became annoyed, which in turn annoyed her. If he could talk to others while they were dancing, so could she, she reasoned. After a while, she felt tired and decided to rest. Kara* came by and asked Jill if she felt all right. Jill said, "Yes, I just wanted a break." Geoffrey appeared and performed some antics to make her smile. Although she said she had a good time, she was relieved when it was time to go home.

Jill had four heme treatments during the first three-and-a-half weeks in October. Since she had had only one attack that month, things seemed to be improving. But then Jill reported that the red abdominal ring was back. A heme treatment was scheduled for the next day. I said if it was still there Jill should show it to the APRN. As it turned out the ring was gone but APRN Gillian* was concerned enough about its reappearance that she scheduled another heme infusion as a safety measure. It seemed NHC thought it was probably connected to the porphyria, too.

Then, I received a jury summons. When the court administrator came in to give jury instructions and details of the civil case for which the jury would deliberate,

I was shaken. The case to be heard was against NHC. The plaintiff was a family member of a five-year-old girl diagnosed with sickle cell disease who had died. Dr. O'Connor had been her hematologist. The administrator went on to list the trial dates and asked those with reason to restrict them from serving on the jury to raise their hands. I raised my hand. I heard typical reasons: business trip obligations, already scheduled vacations, caregiver requirements for very young children, the elderly or infirm. Then it was my turn, "My daughter has a liver disorder and requires regular infusions at NHC. Dr. O'Connor oversees her treatment." I was among those dismissed from the jury pool. As I moved to the elevator with the others, a woman reached out, "Don't let anything you heard in there rattle you. Everything will be all right for your daughter." I thanked her, but as the elevator moved, my head spun. I had just heard about a child who had suffered from sickle cell, a treatable disease. She had been cared for by the same doctor and staff in the same hospital as Jill—and she had *died*. The enormity crashed over me. I made it to the car and the tears came.

CHAPTER 30

Chilly

The purpose of life is a life of purpose.
— **ROBERT BYNE**

The jury summons experience galvanized me—I *needed* to know if there were other children who experienced such extreme symptoms of AIP that regular Panhematin tune-ups were required. I wrote letters to registered APF In-Touch AIPorphyrics members saying that my thirteen-year-old daughter had been diagnosed with AIP through DNA testing a year or so earlier and we were planning to write a book about her story to help others. I explained Jill's lack of darkened urine during attacks and the APF-related doctors' skepticism and asked if they would share any recollections about their own childhood, especially as it related to AIP. Replies from around the country soon began to arrive.

Simultaneously, more and more convinced that toxins in the Littleton schools' IAQ were responsible for Jill's frightening reactions, I turned my attention to proving the theory. I knew discontinuing an "offending substance" was crucial to avoid and/or stop attacks, but before that could be done, the "offending substance" had to be identified. The Benton School's IAQ report had stated that nothing extraordinary had been found. And the middle school building had been built only a few years earlier according to stringent State standards. Yet Jill's episodes had worsened there. Contrary to what had been implied, my research about school IAQ issues indicated there were *no* federal or state guidelines regarding indoor air quality or acceptable levels of various toxins for schools. That word "toxins" got my attention. Jill had been exposed to many public access indoor environments: malls, theaters, museums, retail stores, doctors' offices, hospitals, EDs, Littleton's and neighboring towns' libraries and other municipal buildings. Most of the reactions she had had were at the Benton and the Middle school buildings; her health had improved whenever she left them. And after months of no activity, returning to a Littleton school clearly coincided with ongoing activity. But I wondered, could exposure to school toxins result in "delayed" AIP activity?

As a child, I had a tendency to develop an itchy rash whenever my mother switched laundry detergent so the first "toxin" I thought of was the cleaning product used throughout the district's school buildings. Then, because I could not think of anywhere else where large quantities of dry-erase markers were used, I targeted them too. I had a hunch both products contributed to Jill's behavioral and medical concerns, but I still had to figure out if one product was more potent than another and/or if a combination of them could make it worse.

Mr. Bell, director of building and grounds, had not returned my call. I called again to ask about getting manufacturers' ingredient information, called Material Safety Data Sheets (MSDSs), for the cleaning products and dry-erase markers. "You'll have to request them from the director of student services," he said. So I called Bart and asked for MSDSs for the EPA-approved "green" cleaner and the dry-erase markers used throughout the school system. I also asked about the possibility of coordinating an AIP informational session for Jill's peers, teachers and LMS administrators about how its symptoms might sometimes affect her. I said, "The NHC nurses tell me they often give such talks to school groups."

He responded, "That request is unprecedented."

"Well, Jill's medical condition is *unprecedented*!" I replied and asked him to discuss it with Maria and to put their answer in writing to me and Ed.

Along with the MSDSs, Bart sent the resumes of two potential psychiatrists to conduct Jill's psyche evaluation. After research, I selected Dr. Werrmona.* Meanwhile, Jill was looking forward to celebrating Halloween. In spite of having received the vaccine and the janitorial staff's diligent application of cleaners to all surfaces multiple times a day, Jill missed a couple of school days because of swine flu (H1N1). She rallied, though, in time for trick-or-treating with Chelsea* and Marie.* Marie's mom, Allyson,* had agreed to chauffer the girls. After a few hours, Jill was tired and relieved to come home for the night.

At her last heme treatment of October, I heard Jill tell the nurses there had been a problem with another student in math class and she no longer felt safe at school. She later told me that out of Mrs. Menard's hearing range, egged on by Nellie's* looks, snickers and smirks, Camerin had directed raunchy garbage talk her way. I emailed school psychologist Karen to say it was obvious Jill had been targeted by a group of eighth graders as the "kid to pick on." And since no LMS adult was dealing with it, I had no choice but to get involved. I advised her to beware that I would be in more frequent contact with her.

October gave way to November. On only the third day of the month, the phone rang. Tony said Jill and Camerin had had a confrontation and that Camerin had been reprimanded, but Jill would not calm down. He asked me to come to the school. I went to Karen's office, where Jill was waiting. Though he had not witnessed the incident, Tony launched into his account of what had happened. Jill kept attempting to butt in, which further inflamed him, so I turned to Jill for her version. She appeared oddly flustered, could not remember details, and her account of what happened was fuzzy. Troubled, I said, "Jill, I'm sorry but it's been eleven days since your last infusion; let's go to NHC to get you some heme. You'll feel better and can come back tomorrow." She became belligerent. Tony told her she couldn't "just hang out" in the nurse or school psychologist's office and had to leave the building with me. At that Jill's emotional status plummeted. I tried to get her to go with me to NHC, but she was immovable. She wanted to finish the day *in school.*

I worried that her bout with the flu; her menses; continued bullying episodes; threats made by Kaitlin and Camerin and the Halloween excitement since her last heme treatment appeared to have pitched her into a bad situation, and she needed heme to get stabilized. Things quickly morphed into the worst behavioral school episode yet when Jill snapped, "I want to go back to class."

Tony retorted, "*That* isn't going to happen. You're going home. You can come back tomorrow."

"I'm not going anywhere," she shot back.

The nonsensical dialogue went on for another half-hour until I said, "Look, if you're not going to come with me to NHC, then I'm going to have you brought there." She would not budge. Although I had to get Jill out of the school, I was not able to carry her myself. I asked for the EMS to be called. A Littleton police officer showed up, too. He had been through this with us at Benton school and knew the drill. Jill was adamant that she did not want heme and would not listen to reasoning. The EMTs brought in a stretcher and told her to lie on it. She did but became more agitated. Concerned that she might fall off and hurt herself, Larry and the ambulance crew suggested restraints. What could I do? I had to get her out of the school. I thought a heme treatment would help and she would not come with me. I felt I had no other choice. It was turning out to be a really bad day. I realized it was too late to arrange a substitute for my CCD class so I asked the EMS to take her directly to NHC. I said I would get there as soon as my class was done and left to ready the classroom. But when I checked my cell phone messages fifteen minutes later, Tony said Jill had been sent to MedCity ED. I did not understand why; she had been responsive when I left. Our repeated requests to transport her to NHC were useless. Ed went to MedCity to be with Jill. By the time I arrived after class, she was sitting up but not talking. Ed was standing by her bed and said, "She sees 'something' in the air." I watched as Jill reached for whatever only she could see.

"She's hallucinating; she must really be low on heme," I said. It had been a while since she had had an attack that involved hallucinations. We both watched as she repeatedly grabbed at something in mid-air. Then Ed was called back to work. I realized Jill would not be getting heme that night. If only she had gone to NHC, the heme would have already revived her liver. Over the course of the next two hours, the hallucinations continued. As she regained awareness, her ability to talk returned. She said she saw "pepper" in her line of vision and that "something came out of the light [fixture] and was just hanging in mid-air." Then she accused me of shaking the bed. I was nowhere near it. She claimed the walls were falling in. She complained about being dizzy—very dizzy. It was shaping up to be a long night.

The nurse brought discharge papers at about 9 p.m. Jill refused a wheelchair and walked, leaning zombie-like against the walls, the whole way out of the hospital.

When we got home she complained of a stomachache. I told her to try to sleep until it was time to go for her morning infusion.

During the drive to NHC the next morning Jill recounted what had happened the day before. She said she must have slipped into seizures, which is why she had been brought to MedCity, not NHC. Upon arrival the nurses "were rude to me and pulled their masks over their noses and mouths like I was disgusting or something." She heard the doctor tell them, "You will treat this patient like any other seizure patient." He was getting used to Jill's frequent flying into that ED, and I appreciated his professional demeanor.

I told Jill that I was annoyed with her. "If you had only come with me yesterday you would have gotten the heme, avoided all the stress, pain, restraints and hallucinations you had to deal with and you might have even been able to return to school today instead of missing it entirely." I told her it had been a good lesson she learned and I hoped it would leave a strong enough impression on her that it would not happen again.

Jill went on to tell me what had happened to set everything off. Apparently, while the math teacher had been distracted with a visitor, Camerin slammed her desk into the back of Jill's seat then balled up her fists and lunged at her, threatening to punch her in the "f#cking face." At that point Mrs. Menard saw what was going on, told Camerin off and sent Jill to the nurse's office where she was given Ativan. I asked if Mrs. Menard had sent Camerin to the principal's office. "No," she said.

"Did anyone else hear her threaten you?" I asked Jill.

"Yes, the whole class saw and heard it."

She also said a boy offered to accompany her to the nurse, but she declined. "Aren't you afraid of Camerin?" Jill said he'd asked her.

"No," she'd answered, but I could see she was bothered by the girl's mercurial behavior.

Sick of Camerin's attacks, the next morning I walked into the Littleton police department with Jill and said we were there to file a complaint against a student who had threatened Jill at school. Officer Bennington* came out. I gave a brief review of Jill's illness and the hospitalization the day before that could be traced directly to Camerin's bullying. Officer Bennington knew Camerin's family and offered to pay a visit to her and her parents. Having seen the local press police reports concerning Camerin's family and not wanting to risk retaliation for Jill at school, I said, "I don't want to cause any more trouble for the kid at home than she probably already has; I would rather you visit Tony and tell *him* I was here and registered a complaint. I think it best *he* tell Camerin this is serious." If that didn't work, I said I'd be back to take him up on his offer.

CHAPTER 31

Chill Persists

The genes loaded the gun, but the environment pulls the trigger.
— DR. MEHMET OZ

I received Bart and Maria's letter denying my request to have professionals talk about AIP in the school. Unable to understand how a request made by a parent who was waiving privacy protection was refused, Vanessa and Krista were mystified. "They nixed the opportunity for other students to support Jill? I have another client whose medical staff took the time to do exactly this type of session in his school. Do they not understand the concept of freedom of speech?" Vanessa said. Krista recommended the issue be escalated to the Board of Education.

In the meantime, Jill was still contending with Miranda's meanness and said, "Miranda told me she's mad at her mother for getting married again," and that she now had a little brother from her father's new relationship. Upon hearing that, I said Miranda was likely frustrated by her current home situation and sometimes when children are not allowed to get those frustrations out at home, they exact measures of satisfaction from others.

"But that doesn't mean it's acceptable. Don't let her hit, punch or otherwise hurt you," I told Jill. "You need to find your voice and tell her, 'Enough.'" But in saying that I knew the probability of Miranda retaliating was high. "Just be aware she might become even nastier to you when you stick up for yourself." By then, Miranda had realigned herself with Camerin's clique.

Meanwhile, I received the MSDSs I had requested from Bart and fired up my search engines. I soon had enough information to get head bells sounding again. Manufacturer Environ LLC's product H2Orange2's MSDS for the "green" cleaner listed hydrogen peroxide as a hazardous ingredient. "That's odd," I thought. "Mr.

Bell said hydrogen peroxide is safe so why is it listed as hazardous?" I emailed the question to the manufacturer. A representative responded by saying hydrogen peroxide is considered a biocide because it kills microscopic germs and, as such, the government required it to be labeled as a hazardous ingredient. Biocide (includes pesticides and antimicrobials) was cited as an AIP trigger in one of my favorite AIP research articles. Being savvy enough to know what goes *on* you goes *in* you, I investigated further. There was nothing to be found on the EnvirOx MSDS website under the heading "Toxicological Analysis and Biomedical Investigations" and its subheadings "Toxicological Analysis," "Biomedical Analysis," "Arterial Blood Gas Analysis" and "Haematological Analysis" category subheadings were all blank. The arterial blood gas mention intrigued me. Early on, I had asked doctors about the possibility of measuring Jill's arterial blood gases during an attack. I hoped to see if oxygen in the blood cells could be measured because I wondered if the AIP-related heme/oxygen deficiency contributed to Jill's fatigue when going up and down the stairs at school while wearing her book bag. The section titled, "Clinical Effects" reported symptoms of transient dyspnea or shortness of breath and cough. Jill frequently had an irritating cough when I picked her up at school. It hung on while we registered at NHC. In fact, she was often offered a protective paper face mask. That was all I got from that MSDS because, "The exact composition of this material is a trade secret."[68] Eventually I would get information about the effects of hydrogen peroxide on the human body.

Next up were the dry-erase markers used in nearly seventy school rooms in the building. Ingredients included Special Industrial Solvent 200 Proof, Ethanol, Isopropyl Alcohol, N-Proponal, 2-Propanol and Carbon black. All toxins. As I researched websites of chemical manufacturers, OSHA, EPA and other sites for more information about each ingredient I found known effects on humans included possible CNS effects, respiratory tract irritation, dizziness, faintness, drowsiness, headache, nausea, vomiting, staggering, unconsciousness—eerie reminders of Jill's symptoms. Upon further investigation, I discovered that one brand's black-colored markers contained greater amounts of two specific toxins than the other colors. Actually, it was the only color that contained carbon black as an ingredient.[69] Head bells rang. I was already aware that alcohol, or ethanol, is a known AIP trigger. Given Jill's extraordinary reaction to teensy amounts of Heparin, I wondered if the solvent/alcohol marker fumes affected her, too.

I sent Bart a letter listing the specific products, EnvirOx H2Orange cleaning dilution, Dixon and Artline dry erase markers, and ingredients that concerned me and why, and the symptoms that had been proven to have an effect on humans:

> It seems that Jill might be ultrasensitive to the combination and length of exposure to these agents.... The reality is that her problematic behavioral (i.e. read brain-driven conduct)

---

68 *Material safety data sheet for water dilutions of all H2Orange Products.* EnvirOx LLC. January 2004. Accessed circa November 2009.
69 *Artline Whiteboard Marker MSDS No.AA1004A-9401.* Shachihata. January 5, 2007.

and physical symptoms accelerated at Benton School from September – December, 2007. When she was taken out of that building to be tutored at the library, there were no seizures, no behavioral problems, no nausea, no tremors, no stomachaches.... [Upon] returning to Benton and then entering LMS, her seizures and behavioral concerns not only returned but accelerated in frequency and intensity....Behavior is controlled by the brain. If chemical components such as those used in cleaning products and markers detailed above can cause the symptoms noted, it isn't a stretch to think they could wreak havoc on the neurological-behavioral system in someone so predisposed.... In closing, it is obvious to me that Jill could potentially become very, very ill in LMS. I ask for your recommendations/action plan as soon as possible. Jill's life has already been harshly impacted. Please indicate what information you need from me to take appropriate action to insure Jill's health will not continue to be harmed by returning day after day to the same environment. Heme has been a Godsend for Jill, but it appears it is not able to keep up with the potential poisoning her system continues to be exposed to. It seems foolhardy to keep putting "fuel" into Jill's liver only for it to be depleted so soon.

Bart responded:

As I am sure you are aware all supplies meet green seal qualifications as set forth by the U.S. Department of Health and approved by OSHA. While I appreciate your concerns and the complexity of Jill's condition, without medical verification and documentation, we cannot assume that any physical symptoms are a direct result of exposure to diluted cleaning agents that are approved for use by state and federal oversight agencies. We feel that the current medical response and educational plan (504) in place is appropriate and adequately addresses her needs. [70]

As long as they had EPA-approved and OSHA-safe claims to lean on, I knew my assertions would be ignored. I had no way to scientifically prove these chemicals *were* connected to Jill's repeated fainting and convulsive attacks, but that didn't deter me. I reviewed the book *What's Toxic, What's Not* again and noted "green" hydrogen-peroxide based cleaners and dry-erase markers in schools were not mentioned—they probably were not even being used in schools when the book was written. At about this time I had come across a report about hair analysis being used to determine the presence of chemicals. The article claimed a much better reliability rate than urine or blood testing. I wondered if it might be plausible to have Jill's

---

70 LMS.* Letter from Special Education Director Bart. November 6, 2009.

hair tested for these chemicals and decided to contact one of the *What's Toxic* book authors to see if he had information to share about testing chemicals. He replied,

> [These chemicals] can be tested for in the urine but only very shortly after exposure, within hours. The ingredients in the markers used in your daughter's school are of generally low toxicity and are not amenable for testing in hair or any other body fluid/tissue [and finally], I still do not think testing your child is the answer. If your daughter is sensitive to this exposure, I would just ask the school to limit the use of markers in her class.[71]

It wasn't *his* child collapsing. It would take many more months of research and recording Jill's ongoing symptoms, attacks and treatment regimen before I connected dots in the AIP/school toxin puzzle.

Meanwhile WHACK-A-Jill! continued. The next week brought report cards and parent-teacher conferences. After receiving Jill's progress report a month earlier indicating that all subjects, with the exception of the notation of "Danger of Failing" for Conversational Spanish, had been rated average for academic status and satisfactory for effort and conduct, Ed and I were stunned when Jill brought home a report card devoid of grades. She said, "When Mrs. Booker gave me this she said, 'You basically failed everything but they didn't want to put that on paper.'" At the bottom of the report card was typed, "*Did not earn grades in academic classes.*" Teacher comments ranged from "class absence affects performance to medical excuse to fails to make up missed work."[72] I couldn't understand how educated adults who claimed to be committed to the institution of children's education could let *any* student not only sink, but also be pushed down like this—especially one who is ill. I had picked up Jill from school for heme infusions *eleven* times in less than three months. As far as "missed work" went, not once had any work been left at the front desk by *any* of her teachers. Not one "What you're going to miss this afternoon" sheet of paper, no reading assignment, no homework, no makeup work, nothing. I had given school administration plenty of notice about her treatment schedule. I called Lizabeth and told her about the progress report we'd received that had indicated all was "satisfactory" or "average'" before, only to have been followed by this blank report card. I told her about Yvette's comment to Jill as to why no grades had been entered on it. Lizabeth was genuinely surprised and said that the progress report was "kind of a standard 504 interim report," but she had no idea why grades on a report card would have been left blank. I knew Lizabeth had met with Yvette periodically during the last school year so I asked if anyone from LMS administration had ever indicated they wanted to meet with Jill. Specifically, other than hearing the tutor's academic reports and updates, had Yvette ever implied or stated a desire to meet and to get to know Jill, find out for herself that she was looking forward to getting back to school, anxious about reconnecting with peers and hoping to make friends,

---

71 Connecticut Department of Public Health. Email from B. T. November 23, 2009.
72 LMS.* Jill's 1st quarter report card. November 1, 2009.

at least? "No," Lizabeth said, Yvette had never asked to meet with Jill or expressed a desire to find out anything more about her other than what her grades were at any given time.

I had many questions for Jill's teachers during each fifteen-minute parent-teacher conference: Why had no grades been entered on the report card, especially since the progress report had indicated mostly "average" and "satisfactory" ratings? Why had they waited until the eleventh or twelfth week of the school year to indicate a problem concerning Jill's academics? Why had no assignments been left at the front desk so Jill could do schoolwork during her many infusions? No complete answers were forthcoming. I asked the teachers to be open to the possibility—no matter how slight—that unseen, undetected toxins in the school *might* be contributing to Jill's recurrent attacks even though they were considered safe according to federal and state standards. I asked about the use of dry-erase markers in individual class-rooms. A couple used them infrequently, but the Language Arts teacher used them regularly. I asked if he would be amenable to using the lighter color markers because I had discovered that black markers contained the highest amount of an extremely toxic chemical. He readily agreed to that suggestion. Jill was fine in his room for the rest of the time she attended LMS. However, I missed the meeting time with math teacher, Mrs. Menard, who used black markers exclusively. Not having had that discussion cost Jill. She continued to have fainting attacks in the math room. Mrs. Morrison* and I discussed Jill's fainting episode in the chemistry lab. I shared Jill's recollection of her "worst headache ever" just prior to fainting. We agreed the chemistry lab was not a safe place for her to be and worked out alternative methods for Jill to "do" experiments. She also advised me that EnvironH2Orange2 was used for cleaning the white boards, too.

Thanksgiving was approaching. It had been a year since Jill's AIP gene had been identified. So much had happened in twelve months. Dr. O'Connor and the Hem/Onc crew had worked with us to figure out an infusion schedule that seemed to be working at keeping Jill semi-functioning in LMS. We had settled on her receiving one infusion a week, two on the week prior to menses. I was still trying to find a rhyme or reason for her sporadic reactions and/or attacks since school started. She attributed everything to the stress associated with the bullying. I did not.

When I arrived at school to pick Jill up for the next heme treatment, Tony happened to be in the lobby and opened the door for me. I nervously joked, "She's okay, right?"

He said Jill was fine. "In fact, she's been pretty good for a couple of weeks now," he said.

"Well," I said, "getting the bullying situation under control is helping some."

"You know, you use that word a lot," he chided. "There are two sides to every story in bullying," he said. "Sometimes it appears that Jill is instigating a situation."

I sighed, "Tony, I don't know where you get your training from, but when it comes to bullying there most certainly are *not* two sides to every story, and if you would get *it* under control then *I* wouldn't have to use the word *bullying* so frequently. So as long as *it* continues to happen, I will continue to use *it*. Just so you know."

CHAPTER 32

Microburst

*Any overt acts by a student or groups of students
directed against another student with the intent
to ridicule, harass, humiliate or intimidate
another student while on school grounds...*
— LMS BULLYING POLICY, 2009-2010 SCHOOL YEAR

November shuddered exhaustingly out. During the month, Jill had endured eighteen school days, seven heme appointments and the worst episode she had had at school. Yet, through it all she continued to write songs and sing with Lora. She had tried numerous times to get together with Miranda after school or on weekends but was stymied by one excuse after another. Meanwhile, Miranda had picked up the pace of physically manhandling Jill. I checked Facebook for clues; my attention was drawn to Miranda's penchant for correcting Jill's spelling and grammar and continually putting her down. I noticed she had sent a Facebook message to Jill, who was trying to find out if Miranda was "mad" at her, "No I'm not. Leave me the f#ck alone!" had been the reply.

December came charging in. It would turn out be a December to remember. Near the end of the second day into what should have been a glorious month, the phone rang. Tony said Jill was having a meltdown and to come right away. When I arrived he attempted to fill me in on what had transpired. This time, the trouble involved Miranda. We got to the classroom where Mrs. Menard waited with Jill. She said, "She asked that we call you, but we didn't want to bother you." I knew that Jill asking for me meant she was willing to take the chance I might arrange a heme treatment. Tony proceeded to tell me his version of what had happened. What I perceived was Miranda and Jill had had words. Both ended up in the principal's office where each was given time to speak. I had suggested numerous times to Tony that if and when Jill was involved in a situation with another student, it was best to hear each separately. Obviously, that had not happened. Jill refused to speak, so because school was being dismissed, I returned to the lobby to wait for her.

When we got into the car, I asked her to tell me about what had caused me to be called. Where she'd been "fuzzy" last month, this time she articulated everything clearly. It had started in the lunchroom when Dianna* told Jill that Miranda had called Jill a stalker, a Facebook reference the students really took umbrage to. Jill walked over to Miranda and said, "I'm *not* a stalker." Then she returned to her place in the lunch line, at which point Miranda, Nellie and Tammy started calling Jill's name over and over in a singsongy way. After the others tired of that, Nellie kept it going. Jill pointed at Nellie and said, "Stop it."

This prompted Camerin to hurry over to the "tough boy" table to report, "Jill just stuck her middle finger up at us.

The boys joined in taunting, "Jill, Jill, Jill," over and over again.

As the students left the lunchroom and returned to classes, Miranda ordered Jill to, "Get away from me. Now." Because the hallway was crowded, Jill said she could not move quickly enough, which further annoyed Miranda. Jill said, "All I said to you was that I wasn't a stalker."

"Just leave me alone," Miranda snapped and when Jill began to cry, said, "Get a hold of yourself. I don't care about you and nobody else cares about you." Upset, Jill went to math class where Mrs. Menard ushered her to Tony's office. Jill asked for Ed or me to be called; the request was denied. Miranda was brought into the office with Jill to tell her side of things. She left out calling Jill a stalker, the serenading episodes and everything else she had said to Jill. Jill bolted from the room. When I asked why she had not told Tony what happened from her perspective she said, "Miranda is the smart kid. I'm the troublemaker. He doesn't listen to what I say."

I was angry that Jill's request to call me or Ed at the beginning of the Miranda/Jill flap had been dismissed. As I drove off with Jill sniffling beside me, I said resignedly, "Unfortunately for you, she's able to get away with things."

Jill yelled, "Why can *she* get away with things, and *I* can't?" I replied, "Well, it's not that she's *allowed* to do certain things, it's just that she's sneaky, it's called 'smart enough to get away' with whatever." Jill yelled *"That's what she ALWAYS says!* Today Miranda pointed at me and told Chelsea, 'Unlike Jill here, *I'M* smart enough to get away with it." Upon hearing that, I turned down a side street, debating with myself, "Should I go to Miranda's house and wait for her mother to come home from work?" I no sooner had that thought when there was Miranda, walking along the side of the road. Impulsively, I stopped the car, put down the window, looked directly at her and said, "Miranda, the bullshit stops now."

She looked at me, so cool, calm and collected and asked syrupy, "What?"

I reiterated, "That means today," and drove off, vowing to look into the area's magnet schools. If I could help it, Jill would *not* be going to LHS.

When I got home I told Ed and Kevin what had happened, including telling Miranda off. Ed said it was a mistake to have done that. Kevin said he was "going to tell her off on Facebook," and ran to the computer.

"Oh no, you don't—you let me see anything before you send it," I said. I did not want him shooting from the lip as I had done. He composed a well-worded chastisement, showed it to me then sent it to Miranda.

It was not long before her father responded to Kevin asking why he would have written to Miranda about a bullying situation. After all, he "didn't raise Miranda to be a bully." I advised Kevin to tell Dwight,* to contact me via my business email. His message was in my email box before long. It was easy to see how this was going to go down. Before it was over, I had a good idea of why Miranda's mother had divorced Dwight and confirmation of where Miranda learned her bullying tactics. He started off:

> I am not really sure why I am even being involved in such a minor issue, but now that I am, I have become increasingly aware of some issues needing discussion. I have heard from the principal of the school as well as teachers and other classmates in order to get a clear picture before contacting you...the ball actually lies in your court on this one? What I mean is I believe the issue lies within your daughter. I would guess Jill needs some guidance and some positive attention. Jill is looking for attention she is not getting somewhere that is obvious. Miranda may be many things, but she is not now, nor has she EVER been a bully. SHE is not the issue here. Jill is. Miranda has strict instructions not to approach Jill, provoke Jill or instigate anything involving Jill from myself and her mother."[73]

It was going to be a long night. Miranda, like Jill, was strong-willed. But unlike Jill, she had a penchant for nastiness. I had seen it on Facebook and I had seen the bruises on Jill. I fired up an email and sent my answer. We emailed back and forth until he wrote, "PLEASE NEVER E-MAIL ME AGAIN. I will be at the Littleton police tomorrow to substantiate the claims made by you and am going to let the proper powers/authorities/whomever deal with this."[74] I never did hear from Captain Sullivan.* He knew the score. Shortly thereafter, Dwight sent me a LinkedIn email invitation that I ignored.

The entire fiasco had blown up in only the first week of December. There was still so much left to the month. At Jill's next heme treatment, when asked how she had been she reported on the latest bullying situation that involved Miranda. Emma* expressed concern about the continuing bullying reports she and the NHC staff continued to hear about the Littleton school system. She asked if a school social worker and/or guidance person was taking an active position to curtail the offenders and offered to have the hospital social worker broach the subject with school administrators. I laughed ruefully. "That would be nice, but until recently, we didn't even know there *was* a school social worker—still haven't seen, never mind, *met* the

---

73 Dwight. Emails to author. December 5, 2009
74 Ibid

person! And the guidance counselor? Her duties regarding Jill were reassigned to the school psychologist. And as far as the bullying is concerned, we've exaggerated the whole thing; matter of fact, I have an affinity for using the word bullying. I told her, that at Krista's recommendation I had asked multiple school administrators for permission to discuss AIP with Jill's peers and the teaching staff only to be denied.

Emma was shocked, "Why?"

I said, "Student confidentiality. They say it can't be breached."

Emma asked, "Even with the parent's permission?"

I finished, "Guess so. Her struggles to integrate into the social fabric of the school environment after being out for so long and continuing to miss academic time for treatments, not to mention the embarrassment of routinely falling, fainting and convulsing in front of peers and school adults? 'Get over it, Jill!' is the attitude she faces every day."

On the plus side, letters, emails and telephone calls continued to arrive from the "request for AIP information survey letter" I'd sent to many AIPorphyrics. I spoke with several people about their memories of childhood health issues. We received more clues and many helpful porphyria management tips from wonderful people who had lived with AIP for many years. Support, gracious remarks and best wishes for Jill accompanied every reply and lifted our hearts.

CHAPTER 33

Light Mist

The greatest suffering in our world is that of alienation.
— FREIDA FROMM, GERMAN PSYCHOANALYST

Miranda took every opportunity she could to shoot nasty comments Jill's way. Thankfully, Jill was super about ignoring them. One day she mused, "Lots of people are saying Miranda has gotten mean. I think she's always been mean and maybe they're just getting to see that now."

I replied, "I think since you drifted away, Miranda's world is probably closing in and she's gotta take it out on *someone*. Just continue to be wary of her." Tony said I was making more of the Miranda/Jill situation than I should. I disagreed. This was not the up one day, down the next typical middle school peer relationship, not when someone was routinely being hurt or being made to feel they're worthless. I *knew* it was not just my imagination. Still he insisted Jill and Miranda got along "fine" and had been observed together at various locations. Jill's explanation for that was Miranda was the one who lingered around her. "When she's nice to me, I'll talk with her. I won't be a snot," she said with finality.

Wednesday brought the delight of an unexpected snow day—no school. The building had been closed. Thursday morning arrived and Jill bustled about getting ready for school. Ed dropped her off. Three hours later the phone rang. Jill had collapsed in math class and was on her way to MedCity. Thankfully, the doctors there had the routine down. She had not even needed Ativan, and after an infusion of D10 was ready to go home. But the same thoughts kept running through my head, "How was I going to prove chemicals used in the school building kept triggering Jill's frequent attacks? And why did they often happen a day or more after the school had been closed or she'd been away from the school? Was it the cleaner? The markers? A combination of the cleaner and markers? Something else?" I was as sure about school chemicals contributing to or causing Jill's frequent attacks as I had been about her having AIP. But how was I going to solve it? *What if* the "safe levels" of green cleaners and solvent laden marker fumes were too much for Jill's system to handle? If so, what level of toxicity *could* Jill safely tolerate? Who could help? I decided to take Krista's advice and ask the board of education (BOE) for guidance.

Marie's mother, Allyson was a past member of the Littleton BOE. I contacted her to ask for advice about how to approach the elected officials. She suggested I call the BOE office and request a closed session with them. I made the call and left that message on the answering machine. Maria called a few days later to ask if there was anything she could do because, she said, "The board only hears cases of expulsion or disciplinary action items." I replied since she and Bart had denied my request for medical professionals to come to LMS to discuss within the auspices of the eighth grade health curriculum to students, teachers and others how Jill's ability to function at school might sometimes be compromised, I wanted to address the BOE about it. Another issue was the harassment and bullying Jill had been subjected to for months. To that, Maria said, "Well, I heard she and that one friend [Miranda] got along just fine at the dance and that she's getting along fine in all of her classes." I told her the adults missed a lot to which she replied, "But Joyce, the teachers can't *all* be lying!" I then told her about the blank report card Jill had received, said I would fax it to her to take care of, and feeling like I was getting nowhere, ended the conversation. I also decided a letter would be the more appropriate method of contacting the BOE to address the concerns I had.

Meanwhile, the one bright spot at school was Geoffrey's continued friendliness toward Jill. After a month of her telling me things Geoffrey said to her, I said, "Gee, it seems he might kind of like you."

"Oh, Mom, he's just a flirt. He talks to everyone that way. I don't *like* like him— it's just nice to have a friend." Then, Geoffrey began to communicate with her on Facebook. Ed did not like anything about it. I, however, took Jill's word that he was just a nice boy—and an eighth grade flirt. Then a Facebook message from Angelica* appeared on Jill's "wall" that got my head bells ringing. She posted pictures from the dance, which included Jill and added a note to Geoffrey: "lmaooo seriously this picture is hilarious i love how u were dancing with all the freaks just to be nice!"

Jill took it in stride and said, "Angelica has gotten really nasty. I remember she and I used to be friends, but she's turned into someone I don't want to know anymore." I printed the message and slipped it into a bullying file I had recently created.

Miranda continued to disparage Jill, always out of adult hearing range. Somehow, she'd wangled her way into being the "Language Arts Class Greeter." Jill said Miranda would say hi, hello or a similar greeting to every student who walked through the door, except Jill. Then she would turn to the class and say, "I apologize to everyone I missed, except you," pointing at Jill. Or she would volunteer to hand out papers or books and inevitably "miss" Jill. According to Jill, this occurred frequently but she did an awesome job of not giving Miranda the satisfaction of knowing she was bothered by it.

Karen emailed me to say Jill had expressed a desire to increase her academic performance and requested additional assistance. "We have Guided Learning classes… Mrs. P* is the teacher and Jill is familiar with her because she co-teaches Jill's math class. Let me know if you would like us to put this in place." LMS was suggesting Jill be put into Guided Learning—a special ed class. Of course I approved the change. Jill had been worried about her academics for so long.

The rest of December passed relatively well. Heme treatments seemed to keep Jill on track even though for fully half of them she complained about being nauseous, wanted the hospital room's lights off and stayed under the blankets. An open house for the School For The Arts (SFTA), an out of district magnet school, was scheduled for January. We would be there.

CHAPTER 34

Ice Storm

It doesn't take a talent to be mean...
— AS SUNG BY JEWEL

The new year rolled in, but nothing changed at LMS. From the time Jill had returned in September there had been one problem after another. First was the Beatrice/Mary Ann scenario and Sherilyn's instigation. Kaitlin and the rest of Camerin's hangers-on had their say, nonstop. Then Camerin reenacted her elementary school bullying behavior. Then Miranda began and continued to cause trouble for Jill even after I had told her off and waged an email battle with her father. Now, Jill had accidentally stepped on Nellie's foot while changing classes. She immediately apologized but was met with a barrage of obscenities delivered by Tammy. The next day, Nellie was out to exact revenge. She and Camerin loudly berated and belittled Jill in math class. A substitute teacher let Jill go to Karen's office. On the way back to math class, Jill met Thelma,* who walked with her. As the girls approached the classroom, the substitute came into the hallway and told Jill, "I'm sorry you had to go through that." She also said she would write a report to the principal about what she had witnessed in the classroom.

Nellie and Tammy had taken their turn at the front of a long line of bullies. Whenever Jill "came up for air," someone would push her back down. The WHACK-A-Jill! game was getting old. I contacted Dr. Newton* of the state's education department for advice. She advised me to put every bullying complaint in writing, note the date and time, name(s), location, what specifically had happened and send it to the school principal with a copy to her. So I documented the latest bullying incident, sent it to Tony and copied Dr. Newton:

In accordance with CT C.G.S. 10-222d and 10-222h and Littleton School District's policy 5131.911, this is a formal complaint about a bullying incident that took place on Friday, January 8, 2010 on LMS premises, specifically, math class room #309 during which my daughter Jill was subjected to excessive verbal harassment (bullying) by [Nellie] and [Camerin]...You are well aware of Jill's medical condition and that emotional/mental stress can contribute to negative medical effects...This maltreatment continues to compromise Jill's emotional, physical and academic well-being. It...must...stop.

About this time, Jill had been telling Ed and me about "something brewing" between Nellie and Tammy. The verbal threats between the two might turn physical at any time. In a moment of clarity Jill said, "You know what I think? I think Nellie and Tammy are just trying to get Camerin's attention!"

She was probably right, but we reminded her to stay out of it, "You need to stay as far from those girls as you can, Jill." I restated my opinion that during Jill's seventh grade absence the girls in that clique must have continuously fought amongst themselves—and lashed out at others. "No wonder the administration treated you so harshly when you returned. They didn't know you and didn't connect that the other eighth graders essentially 'threw' you to that group so the teachers and administrators probably thought you were just like them," I said.

The next week Jill and I attended SFTA's open house. It was refreshing to see Jill relaxed and engaged in a school environment. On the way home, she declared she wanted to apply to the magnet school. So when we got home, she went to the computer and applied for part-time status at SFTA for her freshman high school year. She planned to go to LHS in the mornings then catch the bus to SFTA for the afternoon session. I was in a quandary about that. I wanted her away from the LMS/LHS school complex altogether.

The next day was the appointment with Dr. Werrmona. That morning Tony called to say Jill had been involved in a shoving incident with another girl and asked me to come right away. Worried, I drove to school. Jill had never been physically aggressive at school or home. Sure, there were times when she would speak her mind or tell someone off but I had never known her to physically go after anyone. Something was very wrong. When I arrived, Tony and Jill were in the conference room. As usual Tony proceeded with his spiel. He said Jill had been teased earlier in the school day by a couple of boys who had questioned whether or not she was wearing a bra, which she was. Kaitlin joined in the teasing. I had my eye on the clock because Dr. Werrmona's appointment time was approaching. I had come to the school to hear about Jill being involved in a shoving incident, but instead the bra incident had been brought up. Jill was teary-eyed and I could see she was mortified; both she and Kevin are innately modest people. I turned to Jill, "So who was the kid you were in a shoving match with?"

"Tammy," Jill said.

"Oh sweet Jesus—what happened?" I asked. During the past week she had talked about "something" she thought was going to happen between Nellie and Tammy. Now I was there because *Jill* had shoved *Tammy*? I turned to Jill, "Was Camerin in school today?"

"Jill answered, "Yeah." Tony looked uncomfortable.

"So maybe you were right about Nellie and Tammy fighting for Camerin's benefit, but instead of Nellie and Tammy, the problem turned out to be between you and Tammy," I said. Jill remained teary but coherent. She did not comment when Tony recounted how he had separated the girls. Although I had not heard the full story, I knew Jill would tell me later. Then, Tony told Jill, "You are going home with your mother and you won't be coming to school tomorrow." This meant Jill would miss the dance that night, but she seemed relieved about that and so was I.

We headed to Dr. Werrmona's office where the psychiatrist asked to speak with me before meeting with Jill. She asked questions about Jill's birth, infancy, developmental stages, therapies and/or treatments she had undergone through the years. I gave a "Reader's Digest" version of what had happened since Jill started sixth grade. I told her the AIP had been found through DNA testing. I got the distinct impression Dr. Werrmona did not think AIP warranted attention. Then Jill met with Dr. Werrmona. Afterwards, I was called in to hear her assessment which was similar to Dr. Nyeer's. After years of various therapists and specialists offering opinions about what might be wrong with Jill's brain, Dr. Werrmona said in her opinion Jill did not present with any psychiatric condition. "After receiving such a bulky file I wasn't sure what to expect before meeting her. But, I have found Jill to be a bright, well-grounded young lady who just needs to learn to live with a rare, complex disease of which little is known. She needs to become the authority about her body and understand better how it reacts to AIP. And she needs help working through the never ending dramas associated with middle school." She continued, "I asked Jill if she could have three wishes, what would they be? She answered, 'Not to be depressed, to meet a famous person, to become a singer.' To me that is remarkable. She didn't say, 'to never have AIP,' which means she has accepted her diagnosis and is working on coming to grips with all that it entails." Then she turned to Jill, "Some kids have really crappy lives; as a result many get angry and take that anger out on others. Unfortunately, middle school-age is the worst. Working with your therapist, your parents and the school people, you need to find a place in your head that works for you. Just remember—*their* problems are not your problems. It's up to *you* to be the strong one for *you*." She recommended the school conduct a psychological evaluation including an IQ test and said she would include that suggestion in her report.

As we drove home, Jill told me that Camerin had been attacked that morning by Tammy's older sister, a high school student who had violated the rule that middle school and high school students remain on their respective sides of the school complex. Ultimately, Camerin had been bitten by the other girl. The school population was abuzz. Tammy had been counseled to "let it go" but remained weepy. Jill asked her if there was anything she could do to help. Tammy responded by yelling and swearing at her. Jill shrugged it off and continued on her way. That is, until Tammy said, "I'd punch you in the f#cking face—but you'd probably faint!" Jill turned around and purposely hurried back to where Tammy stood sniveling and shoved her. The shoving match was on. Tony appeared and got between the girls. Camerin had been in school, but was suspended early on. That was how the fight between Nellie and Tammy that Jill thought was brewing for Camerin's benefit wound up to be a problem between Tammy and Jill.

"Oh brother," said Jill, "I am so done with their crap!"

Tony's letter came: "This will confirm our conversation regarding the altercation that took place when Jill walked at least 45 feet against the flow of traffic and confronted and subsequently pushed another student. As a result, Jill has been suspended out of school for Friday. Please note that students on suspension may not attend or participate in any school-sponsored activities and may not be on school grounds while suspended."[75] January was over. I could just feel that Jill was nearing the edge.

---

75 LMS* Principal Tony.* Letter to author. December 9, 2010.

CHAPTER 35

Intensifying System

Hope for a miracle, but don't depend on it.
— TALMUD

February sneaked in. After the bra and Tammy incidents were topped off with another suspension, I was uneasy about Jill's return to school. She would be in school only a few hours before I was to pick her up for heme. She made it through the morning okay. Once the infusion had been started, I told APRN Kym about a diagnostic biofeedback technique I had heard about and researched that supposedly could identify imbalances within tissues and cells—something I had been wondering about since I had started researching AIP. I had heard about Computerized Electro Dermal Stress Analysis (CEDSA) from Lora. Since it was not invasive, involved no manipulation and no pain or discomfort, I made an appointment for Jill to hopefully find out how or if AIP was affecting her tissues and cells. Though her fainting spells had reduced, I also hoped to find out why she still frequently felt drained, nauseous, dizzy and headachy. I was not surprised to find one of the first entries provided by an Internet search engine was "Quackery." I was aware that the procedure was not approved by the American Medical Association (AMA) but after further research, still decided to try it. I said, "Who knows, maybe something useful will come out of it."

To her credit Kym said, "Great! Good luck. Let us know if (or what) you find out." Vanessa had a similar response. Before we would meet the couple with the CEDSA equipment, Jill faced another school week.

Mondays and Tuesdays were religious class (CCD) days for us. Jill attended Beth's* Monday evening class after her heme treatment, and on Tuesdays she helped with the afternoon class I taught. For the past two years, Beth had regularly reminded her students of their Catholic responsibility to treat people, especially those who were sick or "different" with kindness. Her teaching style kept things light yet firm. Her classroom was a place where Jill could be just like the others. She sometimes walked from school and usually arrived in plenty of time to help me set up for the Tuesday class. However, one day she was late and unusually distracted during the class. On the way home, she said she had had another shoving incident on her way to the CCD class. "Oh geez Jill! What happened?" Apparently, Thelma had been "talking junk" and they had gotten into something after school. Thelma was the queen bee of her own little clique that included Gina* and Rosa.* Jill and Rosa had always gotten along. But recently both Gina and Rosa seemed to be avoiding her.

"What did I do now?" Jill had worried aloud.

The next day Tony called to say "a girl's parent" had complained about Jill bullying her daughter and said the girl had bruises and a scratch to show for it. Then Tony digressed into remarks about cell phones and text messages. Jill did not have a cell phone so I wondered what he was talking about. He said evasively, "A father got a hold of his daughter's cell phone and was angry about a text message received on it." He had then turned the phone in to Tony.

"We're in the process of trying to piece together cell phone messages from various sources," he said. I was pretty sure whatever happened had involved Thelma, Gina and Rosa, and the messages had been about Jill. Tony would not say anything further. When Jill returned from school, Ed and I asked her to explain what had happened with Thelma. Jill said Stan had been hanging around when she had left the school building and said, "Jill, Thel's talking sh#t about you." Jill was surprised because Thelma had been the one to walk her back to math class after Camerin and Nellie had bullied her that day. She said Thelma had been a distance ahead of her, but before Jill knew it she had approached and Jill found herself involved in her second shoving match in as many weeks. Robbie* came along, pushed Jill and screamed in her face. When everything cleared, Jill continued on to her CCD duties and Thelma and Robbie went off to their respective houses. After hearing her story, I said, "Jill, Thelma's parent told Mr. Dithers that she had bruises and was scratched. How did she get bruised and scratched?" Jill said she had merely pushed Thelma, not enough to leave bruises, and denied scratching her. I told her to write an apology note to Thelma for pushing her and sent Tony an email asking him to arrange a meeting between the two girls so the note would be given to Thelma in his presence.

I also told him that Jill had said that Stan instigated the confrontation between the girls. The next day Tony replied, "In a very heartfelt way Jill orally shared her apology with the other girl. She was very appropriate. It was done well! She then gave her the written note. The other girl was visibly moved and said more than once that she appreciated Jill's gesture!!"[76] I had the feeling that Thelma and probably many other students had never received apologies—or apologized to anyone. Meanwhile, Dr. Werrmona's evaluation results arrived:

---

76 LMS* Principal Tony.* Letter to author. December 9, 2010.

[Jill]…presented no hyperactivity…no psychosis…happy sometimes and sad but not depressed…never been suicidal…somewhat
immature in her relationships with other girls…[adapting] fairly
well to her present medical condition…multiple illnesses, hospitalizations, doctor's appointments and the long periods of time
when she has not be able to attend school have given her a sense of
insecurity in dealing with other teenagers…close and positive relationship with her parents and brother…I cannot give a psychiatric
diagnosis…every effort should be made to have her school day as
normal as possible for her to feel part of the school community…
psychological and educational testing should be done to assess her
present level of intelligence and academic performance….It will be
helpful for Jill…to have the opportunity to meet more creative and
less aggressive children.[77]

Jill tried to salvage the relationship with Gina and Rosa. But in monitoring her Facebook
page I could see neither girl was going to say much. They simply responded that Jill was
"rele [really] nice," but "couldn't talk about anything yet." Jill did not find out what had
caused them to "dis" her but thought Thelma had been involved. She said when a discussion about cell phones came up, Rosa said she no longer had a cell phone. Her father had
had the phone in his possession and was angry about a message that had been received
so he took it from her. She was not going to say anything more. It was time for Jill to
move on. A couple of weeks later she was talking with an older student, Kiera* and the
recent fight between she and Thelma came up. Kiera said she would talk to Thelma since
she knew her quite well. Shortly thereafter, Jill received a note from Thelma: "Jill, I'm
not going to start a fight with you. [Kiera] didn't tell me to apologize. I'm doing it by
myself. So think what you want. I don't know why [Kiera] hates me because I am not
the only one that's mean to you, people do worse stuff than me! Sorry [Thelma]."[78] Jill
took it gratefully and ended the matter.

Meanwhile, Geoffrey's attention toward Jill revved up. She said he had drawn
hearts enclosing his and her initials and showed them to her. He asked her on
numerous occasions if she liked him. She said she told him, "I like you as a friend
but I don't *like* like you." Instead, just to get him to stop, she said she liked Robbie,
which "made him (Geoffrey) mad." She said rumors were going around that
Geoffrey and Shana* were about to "go out" and wondered if that was true why he
would be acting as he was toward her.

Everybody in eighth grade knew Chelsea had a huge crush on Geoffrey; she told
Jill repeatedly that she was jealous that "Geoffrey even talks to you." Geoffrey seemed
even more focused on getting Jill to admit she '*like* liked' him. He had construction
paper signs, allegedly made by Shana, who was on vacation with her family, that read she
missed him and shoved them in Jill's face. She pushed the papers away, told him to stop
it and said, "Good for the both of you!" "Go out, I don't care!" Geoffrey was irritated.

77 Psychiatric evaluation prepared by Dr. Werrmona* to LMS* administration. January 28, 2010.
78 Handwritten note from Thelma* to Jill. February 9, 2010.

Dwayne,* who was in Geoff's clique, told Jill, "Yeah, everybody at our lunch table talks about how you were so obsessed with Geoff in the fifth grade. They all laugh about it."

Jill said she had replied, "Oh brother, that was three years ago. Why can't everybody just grow up? And I wasn't obsessed with him in the way they think. He was just nice to me and I appreciated that." When she told me about this conversation, my head bells began to jangle. What was Jill being set up for? Yes, Geoffrey *seemed* to be nice but if he didn't *like* like her, what was going on?

Still hoping that friendship might be possible at school, Jill reconnected with LHS sophomore Amber.* Jill and Amber had been in Girl Scouts and now that they were older, wanted to catch up.

School vacation started. The CEDSA biofeedback session was scheduled for that week so Jill asked if Amber could join us for the road trip to the session to be held in Massachusetts. "If it's ok with her mom and dad, it is ok with me," I said.

We arrived in plenty of time for our appointment with the husband and wife CEDSA technician team. Lorraine* described what was going to happen. Copper electrodes would be gently pushed down on pressure points on Jill's hands and feet that corresponded with individual organs and tissues located throughout her body. Measuring the connection between the acupuncture point and the specific organ, the brain would provide vital information. The liver was identified fairly quickly as a problem area; Jill's liver was functioning at about 35 percent, Lorraine said, and was surrounded with cirrhosis and further encumbered by the heavy metals: cadmium, arsenic and iron. Jill's spleen and thyroid were working hard. Though to me it all sounded like hocus-pocus, the experience was fascinating. How would I know if any of it was true? Then, Lorraine got my attention, "Did you know Jill was once exposed to TB?" My head snapped up. She was right. She then said Jill's potassium level was depleted and that supplements could help raise it. Then she arrived at the part where questions would be directed to Jill and her brain would supply answers. "This is kind of eerie," I thought, but since I had seen the amazing effects biofeedback had had on Jill and Kevin years earlier, I sat back and took the rest in. Among other things, Lorraine asked if the breathing difficulty Jill experienced during her AIP attacks was due to a physical reason or was it psychological? The monitor registered green (yes) for physical, then red (no) for psychological. She asked about school triggers. Was the reason for Jill's attacks based on something coming through the heating/cooling system? Green (yes). She looked at me and said, "Something coming through the mechanical system is causing Jill's reactions." Our time was up. Other clients were scheduled. It had been a good day. Amber had been delightful. We all enjoyed the biofeedback experience and went out to eat lunch. The final report was rather innocuous, nothing an MD would consider useful. We would have to wait and see if any of Lorraine's "findings" proved accurate.

For a time after that weekend, things went relatively well. Surprisingly, Jill earned a perfect attendance award for the month of January. She was pleased, but not overly impressed. To me and Ed, however, it was a *huge* accomplishment. It occurred to me that in spite of all the negativity foisted on her, Jill had never once said she did not want to go to school. She went off every day to do the best she could academically, tried her best to get along socially and fervently hoped she would not faint that day.

CHAPTER 36

Mammatus Clouds

It's not what you look at that matters, it's what you see.
— HENRY DAVID THOREAU

Marie's mom, Allyson and I shared observations over lunch about our daughters and discussed a common suspicion about Geoffrey's operatives concerning both Jill and Marie. I said he seemed to be flirting relentlessly with Jill, but why? Allyson said she had seen a Facebook chat involving Geoffrey, Marie and Jill, and it sure seemed he *was* flirting with Jill. "But," she said, "Marie says Jill's always saying that Geoffrey is annoying so if I were you, I'd believe Jill when she says she doesn't *like* like him!" If Jill had not gone through so much medically and missed so much socially, I would have happily let middle school antics happen. But my head bells kept jangling—something about this Geoffrey connection did not seem right.

That afternoon, Jill came home with another troubling Miranda story. This time, Miranda had begun "joking" with Jill, then suddenly reached out and slapped her face. Jill was surprised, embarrassed and angry and said some of the students who saw what happened told her to lighten up. I emailed a complaint to Tony and asked him to address the incident. Since the cell phone/texting situation, he had seemed a little more agreeable to things that concerned Jill. He responded he would deal with it the next day and would call to let me know what happened.

When Tony called the next day, Ed answered the phone. I heard him ask if Miranda's parent(s) had been notified about the slapping complaint. I heard him say, "Well, you know damn well if the roles had been reversed and it was *Jill* who slapped *Miranda*, you would've called us in a heartbeat." He had made his point, but it did not seem to matter.

My head bells were going off. "*Something* set Miranda off," I thought and checked Jill's Facebook account. Sure enough, Miranda's "Facebook boyfriend," Manny [or

Benny—he used both names] had left several messages for Jill. "Hey jill I need to talk to u asap plz add meh!!!!" then "Dude, this is me Manny Fernandez we need to talk plz (plus i miss u)." After a while she obviously had not responded because he messaged "ugh...like she said nobody even likes u."

Jill replied, "mhm I rlly don't know u so bye." I thought, "Good girl, Jill!"

Manny was not happy, "I was just tryin to help ya get payback with Miranda."

Jill closed it out. "I don't know you that's all I'm saying yes I've talked with you before but on FACEBOOK. I don't *know* you. Bye." I printed out the communication, emailed Tony and asked to see him when I picked Jill up for heme. He agreed. I showed him the Facebook messages between "Manny" and Jill. Tony made a positive comment about Jill's clear indication she wanted nothing to do with this Manny person. I said, "You can see this guy taunted Jill about how 'like she said nobody likes you.' I give you this info in the event anything else crops up between the two girls."

The next day, an LMS secretary called to set a date for Jill's next 504 meeting. Ed and I wanted to get better organized first. He felt since Dr. Werrmona had essentially declared Jill "psych free," the school would use that as "not having psychiatric issues that could cause behavioral problems" and she would be subjected to whatever disciplinary measures were meted out by "rogue" LMS administrators. After witnessing the CEDSA evaluation, I was now even more convinced that the weird physical and neurological reactions Jill experienced were connected to the school. I also knew that without scientific support, it would be impossible to prove. All of this led my thoughts back to the SE/504 dilemma. I felt Jill was eligible for the special education (SE) other health impaired (OHI) category, and the meeting the school wanted should be a PPT *not* a 504. The SE designation offers better support than the 504 Rehabilitation addendum.

However, it was clear to me the district preferred to keep as many students as possible in the "cheaper" and easier to manage 504 category. Because Littleton chose to ignore Jill's illness, my vigilance could not stop. She needed that OHI designation. I decided we needed to have a representative from the Learning Disabilities Association (LDA) with us at the next school meeting.

February wound down. Jill had been absent only one day because of a cold. She had had no AIP activity even though the building had been closed for winter vacation. Sticking with regular heme treatments, a vitamin supplement regimen, improved diet and exercise and regular sleep seemed to have kept the AIP attacks at bay. Still, the stress of ongoing peer harassment by students and school administrators toward her was disconcerting. Little did we know we were heading into another volatile period and, this time, Jill's sanity would be at risk.

CHAPTER 37

Multi-Vortex Tornados

*So break me down if it makes you feel right...and hate
me now if it keeps you all right...*
— AS SUNG BY SEETHER

March roared in with yet another school problem. One afternoon when Jill got off the school bus I saw Emily* heatedly say something to her. Then she bolted to her father's car. "What was that all about?" I asked.

"Shana was laughing at me on the bus and I got mad. Emily just told me she was mad at me, too and said, 'I always stick up for my *friends*!' Mom, I *really* hate going on the bus." Ed usually drove both children to school in the mornings because the bus on our route was habitually late. However, they took the bus home in the afternoons. As we drove to her singing lesson with Lora, I asked Jill why Shana had laughed at her. She began, "Geoffrey and I were fooling around in the hallway. He said things I didn't like and I told him if he didn't stop I was going to kick him.

He didn't stop and said even worse things, so I kicked him and he fell down." My head bells jangled. I said, "You *kicked* him? He *fell down*? What do you mean he 'fell down?'"

Jill answered, "Well, he was whispering some nasty things about Robbie to me."

"Okay..." I said.

"He kept saying things I didn't like so I play kicked him and he fell on his knees all theatrical-like. Shana and Angelica went nuts. They yelled that I had pushed him down and all three of them ran to Mrs. Menard to tattle." Because it was time to go home the teacher said she would deal with it the next day. Jill went on Facebook when we got home. She did not say much and after dinner did her homework. Things were as normal as could be expected after yet another incident. Never mind that Geoffrey had had an enjoyable time inappropriately teasing her. The reality was

Jill had caused a student to fall—right on the heels of Miranda smacking her in the face episode. I had a sinking feeling.

After Jill retired for the night I checked her Facebook account. My stomach lurched as I read: "Geraldine: "oh Ho no!!!! mess wit my friends nd I'll kick urr ass!

Angelica: YOU pushed me into [Geoffrey], btw STAY AWAY FROM HIM!

Jill: "[Geoffrey] and me were fooling around he fell down on purpose.

Angelica: Stay away from [Geoffrey] He doesn't like you at all he hates you GET OVER IT

Geraldine: Jill watch mee…U prolly will end up in da hospital after I done wit u!! Ndd [And] leave me friends alone cuz they didn't do shitt 2 u ndd ya [Geoffrey] deff [definitely] Dnt like u

Jill: I may like him but only cause he's nice unlike u

Angelica: idc if im not nice to you haha HAHAHA [GEOFFREY] HATES YOU

Jill: [Geoffrey] doesn't hate anyone cause once again he's NICE unlike u and cares about ppl so believe what u want but ur like seriously nasty

Geraldine: hahahaha [angelica] cares about her friends nd she is a nice person hahahahahahahaha@least I got brains nd im fukin smart. Jill…I deff will kick yur ass…nd u don't scare me one bitt…

Geraldine: Jill first of all if u get in my face im gonna offer u a piece of gum buz ur breath prolly stinks…Then im gona fukin kick ur ass

Angelica: LOL [GER] I LOVE YO. ur asss is hot. Jills jealous"

Shana's "girlies," Geraldine* and Angelica, had harassed and threatened Jill—on Facebook. I wasn't surprised about Geraldine—like Camerin, she'd been a trouble-maker for years. But I *was* surprised that Angelica, the daughter of a prominent Littletonite was egging Geraldine on. I emailed Tony and told him about the threats that had been made and by whom and to warn about the potential problem the next day. Then I printed out the Facebook pages I had just read.

I had just sat down at my desk the next morning when the phone rang. When I answered, Larry, the school nurse said, "Things are a bit hectic here so Tony asked me to call you. Jill was just injured in a fight with another student. Can you come pick her up?" When I arrived I chuckled at the irony of keeping the school doors locked to maintain student safety. For a school with only about 200 students and forty or more adults including two security guards, danger came more from the students themselves than from the outside. As I sat in the office another fight broke out. "Must be fight day," quipped the office secretary as she continued her duties. When Tony finally appeared he said Jill was in the nurse's office and that I could go there. He also said he had responded earlier that morning to the email I had sent him the previous night. "Oh, so he got it," I said to myself. Tony motioned Jill and me across the hall to his office. He said the fight had happened in the cafeteria and it had been caught on tape. Evidently, he had not even been there, yet he said Jill had approached Geraldine and threw the first punch.

Exasperated, Jill butted in, "When I walked into the cafeteria Geraldine yelled at me. She said she wanted to give me a breath mint then 'take care of my ass.' I told her I was done with her. She said, 'Well I'm not done with you, get over here' so I walked up to her," Jill said. Geraldine said, 'You know why you're done with me? You're scared.' I told her I wasn't scared of her and she started punching me. Everyone started cheering.'"

Tony said to me, "I sent you an email in reply to yours." I again said I had not seen it. Then he changed the subject and proceeded to tell Jill off about a bullying complaint another student's mother had called in about Jill on the bus the afternoon before. "The girl was *crying* on the phone to her mother!" he snapped accusingly at Jill. Knowing that *something* had happened on the bus the afternoon before, but not exactly what, I let him rant. Jill kept interrupting, trying to tell her side of things but Tony ignored her. Then all of a sudden, he roared, "You keep complaining about people getting in *your* face, but never about *you* being in *other people's faces!*" He crooked his elbow and demonstrated as though Jill had thrust her elbow in such a manner into another student's face. I could not envision what he was accusing her of and between being angry that he was shouting at her just after she had been pummeled by Geraldine, Jill's continued insistence that she had something to say and the fact I obviously did not have the whole story of what *had* happened on the bus, it took all I had not to scream at Tony myself.

Every time Jill tried to talk about the bus incident he brushed her off, "If *you* hadn't tripped Geoffrey, none of this would have happened. Geoffrey is one of the nicest, if not the nicest student in our school," he snarled scornfully. I said it certainly *seemed* Geoffrey was nice but based on some things I had recently become aware of, I had reservations about his motives. I reminded him that Geoffrey was an eighth grade boy, after all. Tony was not about to change his mind so I changed the subject and said I would contact Mrs. Morrison and ask that Geoffrey and Jill be separated in her class for the remainder of the school year. "Or do you want to take care of it?" I asked.

He said it would be all right for me to ask the science teacher to do that. Then he declared, "I've been accused of favoring Jill Gould." I did not pursue that one; I had had all I could take of him. After Jill had jumped to her feet for the umpteenth time, he sent us out, she with a three-day suspension for fighting. On the way out of school I told her the only reason I had subjected us to Tony's tirade was because once again I did not have the whole story.

As soon as we got in the car, I asked her to tell me everything that had happened on the bus. Jill said after the Geoffrey/Shana/Angelica fiasco in the hallway and Mrs. Menard telling her it would be dealt with the next day, she had gone to her bus, sat in the first seat behind the driver and was soon joined by Marie. Shana and Emily had slipped into the seat behind them where Jill heard Shana tell Emily, "Ooh I can't wait! Jill's gonna get in trouble tomorrow!" Jill said she had then turned around and saw Shana leaning forward, very near the back of her own seat and asked what she was talking about.

Shana said, "You pushed Geoffrey down on purpose! Just leave him alone!"

Jill told her to "get out of my face" and noted that Shana got on her cell phone, complained that Jill was bullying her to whomever she was speaking, then got off at her bus stop. Before long Jill got off the bus and that is when I had seen Emily blast her.

"Did you threaten Shana in any way?" I asked.

"No," Jill replied. I said, "Did you have your arm 'crooked in Shana's face' like this?" and demonstrated what Tony had implied.

Jill answered, "Well, mom, when you want to say something to the kid behind you, you turn around in the seat and put your arm like this on the back of it," she demonstrated.

I said, "I think Shana was caught off guard that you called her out about what she'd just said. She wanted to get out of the situation she'd put herself in so told her mother you were bullying her. And tears often work. Hearing that, most mothers would report it. Shana's mom obviously didn't know the whole story. And Shana didn't appear on the Facebook garbage last night so she's off that hook. And as far as Emily goes, now you know where you stand with her, too. It's too bad she's going to stick up for her friends even when they're in the wrong, but that's not unusual in life. And she just let you know you are not and probably never will be considered her friend. And this is the *nice* girl you've told me about?" I asked rhetorically.

I checked email when I got home. There was a 7:29 a.m. reply from Tony, "FYI, I have a call from a parent about a bus incident involving Jill and her bullying of this parent's daughter. It comes from a vantage point. I will obviously have to talk about this with those involved."[79] There was no mention of the previous night's 11:09 p.m. warning I had sent him about Geraldine and Angelica threatening Jill. I was furious. Tony clearly had not been in the cafeteria when Geraldine attacked Jill. He was covering his own butt and, as usual, doing his best to make Jill the instigator. Though he had obviously received my warning email, Tony's response was that *Jill* had a bullying complaint against her. The vantage point he referenced was the bus driver—another point I did not miss. That a low social-status Littleton school bus driver would support Jill, a transplant's child, against a higher socially-ranked Littleton offspring? I did not think would ever happen.

The eighth grade drama theme finally clicked. Shana and Geoffrey had eyes for each other. Jill returned to school. Individually or together, the two of them decided to rope her back into the previous "fifth grade crush." That explained why Geoffrey made like he was interested in Jill, asked her over and over if she "liked" him, drew hearts and pushed Shana's lovey-dovey signs into her face with the aim of provoking a jealous reaction. But the plan fizzled when Jill said she did not "*like* like" Geoffrey. All she had ever hoped for was friendship. It made me ill to think that these so-called "nice," honor roll students had set up an elaborate scenario in order to humiliate a very sick classmate.

After reading Tony's email message that effectively ignored my warning about the threats to Jill and having heard him tell Jill, "None of it would have happened if you hadn't tripped Geoffrey," I told Ed, "We're going to the police department again. If Geraldine had assaulted Jill on the street, in a store or anywhere else in town, the cops would have been called. Why should threats and assault at school be any different? Littleton students, like everyone else in town, are entitled to police protection. When Camerin screamed at and threatened Jill a couple of months ago she hadn't even been sent to the principal's office. Now Jill's been punched in the

---

79 LMS* Principal Dithers.* Email to author. March 2010.

face and chest—with a port in her chest no less—and this time marks were left on her, not to mention we have the Facebook trail. Maybe if enough school assault complaints went to the police department (PD), someone would finally step up and take notice—that's the only way things will change."

According to *Queen Bees & Wanna Bees* author Rosalind Wiseman, that Jill confronted Geraldine was not unusual because she found that many bullying victims actually *do* confront their intimidator, at least verbally. Doing so was just part of Jill's personality and try as they might, she would not concede to their bullying. That made me proud—but worriedly so. A building filled with toxic chemicals and toxic people terrified me. Yet day after day, Jill went off to school, though no longer with a smile on her face.

Years later, Jill addressed the memory: *"I guess it wasn't enough that I already felt like a freak back then. I think Geoffrey, Shana, Geraldine, Angelica and a whole bunch of other eighth grade kids just wanted to put me in the spotlight and humiliate me—ya know, like sometimes you see people on TV who end up on stage in front of an audience in their underwear or naked or something like that. Well they did."* [80]

In the end, it was a well-worn middle school sham: popular boy pretends to like unpopular girl for kicks. But it was one that could have had fatal consequences. As far as Camerin's targeting her for bullying, Jill theorized it probably stemmed from an incident a few years before when Camerin had ordered Jill to kiss her and Jill had refused.

---

80 Jill's journal. October 2014.

CHAPTER 38

Clearing Mist

*Having faith in God does not mean
sitting back and doing nothing.*
— ANONYMOUS

"What's up?" Officer Bennington asked when we walked into the PD. I said, "Jill was threatened on Facebook last night and assaulted this morning at school. I printed these out. Tony didn't even look at them."

Officer Bennington looked at Jill, "What happened?" She explained what had taken place in the school cafeteria.

When she finished I said, "Tony claimed Jill threw the first punch, Jill disputes that. He said everything is on tape but never offered to show it to me. I don't even think he was in the cafeteria when it happened—too busy writing an email to me in an attempt to nail Jill on a trumped up school bus bullying charge the afternoon before. To give you background about the incident, Jill and a kid named Geoffrey were horsing around in the hallway and she tripped him, though not maliciously. The 'girly patrol' that surrounds this boy went wild. One of the girls later needled Jill on the bus and they had words. The girl called her mother on her cell phone and said Jill was bullying her; the mother called Tony to complain about Jill. Tony said that if she hadn't tripped the boy, none of this would've happened. And now Jill and the girl who assaulted her are suspended."

Officer Bennington chuckled at the ghetto talk in Geraldine's Facebook messages then turned to Jill, "Unfortunately, the law says once Geraldine challenged you and you went to confront her, you are as guilty as she is. That's probably why you got suspended, too. If you had walked away and let her grab you, only she would have been charged. Then he looked intently at Jill and said, "Listen to me, *you are better than them*, I can tell. Don't you ever forget it. Hold your head up high.

It's obvious you have a mom who cares about you like I did, and they know it. You have something they don't." Someone from the schools must have gotten to the PD because he then said to me, "This is a school matter so I won't be able to go there. But I am here to serve you, so what do you want me to do?"

I pulled Jill's neckline aside. "See this bruise? This happens to be the location of her port, through which she gets weekly infusions of blood to her liver. A tube goes right into her heart. I'm sick of this BS. This time I *do* want you to go to the kid's house and tell her and the mother there *had better be no next time*. I guess they never got the memo about not beating up sick people."

Officer Bennington said, "Got it. I'll take a drive over there." This had been my second complaint to the police department about issues that should have been handled by the school. Something was very wrong with the whole scenario.

Home again, I called the NHC Hem/Onc department to report that Jill had been assaulted at school and punched in her port area. Nurse Randi* came on the line, "What does it look like? Is it leaking or oozing?" she asked.

"No, but it's bruised and she's in a lot of pain," I said.

"Well, we'll wait until Monday and check it before the next infusion," she said. "But if the pain escalates or you notice anything leaking from it, get her here right away."

Meanwhile, I called Allyson to ask if Marie had said anything about the bus incident. She said Marie had witnessed the entire thing and shared what Marie had told her. Everything she said was in sync with Jill's version. Marie said she was not the only witness and rattled off three or four names of students who had heard and seen it too. "Yeah," I said ruefully, "too bad they're all going to stick up for their '*friends.*'" I could see I was about to join the motor brigade of parents who routinely picked their children up after school every day because they did not want the torment associated with school bus rides.

I had already contacted Mrs. Morrison to request that Jill's and Geoffrey's seats be separated in science class—and asked her to please be sure Jill was not near Miranda, either. Then I called Geoffrey's mother to tell her I had requested the seating change and why. Jill didn't want me to call, "Geoffrey's a nice guy, mom, I don't want to get him in trouble."

"Maybe so but even nice guys skin their knees—that's how we all learn. His family is a good one, so I think they'd want to know what's happened." Thankfully, Monique* had the same calm, rational approach as when we had talked a few years earlier. I said I had asked Mrs. Morrison to separate Geoffrey and Jill in science class and wanted her to know why. She was aware the two kids had been horsing around and that Geoffrey had fallen. She said he had told her there was nothing malicious in the action. She had not known about the chain of events that happened afterwards, so I filled her in. Monique then said, "Geoffrey said Jill was mercurial and sometimes got in his face."

I confirmed Jill's moods could swing up, down or all around and said we had ultimately discovered she had a metabolic disorder. As far as her neediness and sometimes "getting in Geoffrey's face," there was more to tell. I told her about Jill's allegations that Geoffrey frequently poked her with pencils, asked her repeatedly if she "liked" him, showed her hearts he had drawn with their initials in them and once infuriated her because he had "smacked" her behind. I then added Dwayne had told her that a group of students led by Geoffrey regularly laughed about Jill's fifth grade "obsession" with him, which prompted Jill to tell Dwayne the same thing she had told me, "I liked Geoffrey because he was friendly to me." I said I was uncomfortable with what Jill had told me about signals he had been sending her way for the past several months and how just before the tripping incident in the hallway, Jill said he had needled her about her friendship with Robbie by asking, "Did you kiss him?"

She had answered, "No."

"Did you have sex with him?" he asked.

"That was it. I told him to stop it," Jill emphasized. There were a few other issues we discussed, and in the end, Monique expressed regret that Jill had been hurt and said she knew the girls who hovered around Geoffrey could be mean. She reiterated how she and her husband were committed to giving their children the tools needed for a good, moral life and hoped that they would follow the right path. I told her Geoffrey was known as one of the nicer children in school, but Jill needed to experience having girl-friends before she would be emotionally ready for boy-girl challenges. I also said many girls in school were on track with "normal" developmental social growth and at times that was disheartening for her. However, I was proud that for the most part she followed the "niceness" route too, yet was not above sticking up for herself when necessary. Monique said she understood that. Tony's letter regarding Jill's latest transgressions arrived:

> This will confirm our conversation yesterday regarding the altercation in the cafeteria when Jill approached another student. Subsequently, the two engaged in a physical altercation. As I have previously stated, physical altercations will not be tolerated. As a result, Jill has been suspended out of school for a period of three days. Furthermore, Jill admits to tripping a boy in the hallway on Wednesday. After that incident, it has been reported and confirmed that Jill got on the bus Wednesday afternoon and put her elbow into the physical space of a different female's face. In our conversation yesterday, I reiterated the 'hands off' policy that Jill, her father and I discussed as recently as two weeks ago when a girl put her hands on Jill. Please note that students on suspension may not attend or participate in any school sponsored activities and may not be on school grounds while suspended.[81]

It had only been two weeks since the Miranda face slapping incident. I responded to Tony's letter with a formal complaint about Geraldine's assault on Jill, the fact that he had ignored my email about the Facebook threats the night before but how he had championed Shana's bogus allegation by responding to *my* email with

---

81 LMS* Principal Dithers.* Letter to author. March 4, 2010.

a notification he had received a complaint about Jill bullying another student and finally that I had spoken to Geoffrey's mother who concurred that he, like every other child, did not have a halo. I closed with, "By the way, Jill's port was affected and will be inspected at her next heme appointment but hey, she *deserved* it—right Tony?"

The next morning Jill was out of school on suspension but her weekly infusion was waiting. The nurse attempted to access the port but it had shifted and caused Jill so much pain that it had to be X-rayed. It was determined the port's function had not been impaired and the infusion went ahead as scheduled. But the doctor said because it had been jolted, Jill's entire upper chest area would probably hurt for a couple of weeks. The time spent X-raying the port lengthened the appointment time considerably so I called Sr. Marguerite to let her know what had happened and that Jill would not be in CCD class. Allyson called the next day to ask if Jill was still in the hospital. "No—how did you know about that?" I asked. Apparently Sr. Marguerite had told Beth that Jill would not be in CCD class because she had been assaulted in school. Beth then told the class Jill had been attacked in school, was in the hospital and would not be able to attend class that night.

As Confirmation candidates, she said it was time for them to be the adults the Church expected them to be. "If anyone knows anything about what happened to Jill, you must tell an adult in charge or you can tell me," she encouraged them. Allyson said when Marie returned home from CCD she had made up her mind to tell Tony what she had witnessed on the bus.

Marie said, "I have to do this" because, she said, Jill had stood up for her several times. So Marie went to Tony and told what had happened. Not surprisingly, we heard nothing from him about any of it.

As Ed said, "If Marie's story had put more fire on the flame to burn Jill, we would certainly have heard about that."

While Jill was out on her latest suspension she recalled after the tripping incident, that afternoon she and Geoffrey had chatted on Facebook, "He told me he was going to see that nothing would happen to me." Apparently, he did not. It was painfully obvious that Jill had been dealing with the bullying situation known as piling on by others that Rosalind Wiseman wrote about in *Queen Bees & Wanna Bees*. Sadly, instead of serving as responsible models for the student body, Littleton school adults fanned the flames.

CHAPTER 39

Hole Punch Clouds

I was thinking that I might fly today...
just to disprove all the things you say.
— AS SUNG BY JEWEL

I ended up with bruises and aches on my body and had to go to the hospital after all. She hit my port which is an IV in my chest. Every day I get more and more stares from the kids.[82]

Things settled down—for about two weeks. Jill was covering up things well, but inside her hopelessness was festering. The phone rang. "We got drama," Tony said. "Jill wants you here now."

"I'm on my way," I said, thinking, "*Now what?*"

Ed came out of his home office, "What's wrong now?" he asked.

"I don't know. All Tony said was 'We got drama' and that Jill asked for me. Gotta go." I went to the main office. While waiting to hear about the latest drama, I watched three different students go to the telephone on the counter, pick it up and make calls; none asked for permission before doing so. "That's weird," I thought. "A while ago, Tony made a nasty comment to me about how without asking permission, Jill reached for the phone on the office counter to make a call home."

He said he had reprimanded her presumptuousness. When I mentioned it to Jill, she said *Tony* had told her to call home then barked at her for not asking for permission first. I had just witnessed *three* students make phone calls and no one had challenged *any* of them.

As I waited to hear about the latest drama, Camerin came stomping through the main office, flung the door open and sailed into the main lobby. Then Tony came out and motioned me into his office where Jill was already seated. This time, he was

---

82 Jill's journal. March 2010.

cordial as he proceeded to tell me what had happened. During math class Nellie and Justin,* who, according to Tony was "stirring the pot," were laughing about Jill "getting beat up" a few days before. Jill was sitting in front of them and could hear everything.

Totally disregarding my, Ed's, Vanessa's and everyone else's advice to ignore moronic attempts to get her to react, Jill had turned around and announced, "Anyone who says that are bitches."

"Thanks, Jill, keep digging the hole deeper," I thought.

She was sent to the principal's office where Tony read her the riot act once again and during which Jill calmly asked, "*Why* do you always feel the need to yell?"

Later on, Jill was passing in the hallway when Camerin stepped in front of her. Apparently, Nellie, a frequent pot stirrer herself and no stranger to wordplay, had told Camerin, "Jill called you a bitch." Camerin snarled at Jill.

A teacher heard Camerin and sent both of them to Tony's office. Other than Jill swearing about the "bitches" for which she had been reprimanded earlier, the trouble was found to be with Nellie and Camerin this time. She was free to go. As we drove home, Jill told me she had felt insulted yet again by Tony in front of Camerin. I sighed and asked her what had happened.

"I said I would 'play the game' like you said. (I'd meant for Jill to say that *silently* to *herself*!) But Camerin was a jerk. She said, 'I am who I am and that's the way I'm going to be. *I'm not* playing *no* game.' And you know what Mr. Dither's did? He patted Camerin on the back and said 'That's right always be yourself.' *Why* is it that *I* can never be myself?" she groaned. I did not have an answer.

The rest of that week passed without drama though Jill said Camerin, apparently looking to feed her daily need for conflict, snapped at her for "rolling her eyes." Leaving school that afternoon Jill saw Geraldine wave to her while sitting on a bus. Jill pointed at herself. Me? Geraldine nodded. Yes.

Jill kept walking. Once in the car Jill said, "Mom, how weird *are* these people? They're nice one day—or minute—and nasty the next. But either way, they're mean just about every single day. What's up with that?" Jill wanted so badly to understand.

"Remember what Dr. Werrmona told you about kids who have really bad lives and what Officer Bennington told you about people knowing that you have something they don't?" I asked. She nodded. "Well, lots of times angry people take their feelings out on others who have what they don't. Love, stability, kindness—too many people just don't have enough of that in their lives—so they try to make those who do miserable. There is an old saying, 'misery loves company.' When you grow up you'll understand it better. That clique is trying to bring you down. But I know you. I know finding out you had AIP didn't break you. For months and months I've watched you go through things none of those 'all-mouth/no-guts' types could handle—kids or adults. We've just got to keep praying you will be selected in the SFTA lottery for the magnet school so you can get away from Littleton."

After the next heme treatment, a nurse said they might have to keep Jill overnight because her electrolytes were "off" and potassium levels low.

"Wow," I thought, "that CSDE program was right about the TB exposure and now her potassium is low, too." Head bells jangling, thoughts began to come together.

Lorraine had said Jill was reacting to something coming through the school's HVAC system; for sure, hydrogen peroxide cleaner and marker fumes had to move through the mechanical system, but with everything going on with the building's occupants, I just did not have time for that battle. Jill had not fainted in a while in spite of three months of unbelievable stress. It seemed the aggressive heme/D10 protocol was helping but the treatments were beginning to take a toll on her. More and more, she would complain of being nauseous and achy after a treatment. Zofran helped ease the nausea, but the body aches hung on for a day or two after.

In a few hours, Jill's electrolyte and potassium levels had improved, and we went home. But this time she became sicker and sicker and complained of a fever. When it reached 100° I said we had to go to the ED as we had been instructed to do. "No," she adamantly said. "I'm not going." She could be so difficult some times. Within half an hour, the fever reached 102° and I insisted we get to the ED. Once there, lab results indicated strep throat and that she needed antibiotics. Fortunately, the attending physician understood Jill's need for safe drugs and selected ceftriaxone sodium. After rest, we left but she missed the remainder of the school week. Her Confirmation retreat was scheduled for Saturday. By Friday she was still sick so Sister Marguerite suggested she attend another parish's retreat after she had recovered. The next week she was well enough to return to school—and for another heme treatment. While there, the nurse handed me a letter from Dr. O'Connor. I read:

> Jill has acute intermittent porphyria by clinical symptoms as well as genetic testing done in 2008. The clinical diagnosis has been based on a constellation of symptoms that include psychiatric and physical. Her physical symptoms have been intermittent severe abdominal pain, nausea, vomiting, and diarrhea as well as headaches, weakness, intermittent neuropathies. She may have also had seizures, although differentiating neurological from psychiatric manifestations of disease can be challenging in people with AIP. Porphyria is associated with multiple psychiatric and neurological problems. Psychiatric challenges have been depression, anxiety, hysteria, psychosis, or confusion. She receives intermittent infusions of hematin. These periodic infusions are given intravenously in the hospital. They do help lessen the severity of the disease and frequency of episodes. To facilitate the infusions, she [has a] Port-a-Cath in place. Because of [this] she can't participate in contact sports and needs medical evaluation with fevers. My treatment recommendations for Jill when she is experiencing an acute attack:

- Ativan (Lorazepam) orally at 1 mg or intravenously at 0.5 mg every 4 hours as needed.

- Oral or IV hydration with fluid containing sugar. Specifically for intravenous hydration, I would recommend D10 with half normal saline or quarter normal saline to run at 150 ml per hour.

- Immediate application of supplemental oxygen therapy that should be continued until hematin has been started.

- Intravenous infusion of Panhematin at a dose of approximately 330 mg. In order to receive this infusion, she will need to be transferred to [NHC].

- The Panhematin infusion should be done daily for 3 to 4 days until it is clear that the acute exacerbation or attack has subsided.

- It is my recommendation that the school Jill attends will have on site the ability to give supplemental oxygen in the event that she begins to have an attack on school property. The oxygen can be administered as a nasal cannula at 2 liters until she can be transferred to [NHC]. I would also recommend that she have available to her Ativan orally at a dose of 1 mg.[83]

Tears of gratitude filled my eyes. I had waited so long for this letter and planned to present it at the upcoming PPT.

---

83 Dr. O'Connor.* Letter re Jill's AIP. March 20, 2010.

CHAPTER 40

Black Moon

You always thought that I left myself
open/But you didn't know I was already broken.
— AS SUNG BY THREE DAYS' GRACE

When I returned in 8th grade, I had a LOT OF CATCHING UP both socially and academically but it wasn't long till the rumors were flying. I can remember this one rumor that still gives me chills, about me being obsessed with a guy from 5th grade. That was the beginning of the downfall. I remember too that my "friends" would "play fight" and "joke" around with me but I never saw how degrading it really was. Pushing, slapping, punching, kicking, leaving bruises and marks on me, calling me horrible names—fat, ugly, bitch, whore. I was slowing but surely starting to fall apart by the seams.[84]

The Board of Education (BOE) responded to my letter: "Unfortunately, serious concerns regarding privacy and appropriate use of academic time are raised by your request. Obviously, from your communication, many professional educators and health experts are involved in the situation and we encourage you to continue to work through them. If you have not done so, request the MSDS sheets for all cleaning products in the school. Your request to address eighth grade students at [Littleton] Middle School is denied."[85]

A few days later, Jill received an acceptance letter to SFTA's half-day program for her upcoming freshman year. She would get out of the Littleton school system after all.

During that week, as Jill was leaving school, Camerin and Geraldine yelled to Jill that she was going to get her "ass kicked again." Jill reported to Ed what the

---

84 Jill. Circa Summer 2010
85 Littleton* BOE Chair. Letter to author. March 16, 2010.

dangerous duo had yelled and Tony received another complaint/warning call. The fact that Camerin and Geraldine had outwardly joined forces really got my head bells clanging. I contacted the LDA, told the director about the ongoing bullying from peers and administrators aimed at Jill and asked for help. She invited me to attend an upcoming conference about bullying and said we could meet there.

A couple of days later Jill was back in the principal's office. Tony called the house. Ed's worn patience was showing, "Why is it every time you call here about Jill, you always have a story about her 'instigation?' Why is it *always* about Jill *causing* the trouble?"

He went to retrieve Jill. In the meantime, Tony called back. I answered and he began, "I've talked with a couple of people and have some information," he said. "Good for you, Tony. Good for you," I said and hung up. I figured Ed and Jill would inform me when they returned.

When they did, Ed began telling me what Tony had told him on the phone before he had left to get Jill. Tony had said Jill had "gotten into it" with Kaitlin, Geraldine and Camerin. Rosa was involved and he had spoken to Jill about her tendency to be clingy with people and that she needed to stop that. My blood pressure shot up. We had made enough complaints about the Camerin, Tammy, Nellie and now Geraldine alliance that by now he should have called them all together and read *them* the riot act about targeting Jill for their ongoing nefarious activities. Instead, he professed not to know the composition of the cliques among the student body of which as he routinely reminded Jill, "*I* am in charge."

Jill said she and Rosa were on the way to their classes when Kaitlin stuck her nose in on the conversation they were having, then Geraldine and Camerin entered it and a verbal fray ensued. Jill does not involve herself in others' conversations and is not above telling people off when they do it to her. The bully girls did not like that and threatened to beat her again. Jill said, "So *I* got sent to the principal's office *again*. He yelled at me and said I was always over-exaggerating things and wouldn't listen to me about what Kaitlin, Geraldine and Camerin did. Then he yelled at me about being too clingy with Rosa and said I had to stop it. *He wasn't even there*—how can *he* say what happened or not?"

When Jill told him she had the right to speak she said he'd roared, "No. No you don't—*You don't have any rights!*" Jill was incensed. This time I wanted corroboration before I approached Tony so I went to Rosa's home to see if Carol* would allow me to speak with her daughter about the incident. Carol invited me in; she had few good things to say about LMS and criticized the bullying throughout the school system. Rosa joined us.

"Oh that Camerin is just a bully!" she spat out. "She yells at everybody—even the teachers. She does whatever she wants. She runs the show every day!" Then Rosa said not only did other students treat Jill horribly but the teachers were mean when they talked to her, too.

The subject of Jill's frequent fainting spells came up.

Rosa said, "One time Jill had a seizure and she stayed on the floor for the longest time—like 30 minutes before the nurse even came up." One of the reasons I had hoped to educate the students, teachers and other LMS adults was to impress upon them the need to get immediate medical attention for Jill when she had fainting and/or convulsion spells.

When I told Carol our request to do so had been denied by every school administrator all the way up to and including the BOE, she rhetorically asked, "How *do* people like that sleep at night?" I then mentioned my relief about Jill's acceptance into SFTA's part-time program. Rosa had also applied to SFTA, to the full-time program, but had not yet received her reply. Carol said she hoped Rosa would be accepted and could leave the Littleton school system. By then, the Geraldine/Camerin/Kaitlin trouble making exercise had been corroborated. It was time for me to go. Although it was late, I was determined to send my documentation to Tony that night. When I got home, I told Ed about my conversation with Carol and Rosa; he immediately called Tony's voice mail and left a message about the latest threats made against Jill. I checked my emails; Allyson had sent a message saying that she too had noticed threats made to Jill on Facebook again and had emailed Tony about it. I railed into Tony via email to which he responded, "I got the message."

I was looking forward to the bullying conference and walked into it with paperwork and a check for LDA's fee in hand. The speakers included Dr. Newton, who coordinated the State's school bullying programs and an elementary school principal who explained how her school had implemented a no-cost, adult modeling approach developed by nationally known bullying expert and author, Dr. Jane Bluestein who wrote *Creating Emotionally Safe Schools: A Guide for Educators and Parents*. To me, it sounded like common sense and paying attention to what was going on in the school. The final speaker was attorney Jaclyn Troiano, the same lawyer Krista had referred me to a few months earlier. Immediately following the conference, I located the LDA director and handed her the completed paperwork. As we talked, a few parent advisers milled around. It was not long before I learned that Littleton was notorious as being particularly difficult to work with regarding special education cases. The LDA director told me that given Jill's precarious medical condition, she had to meet with her board members to better determine if they could adequately assist us. That meeting would be held in a couple of weeks, she said. As I began to tell her that Jill was fighting for her sanity and physical safety every day, I noticed Attorney Troiano standing beside me. Our brief discussion confirmed my suspicions that Jill's school problems needed legal guidance. I said I would contact her soon and determined the PPT would not be scheduled until I was sure Jaclyn Troiano would be at the table.

Two days later, Jill went off to school as usual. The phone rang and Tony said, "Jill's been in a fight. We have it on tape. I've called the police. Now you'll find out what happens when the police are involved." Ed went to get Jill as I gathered necessities for the heme treatment scheduled for that afternoon. When they returned, Ed said Jill had been assaulted again—this time by Camerin. He confirmed Tony had called the police and we could expect to be hearing from them soon. Jill and I had her heme appointment to get to so Ed went to the PD while we were at NHC.

Jill had already told Ed her version of what had happened. On the way to the hospital, she told me too, "In between classes I accidentally bumped into Camerin in the hallway." She said she then hurried around the crowd on her way to the girls' lavatory, which had been her destination before going to her next class.

Camerin and her gang were yelling at Jill so she stepped out of the lavatory alcove she had arrived at and came face to face with Camerin. She apologized. Camerin yelled at her, "Don't give me that dirty look!"

Jill replied, "I'm not giving you a dirty look."

Camerin then yelled, "Don't give me an attitude!"

Jill said, "I'm not giving you an attitude."

Camerin then turned to the girl closest to her, who happened to be Geraldine, and said, "Hold my books. I'm gonna punch this bitch in the face." She punched Jill in the jaw. Jill grabbed Camerin and tried to pull her to the ground, but Camerin ended up on top of her and began pounding her in the stomach and chest. Jill pushed Camerin off. When they got up, Camerin turned slightly. Jill seized the opportunity to jump on Camerin's back, crooked her arm around the girl's neck and proceeded to punch her as hard as she could. She said onlookers of eighth grade students and some seventh graders were in the vicinity and saw what was occurring. She said at first Kaitlin and Camerin's posse were cheering Camerin on. But once Jill jumped on Camerin's back, things became quiet. Several teachers arrived. Mrs. Menard and Mrs. Elliott* attempted to separate the girls; Mrs. Menard pulled at Camerin and Mrs. Eliott held Jill. Camerin was trying to go after Jill again, but Jill would not back down. Once again, Jill was on her way to the principal's office.

Thanks to LMS' ineffective administration that allowed Beatrice, Mary Ann, Kaitlyn, Camerin, Miranda, Tammy, Nellie and all the others who had habitually harassed her to operate with impunity, Jill was on the brink. Her heme treatment that afternoon went as well as could be expected after having been punched out, but I was truly worried about her mental status. My thoughts returned to what Randi the Hem/Onc nurse told me a couple of weeks earlier when we had talked about the bullying Jill was fending off. At the time, she suggested I Google "Phoebe Prince." I did and learned the chilling story of the seventeen-year-old Irish immigrant who had been bullied so horribly that she had taken her own life. There were only two and a half months left to the school year. I doubted that the LMS troublemakers would stop. Like their depraved counterparts who had continued harassing Phoebe's family after the poor girl's death, conscience was not part of these Littleton middle schoolers' lifestyles.

CHAPTER 41

Cold, Clear

These foolish games are tearing me apart. Your
thoughtless words are breaking my heart.
— AS SUNG BY JEWEL

When Ed returned from the PD, he produced a written summons and reported, "Jill and Camerin were both arrested and charged with disorderly conduct. Their court date's in a week." Officer Bennington had viewed the tape with Tony and told Ed that Jill could be seen waiting in a lavatory alcove, then stepping out into traffic to confront Camerin.

I asked, "Okay, Jill, you bumped into Camerin. Why did you bump into her? Were you moving too fast, twist an ankle, lose your balance?"

Jill responded, "I came out of class and needed to use the bathroom so I was kinda walking fast. Then a kid bumped into me, and I bumped into Cam."

"What kid?" I asked.

"It doesn't matter. It wasn't his fault, it was an accident," she replied. "Okay, then what happened?" I pursued.

"Then I headed for the bathroom and Camerin and her friends were swearing and yelling at me, *'Can't you even say sorry?'*" Jill repeated the rest of what happened, ending with "then she punched me. Then we started fighting. Then I got sent to the principal. Then she got sent to the principal."

I turned to Ed. "There's no sound on the tape?"

"No," he said.

"Okay, what Jill described matches the cop's description of what he *saw* but he couldn't *hear* that Jill was *apologizing* for bumping into Camerin," I said.

Ed said, "The incident *was* over fairly quickly."

"Yeah," I said, "but we know that someone bumped into Jill, causing her to bump into Camerin. No one investigated *how* everything started and there is no way we can confirm that. But Jill can tell the court that she wasn't *confronting* Camerin, she was *apologizing* after which she got punched in the face. Thank goodness Tony called the police. Jill will have her day in court and this LMS bullying crap will be exposed, for all the good it will do." Ed was upset about Jill having been arrested and the court date. My gut feeling was that once the truth had been presented everything would be fine for Jill. Tony's letter arrived to kick off April:

> This will confirm our conversation regarding the fight that took place. Jill and another student exchanged words in the hallway. Jill walked toward the other student. A fight ensued. Both students were referred to the Littleton Police. As a result, Jill has been suspended out of school. This is the third physical altercation that Jill has participated in. Each time, Jill has approached the other student. She has been counseled by me, the school psychologist and others to walk away from confrontation and to report immediately any inappropriate contact or verbal exchanges. If any more physical altercations occur, a request for an expulsion hearing may be forwarded to the superintendent. Please note that students on suspension may not attend or participate in any school-sponsored activities and may not be on school grounds while suspended.[86]

On a positive note, with the signed contract sent via overnight mail, Jill had just become Attorney Troiano's newest client.

Between her suspension and the impending vacation, Jill would be out of the school for a total of *twenty* days. With no school and plenty of time, she turned to Facebook a lot. It was not long before she brought the laptop in to show Ed and me something she had found. Camerin had been busy in the days following the "fight." She had posted messages about her beat down of Jill and that her posse was right with her. A group photo featuring Camerin, Geraldine and Nellie titled "the badasses" was right on top. I printed the pages out, said, "Thanks for the evidence, Camerin," and put them in an envelope with the court summons.

Court day arrived. Camerin and her mother were among the first called to meet with a probation officer. Camerin avoided looking anyone in the eye when she returned to the waiting area. I took that as a good sign but was irritated. If we had known to get there earlier, too, we might have been able to present Jill's story and the Facebook evidence *before* Camerin went in. Jill was called to meet the same parole officer (PO) who had seen Camerin. Marc Zlotowski* said Jill could either tell her story to him which would essentially mean she pleaded guilty to the disorderly conduct charge or she could plead not guilty and present her story to a judge.

---

86 LMS* Principal Dithers.* Letter to author. March 29, 2010.

Then a court date would be set. Ed spoke first. "I think Jill should just plead guilty and tell her story."

I disagreed, "I think we should take this as far as we can and let as many people know about the problems at LMS. Jill's been through too much and this has got to stop." The PO talked about what might happen if we went to court and said Jill would have an opportunity to tell about the mitigating factors that resulted in the fight. I said, "It wasn't a fight. It was an assault. This is the second attack on her in a month; the first one was perpetrated by Camerin's 'friend.' Jill's been a target for the bully brigade and the damn school has done nothing about it. She has a port in her chest," I said as I pulled Jill's neckline aside to show him, "because of a liver disease that requires regular treatments at NHC. And still, they keep at her." Finally, I looked at Jill, who had kept silent, "Sorry Jill, what do you want to do?"

She replied, "I'll tell my story. I want this to be done." So Jill told her story.

As she spoke, the PO typed into his laptop then read what he had typed to her. "Do you agree with what I have typed here?" he asked. She read it and said yes. He printed it out and we signed it. Then he told Jill to sit in the waiting area until he came for her.

After she left the room, I said, "I want you to know Jill didn't give you the whole story." His eyebrows arched up. "She neglected to tell you how everything started. She told me only after I'd pushed the point—I like to get the whole story from beginning to end. Apparently a boy bumped into Jill which caused her to bump into Camerin. Then you heard what happened. What the cop *saw* on the tape was accurate but he never *heard* that she stepped out into hallway traffic to *apologize* to Camerin. Jill has no agenda to get the kid who bumped her in trouble; she said it wasn't a big deal. Well, it sure turned into one hell of a big deal. She took the punch and the other kid got off. And I agree, it was an accident, a mishap. Jill told me if she hadn't stepped out to apologize when she did, Camerin would have tracked her down and hurt her sooner or later. She's been after Jill since the beginning of eighth grade—after Jill missed virtually her entire seventh grade for medical reasons. After the 'fight,' Jill told me, 'I'm sick of being the girl who always cries and asks for help—and no one ever does!' The principal was just happy to have nailed Jill *again*. And neither he nor the police officer got the complete story. I've coined a couple of phrases for how Jill is treated at school: WHACK-A-Jill! and GOTCHAJill!"

Ed pulled out the Facebook pages. "Look at these," he said. "Camerin and her buddies posted these messages on Facebook—and either didn't think about blocking Jill's access as a friend, or more likely, didn't care. She's that arrogant."

He showed the 'badasses" photo first. I pointed at the picture, "This is Camerin, right? You just saw her. This is Nellie, the pot stirrer. And this is Geraldine, who attacked Jill a couple of weeks ago. Now read Camerin's bragging—*and* the responses:"

"Camerin: "WHEN I SHUT MY MOUTH AND WALK AWAY IT DOESN'T MEAN YOU'VE ONE IT SIMPLY MEANS YOUR STUPID, FAT, SLOPPY ASS ISNT WORTH ANYMORE OF MY TIME SO STOP HATIN ON WHAT YOU CANT IMITATE AHA."

Kaitlyn: "no shit [nellie] hahahahahha!!!!! Luv u ... Cam!"

Camerin: "my name must tast good cuz its always in your mouth aha…u needa stop talking smack bcuz its gettin old and imma deff kick ur ass with my gurl [geraldine] ya hard mhhm aha that's wat I fuqqin thought bitcchhhh!!!!!!….I love being me its just so damn great aha!!!!!!"

Kaitlyn: "ya like for real she keeps talkin bout us 4 and it rele is getting old…if she sed suttin more I prolly would have kicked her ass!!!!"

Camerin: "yea I no and like normal we get in trouble aha but I dnt give too shitttssss the next time she openz her mouth my fist will be through it"

Camerin: "aha I told [geraldine] that imma go to school Monday nd be like to [tony d] that I have add aha and tht I need special treatment like jill aha in c what he says lol."

I said, "See that one about telling Tony? That sorry excuse for a principal actually told me and Jill he'd been accused of favoring Jill! That little Facebook snippet just told us where that 'concern' likely came from—he's concerned what the queen bee of the school bullies says? We just hired an attorney to represent Jill's educational needs. I've been to the Littleton PD twice about bullying this year and I've talked to the State's 'bullying expert' who advised me to file written reports to the principal and to copy her. I know bullying is considered a 'school matter,' but when a kid gets threatened and harassed repeatedly and assaulted twice, especially a sick kid, and the school looks the other way yet blames Jill, guess what? I'm going to the police!" I continued, Jill is a good soul and I don't say that just because she's my daughter. She's not meek, she's not phony and she keeps things real, which is what the bullies *and* the administrators don't like because they're too caught up in maintaining a phony image—they want bullied kids to put up and shut up. With Jill, what you see is what you get. She's thirteen and lives with a disease few people in this country even know about. In that respect she is far more mature than her peers ever will be. She tries her best to accomplish academic goals and gets up and goes to school every day even though her spirit is being killed little by little day after day there. Furthermore, a single punch to that port could change Jill's world forever; in fact, with a tube that extends into her heart, one punch could kill her." I was done.

PO Zlotowski said Jill's "record" had been expunged; she would not ever have to report she had been arrested. He said he had told Camerin very sternly she was not to talk to, go near or otherwise bother Jill. He continued, "You're doing exactly the right thing. I'm glad you've hired an attorney and I encourage you to continue to file written complaints and to go the police whenever needed. Do whatever you have to do to protect your daughter."

CHAPTER 42

Arctic Front

*My shadow, it irks me/And I know what I can
see/But it's getting harder to breathe/It's
empty and shallow/This just isn't me.*
— FROM "FIND ME" BY JILL GOULD

With the PO's words ringing in my head, I wrote the latest bullying complaint to Tony as soon as I got home, "This is our third bullying complaint. You know of Phoebe Prince's suicide. Are you waiting for one 'good' punch to Jill's port-a-cath to result in a manslaughter or homicide charge on your watch? We will keep going to the authorities—and to the courts, if necessary."

Tony called to say they had decided to assign a paraprofessional to accompany Jill throughout each school day. Whatever their reason, Ed and I figured no one would bother Jill with an adult present. But when Tony's letter arrived we realized LMS had only 'upped' the GOTCHAJill! game:

> School personnel will be assigned to attend all classes with Jill, [having] the following roles and responsibilities:

- Be omnipresent in all of Jill's classes.

- Document appropriate and inappropriate interactions for discussion later.*

> *Discussion with school counselor, school psychologist and/or school administration.[87]

---

87 LMS* principal. Letter to author. March 30, 2010.

During vacation Jill had two heme infusions. Amber accompanied Jill for one of the sessions and buoyed Jill's spirits. The girls busied themselves with crafts. Near the end of the treatment Amber said, "Mr. D and all those a-holes at school should have to sit through this."

I agreed. "Great idea; but that'll never happen." A representative from Paul Newman's Hole-in-the-Wall-Gang Camp visited Jill to see if she might be interested in attending during the upcoming summer. Jill agreed to try it so I went online and started the application process.

The SFTA Kickoff Orientation for newly accepted students took place during vacation. Jill quickly bonded with two other girls, and within a short time, the trio had commenced singing together. Caught in a fast moving crowd on our way to the auditorium, I caught a glimpse of another Littleton family but did not have a chance to speak to them. Jill went on a group tour of the building. I attended a presentation about the school. Soon, the students returned to the auditorium and Jill said she had seen Alice,* another Littleton student who was "part-time, like me."

A few days later, Jill began to complain that her throat really hurt. Within a couple of hours she had spiked a fever and we were off the ED, knowing and dreading that it would be a long time before we returned home. Before the ED staff could treat her, they had to determine the source of the fever and to do that they had to draw blood. Numbing cream was applied. But Jill's port would not cooperate. Jill told them, "You'll need a 20-gauge, inch and a quarter (needle length) and my port is tilted just so," indicating how with her hand. "It's under the scar and the needle will probably hit the outside wall." After a few tries, the first nurse gave up. Another nurse tried. Finally, one of Jill's favorite ED nurses, Kristin,* took her turn. After some time, she was able to access the port but not before Jill was sobbing. Following the punches Geraldine and Camerin had delivered, the port had slipped again and the pain was too much for her to bear. The lump in my throat was huge and tears filled my eyes. By 9 p.m. Jill finally had an antibiotic flowing through her port. A nurse came in at midnight to say her shift was over and she had to flush the port so we could go home. Thankfully Jill caught it first. "Is that Heparin in that syringe?" she asked.

"Yes," answered the nurse.

"Sorry, I need tpA. I can't have Heparin," Jill said. Three hours later, a different nurse arrived with the tpA flush and asked, "Why don't they just use saline?" I shrugged. I just wanted to go home. Jill's Confirmation retreat was scheduled to start in a few hours.

Jill and I arrived at the retreat center and went in to register. It was obvious that an extensive gathering of youths was expected. With about four hours free, a tour of the grounds seemed like a good idea but it was drizzling so I went back to the car to read. As I finished reading the newspaper, an ambulance, EMS truck and police car pulled into the driveway. "Now what?" I grumbled as I left the car and walked through the thickening drizzle. My heart pounding, I approached the passenger side of the ambulance. An EMT put the window down. "By any chance, is my daughter in there?" I asked.

"No, she's still inside. Just go up the stairs to the left. She's in the first room," she said. I followed the directions and found a man monitoring the hallway, "The EMT said my daughter was in here," I started.

"Yes, she's right in this room," he gestured.

I turned to the doorway and saw a girl—not Jill—seated on a couch with several adults tending to her. My relief was huge. "I'm so sorry you're not feeling well," I said to the girl, "I'm sure your mom will be here soon, and I sure hope your day gets better." I fled to the car where I sat for a few moments to calm myself. A headache began to throb and I left the car to begin a meditative walk through the pathways. By the time I finished, it was raining in earnest and the retreat was nearly over. When Jill came out, I asked her about the girl who fainted. "How do you know about that?" she asked. I described what had happened. She was mortified that I had approached the ambulance. I told her not to worry, that is what mothers do, and said though I felt bad for the girl who had fainted, I was relieved and thankful that this time it had not been her!

When Monday morning came, Jill went to school anticipating the paraprofessional's company. It was heme treatment day, and as I arrived to pick her up the office secretary said hurriedly, "Mrs. Gould, I just tried calling you! Jill has collapsed again!"

I said, "When?"

"Just a few minutes ago. The nurse is with her now. The ambulance has been called." I asked where Jill was. "Room 309," she answered. As I moved toward the stairs, Tony joined me. We arrived at Room 309, which I had not connected was the math room—*again*. Jill was sitting on the floor next to her desk.

Nurse Pam* was there and said, "She apparently just slipped right out of her seat. She hurt her back so we don't want her to stand up." Jill was awake and lucid.

I said, "Jill, you really can't stand?" She shook her head no. "You can't stand because your back hurts?" She nodded. I calmed down a little bit. I had feared she was paralyzed again; the potential for AIP paralysis still unnerved me. The paraprofessional, Mrs. Malcomson,* was seated on the opposite side of the math room. I asked her what had happened just prior to Jill fainting.

"Nothing. She just put her head down and slid to the floor," she said.

Pam said the ambulance would be here any minute.

"She's scheduled for a heme treatment in half an hour," I said. "Can't I just ask them to put her in my car and I'll bring her there?"

Larry said, "Probably not. Once called, they have to transport the patient to a hospital." I called Dr. O'Connor's office, spoke with a nurse and told her Jill had had another fainting episode at school and that we were scheduled for a heme appointment, but she would be arriving late by ambulance. The EMS arrived, put a neck brace on Jill and got her onto a stretcher. I spoke to the lead EMT and asked if she could be brought to NHC since she was expected for a treatment. He said yes, they could do that. As it turned out, he had taken care of Jill before. "We've got oxygen and will give her Valium if she starts seizing," he said.

I thanked him, "But please, no Valium, Ativan is better." I told him she had been given Valium one other time during transport and it had triggered severe flank pain.

"Oh, that's right, I meant Versed. We've used that before on her," he said. I told the EMTs that I would see them in Hartford and left. When Jill arrived at NHC, she wanted to take off the neck brace—now. I hoped she was not going to escalate! The medical staff checked her neck, reflexes, etc. Jill reiterated she was fine and just wanted to sit up. They let her. She sat up. After a while, they cleared her, we left the ED and walked to the infusion center. Jill was okay this time. With plenty of time to talk during the infusion, the topic turned to the paraprofessional. "She's tough, mom," Jill said.

"Well, her daughter was one of LHS's top graduating students last year. She probably thinks every kid could be like hers if only they'd apply themselves—and had parents like her," I said. "If she's tough they probably selected her because *you've* been labeled a troublemaker and they want someone tough to keep an eye on you. Just be who you are, and if she has any intelligence *and* integrity, she'll see *you* are not the problem. Give her a chance, things will get better," I told her. Sadly, they would not.

CHAPTER 43

Polar Vortex

God is just. He will pay back trouble to those who trouble you and give relief to those who are troubled.
— THESSALONIANS 1:6, 7

One afternoon Jill came home from school and said she had attended a mandatory school assembly about cyberbullying "that freaked me out." She said the presentation consisted of a Power Point program and discussions about students who had committed suicide because of bullying. Tony followed with, "Suicide is never the answer. Kids need to think about the people left behind and how hard it would be for them." Jill said Mrs. Morrison had noticed that she (Jill) had been visibly affected and asked if she was all right; Jill had answered, "Yes," and went to her next class. But in relating the story to me later she confided, "I know why Phoebe wanted to end it all; it was just too much for her. I get why someone would want to stop the emotional pain from kids bullying them. Mr. Dithers doesn't have a clue about that. Phoebe doesn't have any pain anymore. It's all over," she said, a little too dreamily.

Alarmed, I said, "Yes, but what he meant is that her parents, brothers and sisters and the people who love her are left behind to handle the pain of losing her. They'll never be able to see her go to college, get a job, get married or become a mother. That's a lot to lose because of some nasty kids."

"Yeah, but it was *her* decision," Jill retorted.

The next morning Jill went off to school as usual. Unbeknownst to us, she had not fallen asleep until the wee hours of the morning because she had been plagued with thoughts of seeing Phoebe hanging in her bedroom closet. That afternoon, as I sat in the car and watched students exit the school, Beatrice came out looking extremely nervous and stood by the curb. She usually walked home, but it was obvious she was waiting to be picked up. I turned my attention to the paper I was reading. When Kevin got into the backseat, I looked up. Beatrice was anxiously looking toward the school exit doors. I looked in that direction, too, and saw Nurse Pam and Jill headed for our car. "Good grief, now what?" I said. Mickey drove up, and casting one last anxious look in Jill's and Pam's direction, Beatrice jumped into his car and he zoomed off. Jill was crying when she and Pam got to the car, "Oh, no! What happened *today?*" I cried.

Pam said, "Tammy said something to Jill at lunch. I'm going to ask why that para doesn't accompany Jill for lunch, too. Then later on she got upset in the bathroom and that's why I came out with her," she said. Jill got into the car. I was riled up, angry at the school again, but more angry at myself because I had not anticipated lunch coverage either. I should have made sure the para would accompany Jill *every minute* of the school day—*why* hadn't I thought of something so simple?

"Thanks, Pam. You're right, but watch yourself or they'll be after you, too!" I said and drove off.

"OK, Jill, what happened with Tammy today?" I asked.

"She stuck her nose in my business." Jill said. "And…," I said.

"I was sitting with Chelsea and Marie at one lunch table and Tammy was sitting with Camerin at another. Chelsea and I were horsing around, and Chelsea held up a book like a shield in front of her as if she was defending herself against me. The next thing I knew, Tammy told Chelsea, 'Don't take that from her, you have a right to defend yourself, Chelsea! You gotta stand up for yourself. You gotta *fight* her.' Then Tammy *and* Camerin came over to my table and I told them to get out of my business." The light bulb went off along with a head bell clang. Camerin! *Another* thing I'd been a dunce about! I should have known since Camerin had been warned by the parole officer to stay away from Jill, she would use others to do her dirty work. Her pot-stirring friend Nellie had moved away so Tammy was doing everything to take her place and stay on Camerin's good side, and that meant going after Jill every chance she got. I had been late about figuring out the probability of that happening and warning Jill. I did not suppose the juvenile courts were set up to communicate to schools about warnings made to students about 'keeping away from certain others' so LMS would claim they did not know and could not be faulted. And they most likely would not connect that Tammy was playing her part in the entire "impress Camerin" game; if I had told anyone that, it would have been ignored or thought or said I was "too involved" with kid politics. But they had listened and *acted* on Sherilyn Martin's boldface lies and mealy mouthed whining!

Steaming, I drove out of the school parking lot. Jill said, "I said something to Tammy and I should have known that it would come back to bite me." I hit the brakes.

"What? What exactly did you say—and why?" "After what happened at lunch, I was on my way to my next class and Tammy was at her locker. She gave me 'a look.' I just said, 'watch your back' to her because I was going to tell you and dad when I got home that Tammy and Camerin had started trouble with me in the cafeteria. No one at school ever listens to me when I make complaints," she said. Then Tammy told Mrs. Menard about what I said to her. Mr. D. called me out of class and asked me if I told Tammy to watch her back. I said yes and explained why I said that to her. Mrs. Malcomson said, 'Jill, no one said anything to you today.'"

"Mom, *SHE WASN'T EVEN THERE!*" "And Mr. D just gave me his usual garbage so I said I was done with him and went to the bathroom. I got really upset in there and punched the door—hard, over and over again. I was so sick of them always out to get me every day. Every—single—day, Mom. Then Mrs. Podurski* came in and said I was making too much noise and to calm down. After about ten minutes, I went to the teacher's room with her, she called Pam and then Pam brought me out to the car."

"Oh Jill! So, all of this *just* happened?" I asked.

"Well, since lunchtime," she answered. I felt horrible for Jill and now there was another reason for the rest of the students and teachers to think she was insane.

The phone rang soon after returning home. Tony was calling to say he had sent me an email report of the latest "incident." I told him I hadn't seen it yet, but Jill had told me about what had happened. He replied he had tried to talk to Jill, too, but she spoke very confusingly. I told him she had just told me her story and it was not one bit confusing. Ever since I had listed "confusion" as an AIP symptom on a school health report, I had noticed a variation of the word was applied to Jill whenever a problem occurred. It seemed to me that the school administrators were the ones who were confused. I told him I was not happy to hear that Mrs. Malcomson had told Jill, "No one said anything to her," when she had not accompanied Jill during lunch or on the way back to class. Very inappropriate, not to mention unfair, I told him. He said there had been five adults monitoring the lunchroom and nothing had been reported to any of them. I said, "*FIVE* adults and not one of them noticed *anything*? What kind supervision do you guys do anyway? Just the fact that Camerin and Tammy were together in Jill's proximity should have been enough reason for someone to get involved. Camerin was specifically told by the parole officer to *stay away* from Jill. And why won't *you admit* that Camerin and Tammy are in a clique?"

"So *you* say," Tony retorted. "Jill admitted she told Tammy to 'watch your back' then told me she was 'done with me' and went into the bathroom." He then said Jill had carried on and caused a ruckus in the bathroom. I made a mental note to get Mrs. Podurski's story, since I trusted her more than Tony. But I was not hopeful of getting anything from her; teachers can be leery about saying anything the administration does not want them to say.

Then Tony said one of the most ridiculous things I had heard him say the entire school year. I am sure he said it with a straight face and in absolute sincerity. "Tammy told Mrs. Menard that when Jill told her 'you better watch your back,' she *feared for her life* (he said it in italics, too)."

I began to laugh hysterically. "You mean, the same Tammy who told Jill 'I'd punch you in the f#cking face but you'd probably *faint*' a couple of months ago?! *Come on Tony! You really are too much!*" No one in authority had done *anything* when Tammy told Jill she'd punch her in the f#cking face and taunted her about fainting, which started the shoving match that Jill got suspended and now Tammy *feared for her life*? Tony chided me about "cackling" then said, "Mrs. Gould, I just don't know how this lack of trust has come about."

"Well, let me enlighten you, *Tony*. It began with the very first 504 fiasco in which you jerked me around. Remember? If not, in your spare time, look up the minutes of that meeting and refresh your memory." I said. Tony said because Jill had made a threatening statement to another student she would not be permitted to attend the dance the following night.

I told him, "Good. We don't want her anywhere near you and that dysfunctional group of kids anymore. She and we have had our fill of all of you."

I forwarded Tony's "complaint" email message to Attorney Troiano and Vanessa and kept Jill out of school. She was nervous about retaliation from students who were connected to the Camerin/Geraldine/Tammy clique. It was obvious that no one in the school, adult or peer, would offer Jill support. She said, "Mom, I would rather take a thousand needle pokes to my port without numbing cream than put up with those kids or Mr. Dithers for one more day." My heart broke and Isabel Allende's words recollecting her daughter *Paula*, paralyzed and in a coma from which she would not recover came to mind: "...for weeks, even months you had been tense and tired...you were suffering...; the porphyria was poisoning you, and neither of us saw it...."[88] I emailed a message to Tony and copied Attorney Troiano, Vanessa and Dr. O'Connor, "Jill will not be in school today. After yesterday's incidents, she/we continue to fear for her physical and mental health safety."

88 Allende, I. *Paula.* (New York: Harper Perennial), 20.

CHAPTER 44

Killing Frost

My heart sinks deep down inside my soul.
— JILL GOULD

Vanessa and APRN Kym each laughed when I told them about Tony saying Tammy had "feared for her life" when Jill told her to watch her back. They saw what Tony had missed. I was pleasantly surprised that teacher Elena Podurski emailed me her account of what she had witnessed the previous afternoon. She said she had walked Jill back to class after lunch but hadn't actually heard what was said to Tammy. After Tony confronted Jill in the hallway, things escalated quickly. She wrote,

> When I entered the girls' room she was locked in a stall, crying and banging her fists on the wall. I tried to talk with her and convince her to come out. She yelled back she would not. I told her she was going to hurt herself and she said she didn't care. [When she came out, I] checked her arms to make sure she had not hurt herself. She said that you "hired an attorney." I told her to focus on what happened here in school. Jill eventually left with the nurse to get out of the hallways before the bell rang to avoid other students. I did not see her again after that.[89]

It was ironic that Elena had told Jill to "focus on what happened here in school" meaning schoolwork because that was what Jill had been trying to do since the first day of school. But most days it turned into a "Schoolwork Interrupted" movie with "Mean Girls, Guys & Adults" sub-plots.

---

89 LMS SE teacher Ms. Podurski.* Email to author. April 4, 2010.

That weekend I was so worried about Jill. On the heels of the mandatory bully-ing presentation, I felt the Camerin/Tammy lunch incident had pushed her closer to the edge. I had copied Dr. O'Connor on my message to the school about Jill's physical and mental health. It hit a mark because a hospital social worker visited with Jill and me during the entire next heme treatment.

I reviewed the log I had been keeping and discovered that the most recent heme treatment had been Jill's *39th* of the school year. Dr. Piersen had recommended Jill eventually reduce them to one or two treatments a month. That meant at most she should have had eighteen treatments. Since there were still a few weeks of school, she would have more treatments. Too much heme could be toxic, but she had gotten the treatments primarily because she kept exhibiting symptoms at school, and *symptoms* were the only thing we had to go on. Head bells were clanging again. Dr. O'Connor kept a sharp eye on her iron level. But he said he did not know if heme helped strengthen her liver or if a "heme-filled" liver could override poison-ous toxins that by this time I *knew* were messing up Jill's life. Additionally, the heme treatments seemed to becoming harder for Jill to handle and less effective. What was going on?

Still awaiting a PPT, Jill was desperate to return to school. Like most profes-sionals, Dr. O'Connor's and Vanessa's opinion was that children should return to "normalcy" and if she wanted to go to school, she should. For Jill's safety, I had to get Dr. O'Connor's letter to the pertinent people at LMS quickly so I sent it to Tony. I also told him to immediately arrange "adult support" for Jill *during the entire school day* including lunch periods. I also said he needed to redefine his position of the para's role from being one of "catching" Jill saying or doing something wrong to one of assistance and protection from predatory students. I further demanded that anyone fulfilling said role be told to refrain from talking to Jill in dismissive tones, *particularly* when that person did not hear or see what had been said or done to Jill. I closed with, "It is clear the continued climate of no respect and escalating recent activities at [LMS] have damaged Jill's spirit. Please advise when full and complete adult school day coverage for Jill has been arranged. And before discussing any peer complaint with Jill, as we've asked numerous times, *dispense* with verbally attacking her with inflammatory questions and statements."

Jill's mental health continued to decline yet she insisted on going to school. If she was enamored with black clothing before, her signature dress became black long or short sleeved T-shirts, black long pants and black boots or shoes. She had also begun to rim her beautiful brown eyes with thick black eyeliner. She became enamored with the band *Seether* and started posting disquieting messages on Facebook. Her postings were noticed by others, so much so that as she was gather-ing her belongings for a sleepover at Amber's house one afternoon, the phone rang. It was Carol. She said, "Rosa is very concerned about some of Jill's Facebook post-ings and showed them to me. They are very alarming and I wanted to make sure you were aware of them."

I told her about Jill's recent interest in the band *Seether* and that their dark lyrics had really gotten her attention. I told her we had hired an attorney, that a PPT was pending and that I had thought about keeping Jill out of school until that meeting, but Jill was insistent about going back to school. "If we take it day by day, I think she'll be okay; there are only a few weeks left to go. Besides Jill wants to finish the school year. It means a lot to her but I do plan to keep her out intermittently."

Still waiting for a PPT to be set, April ended. Of the only seventeen school days in the month, Jill had had three heme treatments; seven absences due to suspension during which the juvenile court hearing had taken place; a week's vacation from school followed by *another* fainting spell upon returning and yet another incident of her being harassed that had escalated into a breakdown in the girls' room. She had spiked a fever and wound up in the ED where she was diagnosed with strep throat. Then she completed her Confirmation retreat obligation the day after spending the night in the ED. Through it all, she continued to sing with Lora and to write songs, her only coping mechanism. The month of May could not be any worse, so I thought.

CHAPTER 45

Deep Freeze

*They cut me down with sharpened tongues; they aim
their bitter words like arrows straight at my heart.*
— PSALM 64:3-5

I'm starting to think this place we call earth is hell. I am suffering and in pain every single day. No one understands how I am feeling. It's horrible and hard not to not give up. I saw the most horrible video about Suicide because of bullies. My prayers are with them every day because I know what they were going through. In fact they got to break me so much that I started giving up. In the bathroom crying so loud that they said I was disrupting the classes. I couldn't take it anymore, punching the stall so I could feel a different kind of pain. And let out some of the other pain and anger. I cannot explain this kind of pain other than it can make you do crazy stuff. I don't know how much longer I can take it. I am breaking slowly and it hurts. It's just like dying slowly. I need the pain to go away and the only way I know I promised myself I would never do because it's cowardly but I am afraid they will push me to my limit and I will end it.

If I do not make it, I want my songs to go out to people to make them see it's not the only choice. I am suffering from bullies and I can do it but I don't want to end it all. It's all about my choice in the end. But I'll be in a better place. If I leave don't cry cause I'll be happier we will meet again one day. Love, Jill.[90]

May arrived and our flower was wilting. She had been looking forward to the eighth grade end of year activities. But every eighth grade sendoff activity was about to disappear just as the sixth and seventh grade year-end activities had.

Bart responded to my letter to Tony about Dr. O'Connor's letter:

---

90 Jill's journal. April 22, 2010.

I am in receipt of your correspondence to [Tony]. I am aware that at the present time a PPT is pending. However, I request that we hold a 504 meeting at your earliest convenience so that we may formally develop an appropriate interim plan, as well as discuss the use of the adult support that the district is now providing for Jill. In addition, the team will review the results of the recent psychiatrist evaluation from Dr. Werrmona. I wish to clarify that although [Dr. O'Connor's] letter will become part of Jill's permanent file, the district cannot act on any of his educational and/or environmental recommendations or suggestions as they are not specific doctor's orders.[91]

Bart knew that Attorney Troiano was now representing us and that we would not meet without her. Also, we were holding out for a PPT, not a 504 meeting.

Jill's first heme treatment of May turned out to be tough. After the port was de-accessed it sprung a huge blood leak, leaving a substantial stain on the front of her shirt. Then she began vomiting outrageously. It was one of those times when I wondered how well bullies would handle such things. She had the usual complaints of aches, pains and nausea following the treatment, yet she went to school the next day. Jill said Tony could not pay her enough compliments. "You've done far more good things than bad this year," she said he told her among other things. I guess he figured backhand compliments were better than nothing. Or maybe he did not know how to deliver a real compliment. Anyway, she was not in the mood for his blathering and said to herself, "Blah, blah, blah."

I thought, "Maybe she *will* make it through to the end." Then, in mid-May as I was getting ready to take her to her after school singing session with Lora, the phone rang. The caller ID registered LMS. I answered the phone. This time it was nurse Pam. "Joyce, Jill had a meltdown."

"Oh no! Where?" I asked. "At lunch. In the cafeteria," she answered.

"How is she now?" I asked.

"Not good." I burned tracks to the school and Pam escorted me to the cafeteria. Jill was sitting at a table with Tony, Larry, Mrs. Menard, Mrs. Malcomson and other adults. Tears rolled slowly down her cheeks. I sat down and asked what had happened. Jill said, "I don't care. I don't care anymore." Tony told me that Jill had been sitting with Chelsea and Marie at lunch when she inexplicably started crying. Mrs. Menard had written a report that she handed to me. It said, "At lunch, Jill started to cry and claim that she was going to 'end it all.' She said, 'I can't take it anymore, I'm going to kill myself.' She and I talked but I could not calm her. She repeated she wanted to 'end it' and said again, 'I want to die.' Marie and Chelsea overheard everything."

Tony continued the story, "She grabbed her sweatshirt, wrapped it around her neck and began to pull it tightly as if to strangle herself. She made a comment about 'not caring anymore.'"

---

91 Littleton* school district SE director. Letter to author. May 4, 2010.

"That's enough from you!" I said, "It was recommended that Jill should have had two heme treatments a month since September. That means *eighteen*. As of Tuesday, she's had 42! That's well over twice the number recommended—and those are *adult* dosages—yet *no one* can tell us what that much heme actually does to a kid other than to warn us about potential kidney damage and to tell us to check her labs to make sure her electrolytes are okay and her iron isn't too high. And no one can tell us what in the hell the damn toxins in this school are doing to her, either. From what I've figured out, the toxins must somehow destroy the 'good heme'—I don't know how and I don't know why. But for three years, I've seen it happen over and over. So what's all of this doing to Jill's body? Her brain? *Do you even give a sh#t?* But then, it's only Jill. *The Greatest Littleton School Troublemaker of All Time, RIGHT?*"

Then Tony said something about understanding "how much your family has been through."

I snapped, "*You stop right there. You* don't understand any of this—and *You* choose to ignore what's really going on in a school *you claim* to be *in charge of!* In addition to having to live with this 'unknown' medical condition, Jill has been subjected to cruel kids and idiot adults like you for months on end." I told Jill it was time to go. Tony said clearance from a mental health professional was needed before Jill returned to school.

I retorted, "You mean *if* she returns to school. As far as I'm concerned, she'll *never* set foot here again." My last experience with Tony turned out exactly as the first one had. I was disgusted by everything he was and stood for.

I called Vanessa who said, "I'm really concerned about what Tony said about how quickly her affect changed at lunch. I just saw her last night and she was doing okay but I really think she needs to be hospitalized."

"Right now?" I asked.

"Yes, I'm so sorry. Please. Bring her right to NHC's ED. They will know what to do and keep me posted." Jill and I immediately went to NHC's ED. We were ushered to a room and told a clinician would be in to see us. We were back on hospital time.

CHAPTER 46

Bitter Cold

The Lord is near to the broken hearted
and saves the crushed in spirit.
— **PSALM 34:18**

I look back on that little girl who was actually smiling every day who had something to look forward to. But when she was struck by the sickness she was shocked. Falling down all the time not knowing what was wrong with her, she was just a little girl waiting for answers. She was lost in this world of questions, hurtful words, fists and so much more. I remember her very well because that girl was me. I was once so happy and now that girl has died. That part of me is gone. Who I am today is nothing but a lost soul in this big world. Where did I go?[92]

Alone in a sparse ED room, I said, "Jill, did anything happen to upset you this morning? Did anyone say anything to you? Push you aside? I'm just trying to figure this out."

She was quiet for a moment. She said, "Well, there was something. It probably shouldn't have bothered me, but it did. Camerin's mother was parked in front of the school. I happened to see her and she gave me the nastiest look ever." Jill had been pushed over the edge by a single look from a bitter and petulant woman whose daughter was a combative bully.

"So what did you do?" I asked.

"Nothing. I just looked at the ground."

"I'm sorry that you didn't feel strong enough to just look her straight in the eye—*you* have nothing to be ashamed of, but I realize you've been beaten down.

---

92 Jill's journal. May, 2010.

Camerin's mother should be ashamed of herself, but she isn't. That's how it is with people like her."

Around 10:00 p.m. a clinician came in and asked to speak with Jill alone. About 45 minutes later she told me Jill was depressed and suicidal and needed to be placed inpatient and they would look for a placement the next day. We discussed Jill's medical conditions and the school bullying she had endured for so many months. She said both had undoubtedly contributed to Jill's present condition. She said Dr. Marlone would be in the next morning and suggested I go home to get some sleep. Jill would be watched through the night to insure she did not harm herself. "So that's what those people seated at desks in front of the rooms are there for?" I asked.

"Yes, they're our 'psych sitters,'" she answered. I was exhausted. Jill was exhausted. I told her I would be back in the morning, kissed her good-night and went home.

No food from the outside was allowed into the ward. The "psych sitter" took my purse and said I could bring only books in with me. I brought *The Outsiders* for Jill, because it was being read in Language Arts class and had *Queen Bees & Wannabees*, which had captured my attention, for me. As I sat in the room and looked around, it occurred to me we had been in this portion of the ED before. I asked Jill if she remembered. "No," she answered. But I did. It was the time she had complained about excruciating abdominal and back pains that felt as though they were on fire. She was certain she had kidney stones. It had been yet another fruitless ED visit. Now, after all this time, I understood. Because they had not believed Jill about the extraordinary pain, she had been moved closer to the psych ward.

The next morning when Dr. Marlone introduced herself, I said, "I remember that you diagnosed Jill with conversion disorder a year or so ago. As you can see by her chart, she was found to have acute intermittent porphyria. No disputing DNA testing." She led me to a quiet place to talk. She asked questions and this time really listened to my answers. She said it was not prudent to consider sending Jill back to LMS. Knowing that mental health assistance for juveniles was dire throughout the country, I knew we were in for a challenge. I told Jill she would not be returning to LMS and the news about the doctor's inpatient recommendation. "That's the good news," I said. "The bad news is that it could take a while to find a hospital placement for you."

"Why?" she asked. I explained about the extraordinary number of kids who need help. "And, on top of that, you have AIP. Not enough people know about it and it could prove tricky to get a place to agree to take you. You had two heme treatments this week, and you're due for another on Monday. That should hold you for a while since you won't be going back to Littleton and when you're not in school, your symptoms are far apart." She was cheered, if one could be cheered sitting on a bed in a tiny windowless hospital room all alone for hours with nothing to do, and immediately set her hopes on moving from NHC to another facility, "Where I can get help," she said. Every few hours she begged me to approach the clinician on duty to see about the status of securing a facility to take her. She bonded with Jake,* a psych attendant, who kept up a bantering dialogue with her and spread a sheet on the floor to encourage jigsaw puzzle-solving. I alternated between reading *The Outsiders* aloud to Jill and reading *Queen Bees* to myself. It was as though Rosalind

Wiseman had a vantage point within LMS. I read bits and pieces aloud to Jill. "See Jill, this stuff goes on in every school. It isn't only LMS. And the woman who wrote this book is a teacher—someone who cares about kids enough to have figured all of this stuff out and write a book about it to help other teachers understand what's going on right under their noses."

The next day, a facility in western Connecticut considered taking her but had concerns about the AIP. I answered their questions, offered to fax information to them and suggested they obtain Dr. O'Connor's medical opinion. In the end, they decided not to take the chance. I understood, though it meant Jill was there for another night. *"How is this helping me?"* she demanded. "I'm getting more and more stressed every minute. This is *not* a good way to help someone get over being depressed." The adolescent mental health crisis was upon us. Jill was stuck at NHC. This time they said she had a medical condition compounded by depression and suicidal tendencies—180° from the conversion disorder diagnosis. Before leaving that night, I asked the attending doctor to give Jill something listed on the safe drug roster to help her sleep. Then I hugged her good-night and said, "I'll see you in the morning. Try to sleep. Maybe something will pop up tomorrow."

When I arrived the next day, Jill was sitting on the floor in her room, working on a puzzle when she suddenly yelped, "*Ow!* My stomach hurts!"

I asked nervously, "Like what kind of 'hurt'? Nauseous? Period? How does it hurt?"

"Porphyria hurt," she said and doubled over in pain.

I went to the nurse's station and said, "Jill has started with a porphyria attack. She'll need D10 as soon as possible. The pain could get worse—fairly quickly, too." A nurse returned with me to Jill's room, where she was still sitting on the floor, incapacitated.

"Jill, is it any better?" I asked.

She was having trouble talking, "No. I just need carbs, Mom."

I turned to the nurse, "Do you have anything sweet, sugary, maybe cereal?" An aide brought a bowl of Frosted Flakes with milk for Jill. When the doctor arrived fifteen minutes later, Jill's pains were subsiding. The sugar had done its magic. I was impressed and said, "It looks like Jill's getting a handle on managing this AIP stuff. Thanks so much for coming to check her out, but she won't need D10 after all." I had received letters from adult AIPorphyrics who swore by the "sugar treatment." It had just helped Jill.

As the day wore on, a clinician came to talk with Jill so I went to the family room. When I returned, a different psych sitter was outside the door. He must not have seen me enter Jill's room because I heard him snap, "Do you have a *problem* with that blanket?" I looked at Jill. She had a set look on her face. While I did not like that look, I liked the tone of the young man's voice even less. "Because if you don't want it, there are a lot of other kids who would appreciate having it," he continued.

I stepped to the door of the room and asked, "Excuse me, what's your issue with her and that blanket?"

He was surprised to see me. "She's unraveling it. She could pull it apart and use the string...," he stumbled.

"Your tone of talking to a kid who's here for suicidal tendencies because of bullying doesn't work for me. Please get your supervisor in here right now," I said. Within a few minutes, the supervisor arrived. "Look, my daughter is here because of the severe school bullying she's endured for months on top of horrific medical conditions. She certainly doesn't need any crap from someone who's supposed to be *helping*, for goodness sakes." She was apologetic, said the psych sitter had been replaced and would not be assigned to Jill again. I went back to her room. "Someone else will be sitting with you tonight; before I leave, I'm going to ask for your sleep medication and we'll pray that tomorrow will be your last day here." The next day, we were notified Jill would be transported to the Institute of Living's (IOL) child & adolescent program. I went home to get some clothes for Jill. Then I returned to NHC to wait for the ambulance that would transport her to the facility. Soon enough, she was being prepped on the "rules and regs" of the IOL program.

IOL's supervising psychiatrist, Dr. Roberts* is perhaps the most serene individual I have come across; his calm, caring demeanor was beneficial to both Jill and me. Near the end of the week, a partial hospitalization program (PHP) placement was arranged at Mountford Center, about thirty minutes from our home and Jill was discharged from IOL with the following diagnostic description used by mental health professionals, "Axis I: MDD w/psychotic features; Axis II: none; Axis III: acute intermittent porphyria, von Willebrand, thalassemia."

The clinician impressed the importance of setting up the outpatient therapy because Jill still had suicidal thoughts. The next day we met with a Mountford administrator who said the program would include a daily group therapy component that Jill was looking forward to. Tony called to see what was going on with Jill. I told him, "She's in Mountford and won't return to LMS. I've been told Littleton is to provide tutoring through the end of the year."

"Well, I guess I have to arrange for tutoring. I'll get back to you with a plan," he said. He never did. It did not matter so much because my priority was to help my daughter survive and find herself again.

It had been a long spring. I was angry about having had to hire an attorney to get Jill the public education she was entitled to, but at least a PPT had been set. We knew Jill would not be going to the Hole in the Wall Gang Camp; I had not completed the online application and she wasn't in the frame of mind to go. Her heart ached and her songwriting had dwindled considerably, but Jill had found a place where she was accepted for herself in the Mountford outpatient therapy group. But, she had also learned a new coping technique that many, if not most, of the youths in the group resorted to for releasing emotional pain—self-mutilation.

CHAPTER 47

Embedded Thunder

...don't wanna play the victim anymore...
They cut me open, now I'm broken.
— FROM "BROKEN" BY JILL GOULD

The beginning of summer finally brought the PPT which was needed before Jill could advance to her freshman year, regardless of what school she would attend. Attorney Troiano called to say, "Littleton wants another psychiatric evaluation for Jill. Would you agree to see Dr. Werrmona again?"

I replied, "Why not? She'd have to be a moron not to see Jill's mental status has deteriorated in five months." So the PPT was postponed until after the school received Dr. Werrmona's re-evaluation report. Nervous about Jill's liver status, I made sure to keep her next infusion appointment. As the infusion was winding down, the APRN brought up the subject of setting the date for the next one. I said, "Why don't we let her liver decide? She's not going back to LMS so there won't be any more toxin exposure, no stress from kids harassing her every day, no bullying administrators or teachers, no whatever else makes her sick there. We're supposed to have a PPT soon so as long as she has no liver pain or other significant porphyria symptoms, why don't we just wait? Of course, if anything starts up we'll have to get the heme flowing pronto, but if Dr. O'Connor is okay with that, let's say 'It's up to her liver.'" It was a gamble. But I had seen how the "Frosted Flakes" AIP episode had been very different from the ones that originated at school with the bizarre abrupt fainting and convulsive symptoms. Dr. O'Connor agreed to give the heme reprieve a try.

Jill's outlook began to improve. But rescheduling the PPT meant no summer tutoring. And doubts had been creeping into her head about the SFTA magnet school commitment. If she was tired out by Mountford's four hour daily time frame, she worried, how could she handle going to LHS in the morning and SFTA all afternoon in September? It did not help her frame of mind when she got her yearbook and studied the photos of activities she'd missed. She was particularly perplexed to see she had been voted by her peers as one of the students with the *Most School Spirit*. "Why do you suppose they picked me for that?" she mused. Then she saw the photo of the *Most Likely to Succeed* group and said, "Oh, I get it. I *hate* it when they vote for someone just to make fun of them. See this kid here?" She pointed to one of the boys in the *Most Likely to Succeed* picture. On vote day, I heard a bunch of kids saying they were going to put his name down just because he's a kid who doesn't try and everyone knew that. I hate it when they do stuff like that!" But she later told me, "I don't care if they voted for me just to make fun of me. I look at it as a compliment. I know I tried harder than anyone in the whole eighth grade to get to school every day and to do the best I could." Just then I looked more closely at the school spirit picture in the yearbook and was horrified to see the kids had been lined up in front of the "STOMP OUT BULLYING" bulletin board. It looked as though LMS students had voted Jill as having *Most School Spirit* as a joke. It seemed that the photo had been positioned in front of the anti-bullying pledge as the final GOTCHAJill! of her eighth grade year.

As Jill continued to keep an eye on Facebook and saw references to all the year-end activities her peers had enjoyed, her mood understandably fluctuated. The trip to Ellis Island she had hoped to attend; the eighth grade semi-formal dance she had planned to shop for the "perfect" dress for; the pre-dance photo session set up by a couple of parents "because many of these kids have been together since kindergarten"; the action-packed final field day; the exciting, multi-activity resort destination day and the talent show she'd hoped to sing in were not to be for Jill. On top of everything, her last eighth grade report card came in the mail. Of the 180 school days, she had been counted absent for sixty-two, tardy for four and dismissed from twenty-seven. A total of ninety-three school days had been impacted due to illness; mild, moderate and severe AIP attacks, heme treatments or bullying/suspended-related issues. Miraculously, where they had been blank in October, first quarter grades appeared on the final report. There had not been much improvement from first to fourth quarter grades. Jill's self-esteem plummeted again after seeing the yearbook and report card and she said she wanted to repeat eighth grade. "You can't stay back!" I shouted. "I won't let you be in a school that makes you sick or deal with that misguided group again. You can't survive another year like this and this family cannot go through another year like it either! Besides, Littleton wants you out altogether."

Even though she no longer was in their midst, there was one more nasty LMS-related surprise. Jill had been checking Geraldine's Facebook wall to see if the girl had changed the privacy block against her. In mid-June, it had. Jill scrolled through postings until she reached the day Geraldine had assaulted her, then her emotional state nose-dived. She showed me the nasty, cheering comments made by a number of students. I felt sick when I saw that Dwayne had posted a comment. Jill was devastated that he, too had turned out to be a "false friend." I decided I would bring the subject up the next time his mother, Lia* and I spoke. Jill said not to. "Dwayne just wanted to fit in." But I could see his posting had cannonballed her. And Lia had been adamant that if Dwayne was ever anything but nice and supportive to Jill, she wanted to know about it. Coincidentally, a few days later, Dwayne contacted her on Facebook Chat. Concerned that her "chat messages" were gloomy once again, Dwayne called her on the cell phone. When Jill began sobbing, he got his mother. Jill came to me and said, "[Dwayne's] mom is on the phone. She wants to talk to you."

Lia began, "Dwayne and I are very concerned about Jill. I told her if she didn't get you on the phone right now, the police would be at your door to check on her. I am very concerned about her!" I acknowledged that Jill was still fragile and said we were awaiting medication to help her mood improve.

I said, "Lia, I thought you should know Jill happened to be checking Geraldine's Facebook the other day and found a lot of messages other kids posted on the day she attacked Jill. And I have to tell you, Dwayne posted a comment—not directly to Geraldine—but to Shana who had messaged 'That's how we do it bitch!' to which he had replied, 'lmao shana.'" I could tell Lia was horrified and embarrassed that Dwayne had put himself into "it." She had said to tell her, so I had. That was the last time we heard from mother or son.

In spite of the setback, Jill continued to make progress in the Mountford group therapy program. The clinic's psychiatrist Dr. Curtiss* and I worked together to identify a safe antidepressant. Using the American Porphyria Foundation's website, one night I plugged the names of thirty-two antidepressants into the APF drug data base and came up with two that were rated OK! for porphyria patients: Celexa and Prozac. I was uneasy about Prozac because its generic name, fluxotine, had been rated only "OK?" We decided to go with Celexa.

CHAPTER 48

Ball Lightning

The question was how I could keep sane
trying to find a way out...
— AS SUNG BY PHIL COLLINS OF GENESIS

Annoyed about not having heard from Dr. Werrmona for the re-evaluation, I contacted Attorney Troiano: "What's going on? It's been a full month since Jill has had any schooling and Littleton never coordinated summer tutoring. We need to get things moving along." She called Bart and shortly thereafter Dr. Werrmona called me to set up an appointment. We sandwiched the session in between Jill's singing lesson with Lora and her Mountford group therapy session. Dr. Werrmona's demeanor was very different from the first time we had seen her. My head bells jangled. Jill went in first. As the time wore on I became uneasy. Then Jill came out and it was my turn. The psychiatrist began with, "Your daughter has a sort of histrionic personality. That is, she likes the drama associated with what may be going on at any given time." Clang, Clang, Clang. I got it. "Of course! She's being paid by the school district! This time, she'll be fully on board with that despicable bunch." It was obvious the school had given its version of Jill's problems and expected the doctor's report to reflect that. I replied, "I wouldn't necessarily completely disagree with that but given all she's been subjected to, I would say that statement is not wholly accurate. I'll tell you what I told the school principal. As far as bullying is concerned, there is *NO* instigating on a victim's part. Jill won't play the role or the games some kids and some adults expect her to play and they don't like that. They want her to put up and shut up, to accept intimidation and just become invisible. She didn't so she was assaulted—I will not use the word "fights." They were assaults on a kid who is *sick*—with a port in her chest no less and I involved the police because the school did *nothing*."

Dr. Werrmona then said Jill was "depressed" but did not believe her claim she was seeing images as she sporadically complained about. "Only people who use drugs and have serious psychiatric issues see and hear things," she said. Later, Vanessa disagreed, saying it was indeed possible for such things to happen when someone had been traumatized and said Jill *had* been traumatized—over and over again.

My head was screaming but I replied as calmly as I could, "I don't mean to be disrespectful, but I have letters on my desk right now from AIPorphyrics who indicate they suffer from agitation, mania, depression and hallucinations, the latter mostly during acute attacks, but I also have information that states for some porphryics these psychiatric problems can persist between attacks[93] and that hallucinations can be the seeing of lights, object or people that are not present.[94]

So, can *you* explain why Jill appears constantly irritable and over anxious and is prone to falling into convulsive attacks, after which she sometimes has hallucinations at school but nowhere else?"

Dr. Werrmona replied, "Well, it's because her AIP is not being managed correctly!"

I said, "Jill's AIP is managed based on *presenting* symptoms of which she's only had *one* attack since leaving Littleton schools—and that one didn't involve fainting or convulsions. Now, do you think that's a result of the frequent 'preventative' heme treatments or is it because she's been out of the school building for a while? Her porphyria specialist had recommended a total of eighteen treatments for the nine-month school year period but she had over forty Panhematin treatments just so she could be in the school. I believe that something in the Littleton schools has been wreaking havoc in my kid's neurological system for years now, causing these weird symptoms." To this, Dr. Werrmona said I was an overprotective mother.

She evidently had not been told that Jill was at Mountford or why she was there so I filled her in. She responded, "Well, isn't the doctor there giving her something for the depression?"

I replied, "He's concerned about the AIP because the wrong medication can set off AIP attacks."

She snapped, "Oh, that AIP shouldn't be a concern! He should just be calling the doctor who's treating the AIP and ask *him*! He should know what drugs can and can't be used!"

I said, "Sorry, but that's just not true or fair. To begin with, there are *few* doctors who know AIP. Dr. O'Connor, who is treating her at NHC, *wouldn't* know offhand which antidepressant medication to give to her—he'd have to do research, too. And the doctor at Mountford has been exploring which antidepressant medications *can* be used safely where AIP is involved. I've been helping him by checking with the American Porphyria Foundation's website's drug database."

---

93 Wright, Michelle D. original author: and Tidy, Colin Dr., current version author. *Porphyrias.* http://patient.info/health/porphyria. Published online in "Patient." August 17, 2015 and Bylesjö, I. *Epidemiological, Clinical and Studies of Acute Intermittent Porphyria.* Medical dissertation, Umea University. www.diva-portal.org/smash/get/ diva2:141227; FULLTEXT01.pdf. 2008, 10-11
94 Carlson, Dr. K. *Hallucinations Can Occur in Porphyria.* http://porphbook.tripod.com/Mar2004.html. Published online in PES Newsletter. March 2004.

She interrupted, "*You* should not be doing that! There are too many dangers, too much wrong information on the Internet!"

I shot back, "Well, I *am* doing that. And the APF is a recognized site for learning about porphyria. From that, Dr. Curtiss and I have identified only *two* meds that are rated safe for use with AIP and one of those, Prozac, has a questionable APF rating, so there is only one we are considering using at this point. You see, treating my daughter is a *team effort*, as it should be. Dr. Curtiss is working *with* me to help Jill." She had calmed down and was now engaged, "Which drug is that?" she asked.

I answered, "Let's see, C-e-l-something."

She jumped in, "Wellbutrin?" I said, "No, Wellbutrin is listed only as 'OK?' The one I found was C-e-l..." She said, "Z? Zoloft?"

I replied as patiently as I could, "No, 'C.' Zoloft is rated by APF as only 'OK? And because of that Dr. Curtiss decided not to risk it. Jill's condition has been 'fickle' to manage and we wanted as sure a bet as we could find. Let's see, Cele...something."

"Celexa?"

"Yes, I believe that's it," I said. "Oh, Celexa is a good drug! Works very well."

"It may work wonders for some adults but this is a child. I still have trouble reconciling the practice of too many psychiatrists routinely giving adult meds to children without benefit of significant testing. And this kid has the acute porphyric gene for goodness' sakes. The NHC doctor who treats Jill has never had a case of AIP before and there doesn't seem to be any other juvenile-onset AIP case requiring infusion treatment he can refer to, consequently, no other doctor to ask. Doesn't that tell you something? And AIP attacks can be deadly—but then, you know that, right?"

The subject of schools came up next. She said Jill told her she did not want to go to SFTA because she was afraid she would not be able to keep up with the academics. I said I understood that.

"If she can't handle one school socially, how do you think she'll be able to handle two?"

I responded, "First of all, there is something or a combination of somethings in the Littleton school buildings that seems to render my daughter unable to function. What? I don't know. How? I don't know. But I do know that since 2007, she's suffered severe, observable neurological and physical reactions to *something* in those buildings for which she receives treatment from Dr. O'Connor at NHC. So *Jill, her therapist and her father and I* will decide where Jill ends up for school."

She strongly recommended Jill get off Facebook and questioned whether her therapist had ever mentioned that. I said, "Of course she has. But I'm glad Jill is on Facebook *and* that I monitor it. That's how I discovered the first girl was planning to attack her and that the second girl bragged about beating her up. Both printouts provided proof as to their intent and execution and were given to the proper authorities. After that, no, she won't get off Facebook completely. If those kids want to keep her on their 'friends' list, so be it—she doesn't communicate with them anyway, but it's a way for *me* to keep up with what *they* are up to. And if you think that's being overprotective, you're entitled to your opinion."

Dr. Werrmona brought up the issue of Jill sporadically cutting herself as a coping mechanism and told me about another of her patients who frequently cut herself. She said, "I told her that it was stupid to cut herself, that it could lead to infection!" I was appalled that she'd called a patient in severe distress *stupid* and told her so. Thankfully, the session wound down. She said Jill needed a smaller, quieter venue where she could concentrate on her academics. She recommended Jill attend a "therapeutic day school," which is what Vanessa had been saying all along. Then she asked about the results of the psychological testing she had suggested months ago. "Littleton never did anything about that," I replied. It was time for me to leave. I would not know the full ramifications of that session for a while, but when I picked Jill up at the end of her group session that afternoon, I should have guessed when she announced, "I want to get discharged, I'm done with this." I told her that Dr. Curtiss and I thought medication would help and that it had taken too long to get that arranged. The least she could do was to give everything a chance to work together *for her*. She decided to stay with the program. She insisted she no longer wanted to attend SFTA. "I won't be able to do it. I'll fail the academic parts and they'll kick me out of the afternoon arts program."

I tried to reason with her, "No they won't. You'll be at LHS for the morning or maybe you could do tutoring. You'll be okay."

She was adamant, "I won't be able to do it. I have to give up my spot. I'll try to get in again next year." I was angry at the whole situation all over again—the sickness, something in the school building making Jill faint and convulse, the bullying administrators, teachers, students and everyone in between who had contributed to the situation we had found ourselves in. Winning a place in the magnet school lottery was not something to be taken lightly. I doubted Jill would get another chance. But nothing would dissuade her.

June was over. It had been a long, slow and painful ride through a month of unbelievable stress; one heme treatment and *no* AIP activity for Jill, which was, in itself, worth cheering about.

CHAPTER 49

Instability

When you hear thunder, seek shelter.
— WEATHER FORECASTERS' MANTRA

Jill graduated from Mountford's program. Her summer vacation finally started. She had worked hard and made progress in the program though her emotions still varied. She had developed new friendships, and it was good to see her connect with peers, spend time at the mall and talk on the phone or via Facebook to supportive individuals. Dr. Curtiss started Jill on the lowest dose of Celexa. The PPT was still pending; where Jill would start her freshman high school year was undecided. She desperately wanted to "catch up" academically. "I just want to do my work," she said. Mountford, too, recommended that Jill attend a therapeutic school.

Dr. Werrmona's report arrived. Holding back mounting bile, I read the evaluation. It was clear she had not gained any knowledge of AIP before making her assessment and recommendations, and that she was now fully on board with Littleton. The same psychiatrist who only months before deemed Jill "...happy sometimes and sad but not depressed...never been suicidal....I cannot give Jill a psychiatric diagnosis..."[95] this time, among other things, labeled her with histrionic personality disorder. She said Jill did not want to go to SFTA because it was a big school which, according to Jill, was not what she'd said at all.

Lizabeth's last report had noted, "Jill's strength is her vocabulary."

Now, just a few months later, the psychiatrist's report claimed, "She may have a somewhat limited vocabulary."[96] Littleton had paid the fee—and Werrmona's

---

95 Werrmona.* Psychiatric evaluation report. January 28, 2010 session.
96 Werrmona.* Psychiatric reevaluation report. June 20, 2010 session.

report proved that the school-paid doctor provided exactly what was expected of her.

August came in as a continuation of July's hot and heavy dog days. "How long are they going to drag out the wait for Jill's PPT?" I rhetorically asked myself. I knew the answer—they would drag it out as long as they could. I asked Attorney Troiano to contact Bart—we wanted Jill's freshman plans settled. Shortly thereafter her assistant, Meggie,* called, "Can you make a PPT on Thursday?"

"Absolutely," I responded, "we'll be there." Jill had had only one heme treatment each month in June, July and August—exactly what Dr. Piersen had recommended she get down to more than a year ago. She had been in multiple public-access buildings since June with no hint of symptoms. Attorney Troiano called before the PPT to confirm which therapeutic day school(s) we would consider for Jill. She had thought much about where she might go. She mentioned either NHC's or Mountford's school, the latter mostly because Jasmine* was hoping to go there, too. Jill and Jasmine had met in the Mountford program and clicked. Like Jill, Jasmine suffered bouts of depression and was smart and funny. If neither school was a possibility, Jill hoped for tutoring again.

Although Jill had her heart set on attending Mountford's school, I told Attorney Troiano my preference was NHC's therapeutic day school because of its connection to the hospital and should Jill resume fainting at school, it would stop the "transference game" between MedCity and NHC. She said, "Well, their attorney told me they're going to pay for whatever school you want. I told him we disagreed with the psych eval Werrmona did. And furthermore, if they hadn't agreed to an out-of-district placement, we would have fought for an independent evaluation. But I wouldn't recommend putting Jill through another evaluation right now; she's been through too much. I'm not a doctor, but I've represented a lot of kids, and think she might have PTSD from all the trauma she's had. Let's see how the new placement goes. If we feel another evaluation is needed, we can always ask for it."

When we arrived at the PPT Attorney Troiano told us she had discovered that NHC's school was not an accredited high school. That meant Jill would have to transfer to another school after ninth grade. She said Littleton recommended the Nette* School for her instead which was located in NHC's neighborhood. Littleton's "team" filed in. Bart gave a brief overview of the Nette School, said NHC could still be an option and encouraged us to visit both before making a decision. Tony presented an overview of Jill's fourth to eighth grade Connecticut Mastery Test (CMT) scores. She had earned mostly "proficient" levels throughout. The school's attorney weighed into the conversation, "Certainly says she's capable of achieving good academics." Bart said a special education classification would be necessary for Jill to attend the Nette School and made a show of filling out the necessary forms to formally move her into the Special Education-Other Health Impaired (SE-OHI) category.

Bart had been part of the problem all along starting when Jill's weird symptoms first appeared in Benton School. And once he had the DNA report and an MD's letter confirming the diagnosis, he should have called a PPT to designate Jill as SE-OHI because everyone involved knew her medical condition severely impacted her ability to learn. Bart began to define Jill's eligibility by listing her deficiencies. Primary, of course, was the medical impairment that rendered her at times unable to perform in the academic setting. And technically, legally, he was supposed to make "reasonable" accommodations in the school setting for Jill and, with Tony, to effectively manage (*not* ignore, inflame or contribute to) the bullying climate directed Jill's way. The state of Connecticut requires all of its school districts to "...provide for...ongoing maintenance and improvement of the indoor air quality of its facilities."[97] But my pleas to review the data I had amassed that showed the connection between Littleton schools' IAQ and Jill's AIP reactions to school attendance had been ignored. Improving IAQ through substantially increasing fresh air intake was, I thought, an easy accommodation that would improve Jill's overall performance, but that was apparently out of the range of accommodations they would consider.

By the time Bart reached the "social/emotional" section of the form, my eyes welled up. I had waited so long for the special education designation to be restored to her and it had been handed to us just like that. But it seemed to me Jill was being essentially "banished" and, that in using it, Littleton would get away with not addressing its bullying school climate or IAQ. Had both been resolved, Jill might have a chance at remaining in the school district she had attended since preschool. Finally, memories of months' of negative and unpleasant actions by and interactions with the people in that room made me want to scream.

Attorney Troiano noticed my distress and whispered, "Do you want to take a break?" I nodded. We went into the hallway.

"Thank you, I've waited so long for that classification to be restored and now here it is," I said dully.

"This is called victory!" she said, trying to cheer me up.

I replied, "I guess, but it's a hollow one. Jill's sick. So many things could have been avoided if Littleton only had a modicum of ethics!"

"Well, let's look toward Jill's working on getting her academics in place where she's happy with them once again. *That's* what's important," she said. We went back to the meeting where it was decided the next PPT would be held at the "new" school in October to set the IEP (individual education plan). Ed and I thanked the attorney and said, "It's finally done. Jill has the designation she needs though it took bringing in 'legal guns' for that to happen." She accepted our thanks and then said, "Let me know if you need anything else. If they don't go along with what they agreed to in there, we'll see them in federal court. School districts don't usually want to end up there."

A few days later a Nette School staff member called to say the principal was on vacation but she could start the process and set an appointment with Jill and me. It soon became clear to me that Littleton had not disclosed what I considered to be the most important document in Jill's "cumulative" file—Dr. O'Connor's letter regarding Jill's AIP. I asked if they had received it with the package. They said no. A

---

97 State of Connecticut. Act Concerning Indoor Air Quality in Schools. www.cga.ct.gov/2003/act/Pa/2003PA-00220-R00HB-06426-PA.htm.

slow burn started; the letter Bart assured me in writing would become part of Jill's "permanent file" had not. The Littleton school district was putting my daughter's life in jeopardy once again. I said I would bring copies to the meeting when the principal returned. After a tour of the premises during which I took note of old-fashioned chalkboards in the math class and a fully equipped nurse's office, we said good-byes. Jill was impressed with the school and said she thought she would be happy there, even with all the restrictions they had in place. In fact, the restrictions gave her a sense of security. As we waited for the meeting with the Nette School principal to be arranged, Littleton's completed PPT report arrived in the mail. Reading it roiled me. Ed and I were astonished to see that the *Checklist for Other Health Impairment* form, which Bart had asked us to sign blank had been filled in with descriptions—particularly, Histrionic Personality Disorder—taken directly from Werrmona's report. Yet there had been no discussion about that or any other psychiatric states/conditions/influences mentioned during the PPT. It was clear that Bart under the guise of "the district" intended to label Jill a psych case and catapult her out of Littleton.

Near the end of August, Jill's emotions tumbled, and she again posted suicidal thoughts on Facebook. She ended up at MedCity's ED then was transferred to St. Michael's inpatient adolescent program. She stayed for only a few days before suffering a stress-induced AIP attack and was transported back to NHC for a heme treatment. While there, with plenty of time to talk, she confided she'd begun "slipping" right after our last meeting with Dr. Werrmona. Evidently, not only had she offended me that day, in their private session Werrmona had unnerved Jill by telling her that problems with peers and subsequent suspensions were *her* fault and she had become a bully "just like them." I was furious. Jill was back in Mountford's program for another go 'round. With a heavy heart I wrote a letter to SFTA saying Jill would not be attending the school as a part-time freshman after all. The battle to convince Jill once again that she had worth was on.

CHAPTER 50
Stalled Frontal Boundary

If there is no struggle, there is no progress.
—FREDRICK DOUGLAS

As September came, Jill worried, "Is Littleton going to blow me off again? Because if they do, I'm going to be a retarded adult! Am I supposed to teach myself? I don't know how to do that." Shortly afterwards, we met with the Nette high school principal, school nurse and social worker. I asked if they had received Dr. O'Connor's letter from Littleton. They said no, so I distributed copies. I also asked if they knew what brand or type of general cleaner was used throughout the school and noted there were few white boards, which I took as a positive in managing Jill's symptoms. They didn't know what cleaning products were used, but I reasoned aloud, "If you use the same products as the other hospital-related buildings, Jill should be ok because she's spent time in buildings that share the same parent company as this school without symptoms." The Nette team asked Jill to describe her fainting and convulsive episodes, her latest hospitalizations and treatment programs and her perspective of peer and adult relationships at LMS. They asked about the bullying incidents and administrators' reactions to same from Jill's point of view. She reiterated several times all she ever wanted was to do her work and to make friends, but neither had happened. In the end, Jill did not fit the "profile" of a Nette School student and we were left to try to find a school safe from bullies and potential toxin-triggering elements *and* equipped with a staff of adults committed to getting Jill up to speed academically. The task would prove harder than we thought. By mid-September Jill had resumed tutoring with Lizabeth at the library.

October crept in and with it came a letter from Attorney Troiano explaining that the tough economic conditions had produced a backlash on special education programs, resulting in a substantial increase in the number of parents seeking legal representation and introduced new professionals to her legal team. I had enjoyed working with Attorney Troiano and knew if she had selected new staff members, they were top-notch. But the memory of meeting people at the bullying presentation who had commented about Littleton's notoriety for being "extremely nasty to work" with and "super tough" on parents of special education kids and with Jill's situation being so unique, I was rattled. Knowing we needed continued legal guidance, I decided to talk with a local mom I had heard of whose child had for years been represented by a different, "tough" SE attorney. Within the day or so I had the name of Klingberg and Company* and while talking with my friend Anna,* I mentioned the firm. "Oooh! He's the one who makes school districts *quake!*" she said. It was settled; I would see if Attorney Alton Klingberg* would take our case.

One day it occurred to me that while Jill had had two "classic" attacks, both due to stress—she hadn't had a fainting or convulsion episode for six months! She was finally down to the single heme treatment per month. It was time for a Dr. Piersen update. I wanted her to see Jill in a much better physical state than when we had first met and to thank her for helping us with the heme regimen that had given us hope for Jill's future. I also wanted to talk with her about the odd fainting/toxin/school predicament and the inordinate number of heme treatments Jill had had during the school year. Jill was deliriously happy when I told her she could invite Jasmine to join us on the trip to the Washington, D.C. area.

However, before leaving I wanted to tie up the legal aspects of Jill's educational needs and made an appointment to meet with Attorney Klingberg. He described how his own child had suffered irreversible brain damage because of a kidney disorder that resulted in a significant change in her educational needs. School services were not being addressed according to the law so Attorney Klingberg had expanded his service offerings to include special education representation. More than any professional I had met so far, he *understood* what we were up against. Though his face remained mask-like as I told him about Jill's porphyria/school fiascos, his questions belied his calm demeanor. I told him that Attorney Troiano had helped secure the SE-OHI designation for Jill and we were in the process of finding a suitable school placement. He said his firm would take our case. It was time to respectfully say good-bye to Attorney Troiano. As always, she was professionally kind, wished us well and agreed to make the transition a smooth one.

Jill and Jasmine were thrilled when Jasmine's mother said she could accompany us to the D.C. area. Dr. Piersen was happy to see Jill and, as always, her examination was thorough. We discussed Jill's propensity toward bouts with depression and the suicidal ideation born of the LMS bullying, her hospitalizations and subsequent treatment programs. At the time, Jill was taking 40 mg. of Celexa daily. I explained how Dr. Curtiss and I had settled on Celexa and how it had appeared to be helping though I had recently noticed some mood fluctuations. I told her Dr. Nyeer had agreed to supervise her medication needs because she had been discharged from Mountford's and, therefore, Dr. Curtiss' care. I asked her opinion about the potential of commonly used, low-level toxins affecting Jill's neurological system. I also said I had specific concerns about the combination of the hydrogen peroxide-based cleaner and the solvent/alcohol ingredients of the markers used throughout the school as being problematic for Jill. She said she did not know enough about toxicology to address those questions and thoughts so could not rule out whether such products might cause problems for Jill. She agreed that comparing the school's cleaning schedules to Jill's attacks and reactions would be helpful. I told her that was not likely to happen because the school district had steadfastly either ignored the request or repeatedly shut me down when I brought the subject up. I told her the school trivialized the physical aspects of AIP, tolerated the neurological aspects and amplified the psychiatric component. She responded, "Not at all surprising. As it is, AIP is very misunderstood in the medical field, never mind the educational environment!"

The subject of heme came up. I said since she had left the LMS building, Jill had been receiving only one heme treatment a month and feeling the best she had in a long time. The doctor recommended we work with Dr. O'Connor to start "weaning her off the heme" by incrementally adding two weeks between treatments from that point forward until she only needed heme to resolve an attack. We left and visited DC before catching the train home.

CHAPTER 51

Cloud Bank

The eyes of the Lord are in every place
beholding the evil and the good.
— PROVERB 15:3

Back from Washington, Jill was in regular contact with her newest Facebook friend, Clinton, a California teen she had met through Jasmine's neighbor, Bella.* In addition to Facebook communication, Clinton and Jill had begun talking on the telephone. Clinton's interest in anything sports sparked that interest in Jill, too. They rooted for different national sports teams and talked about various rock performers and groups. Clinton listened as Jill sang the latest song(s) she had been writing and bolstered her during the times she was down. Ed and I told her as long as the communication between the two stayed on the up-and-up, that is, no discussion about plans to meet and no sexual, illegal or dangerous talk, they could continue communicating. She knew we periodically monitored her phone calls, Facebook and email to insure that those expectations were met.

Because the files Littleton had turned over to Attorney Troiano were so skimpy, in contrast to Dr. Werrmona's comment about the *bulky* files she'd received, I spent days going page by page through my own files to create a chronological compilation of Jill's medical and educational documents, and delivered the package to Klingberg and Associates. Caring, supportive educational consultant Miriam Adams* came into our world and asked for a copy of Jill's most recent IEP. I told her since the Nette School had not worked out, the IEP had not yet been developed and Jill was back in tutoring without an IEP, but everything considered, was doing well. Her attention and focus was very good; Lizabeth saw no signs of physical distress, anxiety, irritability, confusion, problem concentrating or inability to focus; she was averaging Bs in all her subjects. Lizabeth was aware we were seeking a new school for her and was doing an excellent job of keeping Jill engaged in her academics. The PPT was held in late November; this time, Miriam was with us. Lizabeth presented an overview of Jill's progress, the same information she had already shared with me. When we left the meeting, the plan was to maintain tutoring until such time as a "permanent" school placement was secured. An online, computer-assisted science course to fulfill a science credit requirement was added. As weeks went by and Littleton presented little or no options, Miriam advised Bart that a local Catholic high school that annually garnered a good percentage of Littleton's high school students should be considered. Bart ignored the suggestion. Then two schools called with interest in possibly accepting Jill. Having been turned down by schools who, according to Bart, felt they could not accommodate Jill's medical needs, it was a relief to have two possibilities. Tours and intake meetings for the Havencrest School* and the Kathryn Prixe School* were arranged. Still wary about the potential of toxin triggers, I was determined to observe Jill closely during and after the tours and meetings. Just before Christmas, we drove through an upscale neighborhood of old Victorian homes-turned-commercial buildings and entered the Havencrest grounds. Jill said, "Ooh, kind of creepy," but once inside, fell in love with the character of the place. Her initial "creepy" turned to "I like it, I really like it," and she left with a date to "shadow" students at the school. "What's that old saying, 'Don't judge a book by its cover?'" I teased as we drove away. We set our sights on the upcoming tour of Kathryn Prixe School (KPS). Looking at the website, I quietly had misgivings about KPS being a good match for Jill. Two days later, a KPS student chaperoned us around the school. Tour done, Jill waited in the lobby as I talked with principal Doris* and assistant principal Lillian* about Jill's health, stressing the lengthy latency period she had been enjoying. I said Jill seemed to like KPS, but she had liked Havencrest, too. We left with a shadowing date planned. By then, Jill was on 60 mgs of Celexa daily (an increase from the 40 mgs because depression continued to plague her), was working diligently with Lizabeth and looking forward to moving to a more standard school environment. It had been more than seven months since her last fainting and convulsive symptoms and more than four since her last significant bout of AIP activity.

Jill enjoyed the KPS shadowing experience and looked forward to the Havencrest encounter scheduled for the next day. However, when I picked her up at day's end, she said scornfully, "What a rip-off. I just sat there the whole time. Nobody asked me anything about my schoolwork or what books I use at school now." She continued, "And at lunch some kids started talking about a kid who was absent. I hate that. I'm gonna go to Kathryn Prixe School. At least they were interested in what I was doing in my schoolwork."

We headed to our appointment with Vanessa who was anxiously awaiting Jill's assessments of both schools. After hearing Jill's thoughts, Vanessa turned to me, "And what's your opinion?" I said if Jill preferred and felt comfortable with KPS that's all that mattered. We called to say Jill accepted their offer to attend school there. Doris* was pleased with Jill's decision, said she would notify Littleton, and paperwork would be sent to me for signature. A start date was set for the first day of the new marking period. There was hope after all.

Jill received her report card, a positive review and best wishes from Lizabeth when she left to finish her freshman year at KPS. She was still singing with Lora, meeting regularly with Vanessa and continued taking Celexa to battle ever-present depression. She had also recently begun requesting a sleeping tablet at night. Thinking nerves about starting at a new school were at play, I missed emerging symptoms that the AIP fiend was back in another guise.

PART IV

Small Craft Advisory

You're going to come across people in your life who will say all the right words at all the right times. But in the end it's always their actions you should judge them by.

— **NICHOLAS SPARKS**[98]

98 Sparks, N. *The Rescue*. http://www.goodreads.com/work/quotes/1268663-the-rescue

CHAPTER 52

Full Moon

I was lost in the middle of my life...
— AS SUNG BY THREE DAYS GRACE

I heaved a sigh of relief when Jill ate breakfast and excitedly hopped on the school van for her first day at KPS. But a few hours later, the phone rang, the caller ID registered KPS and my heart skipped a beat. The receptionist, Emma* said, "Jill has a bad stomachache and a sore throat, could you come pick her up?"

"Oh dear God, it can't be happening *again*!" I thought and drove the fifty-minute route to pick her up, wondering the whole way what I had missed. It could not be first day jitters; in all the years Jill had gone to the first day of any school year, she never expressed nervousness, only excitement about going to school.

Jill was mystified, "I don't know why my stomach hurts. It just does. I think I must be coming down with something. My throat's killing me, too." Tylenol and some rest would take care of it, I assured her. They did not.

The next day KPS' nurse consultant called to say she had done some research about AIP and expressed concern. I spent considerable time talking with Wanda* about triggers and Jill's attack presentations. It was ironic that after all the times I had tried to talk to *anyone* at Littleton about AIP, here I was attempting to calm a school nurse about it. I told her there was no standard AIP attack profile but said I would put together information based on our experience for her review. Before faxing it, I re-read it and thought, "If I hadn't lived it, I'd think this was preposterous." Jill made it through the next few days, though continued complaining that she was "coming down with something." We met with Dr. O'Connor for her annual von Willebrand/ thalassemia/AIP exam. He pronounced her throat "looking fine." Then said he had received the letter from Dr. Piersen about suspending heme until it was needed and agreed to give it a try but recommended we meet in three months to re-evaluate the plan. We updated him as to her daily dosage of Celexa after which he reviewed her latest lab results and said her iron was on the low side but not overly so.

As freezing winds whipped and snowfalls intensified, Jill missed several school days because of health complaints. Her attitude at home became increasingly intolerable. I felt a foreboding feeling. Clinton and Jill talked regularly on Facebook and by phone. It seemed the relationship was supportive for Jill. Still, I watched what was going on as best I could. From what I had seen, their disclosures were no worse than what I had seen between her and other Facebook "friends."

During the second week, KPS called to say Jill was on her way to Haven City hospital with what was described as a "slight" AIP attack including a stomachache, shaking, aches and pains. Head bells ringing, I set off for the hospital, trying to grasp what was going on because she had been asymptomatic for so long. When I arrived at the ED, oxygen had already been administered and a D10 infusion ordered. As the dextrose pumped into Jill's liver, her abdominal pains dissipated. On the drive home I asked how the online science course was progressing. "Oh, I don't have to do that anymore," she replied.

"Why not?" I asked.

"Cause Tori* said I don't need to do it and to just throw it away because I'm going to do their science."

Shocked, I said, "Wait a minute. KPS has no homework, no tests, no quizzes (which Ed and I had just discovered) so there's *no reason* for you not to take advantage of this opportunity. I'm surprised a teacher would say something like that."

Jill answered, "Well, Tori *is* the teacher and if she says I don't need it, I don't need it. You're going to argue with a *teacher?*"

"Teacher or not, I will let her know my feelings about this," I replied. As it turned out, Tori called that evening to check up on Jill. She asked if I knew whether glazes or fumes relating to the pottery kiln firing they used in the school could trigger problems for Jill. I told her I did not know, but recalled reading something about that and said I would look it up. I brought up the VLA (online) science program issue and repeated the conversation I'd had with Jill.

"Oh, I would *never* tell a kid that. *Of course* we can work it into our program," Tori said. The next day I talked to Dr. Nyeer about Jill's brooding demeanor, complaints about being sick and ongoing depression/melancholy. She'd been on 60 mgs of Celexa for about three months. "Shouldn't she be perking up by now?" I asked. He said to watch her carefully. I replied that I had begun recording her complaints of sore throats, stomachaches and other symptoms on a calendar. I found the article that mentioned ceramic pigments inducing AIP attacks and faxed it to Tori. But I did not think that was the problem.

School had been in session for seventeen days and Jill complained about sore throat, aches and pains, coming down with something, stomachaches, feeling feverish or some other ailment for almost all of them. Though her enthusiasm for songwriting and singing had waned somewhat, she was still singing with Lora. Late one night, Kevin told me, "Jill's crying." I went to her bedroom door.

"Go away, Mom, I don't want to talk about it," she said.

I returned to my home office where Kevin asked, "Why is she crying?"

"I don't know, maybe she had a fight with Clinton or something. She's going to have to work it out with him," I said.

Monday morning Jill went to school. The phone rang a few hours later. The caller ID indicated KPS. Emma said briskly, "Jill is suicidal and has been cutting herself, she needs to be picked up as soon as possible." I got to the building and headed towards Lucy's office. Jill was agitated, her attitude horrible. The head bells clanged loudly and I worried aloud, "What in God's name is going on?" The drive home was unbearable. Attempts to make conversation went nowhere. We ended up yelling at each other. I turned the radio on. Jill changed the channel to a station with loud, metal music and ratcheted the volume up. I would turn it off; she would turn it back on, louder each time. Finally, I had had enough, grabbed her hand and shouted at her to knock it off. For the umpteenth time, she reached for the knob. I grabbed her hand again, "If you put your hand on that dial one more time, I swear I'll break it!" I yelled. I pulled off the highway with traffic flying by us at breakneck speed and screamed, "*STOP THIS! I'VE GOT TO DRIVE! IF YOU TOUCH IT AGAIN I WILL F—ING HURT YOU!*" She calmed down and I got back into the driving lane and headed home.

Saying she did not want to go to her final CCD class scheduled for that evening, Jill spent the remainder of the day in her room. Then at 5:00 p.m. she came bouncing down the stairs, seemingly renewed, "I guess I'm going to go after all. Can we get flowers for Mrs. L and can I bring snacks for the class?" We stopped at a local market. Jill selected a floral arrangement and snacks to share with the class. Kiera was cashiering that night. Jill insisted we stay in her line though it was long. The girls exchanged pleasantries. Keira told her she looked "great" and asked how she had been. Jill replied, "Thanks...I'm okay." Off we went. She returned from CCD with her Confirmation gown in hand, yelled, "I've got to try this on," and raced upstairs to do it. Perplexed, I thought, "This after a day of suicidal thoughts requiring she be picked up at school?!"

CHAPTER 53

Winter Thunder

Disappointing change of season/Cold has come again...
— AS SUNG BY BLACK STONE CHERRY

Just pretend everything is alright [sic]. Put a smile on your face. It works every time, don't you know? I get on the bus for school and when I get there I pretend like everything's o.k. I have to have the best behavior and not let anything get in the way of that. Yep, it's like I have to be perfect, because if you don't people will jump down your throat for not doing the right thing. But it's nearly impossible to be perfect.[99]

During a therapy session Jill told Vanessa she hated KPS because "They aren't teaching me anything" and did not want to go back. I told her too many people had worked too hard and too long to get her into a "real" school that Littleton was paying lots of money for, and reality was what it was—by law, she *had* to go to school. Many nights, Ed worked with Jill on math problems she was unable to understand in school. He would take her step-by-step through a process and after a few trials she had the concept and "got it." "That's what I wish Tori would do," she would sigh. Something was wrong. Because her last heme treatment had been so long ago, I wondered if maybe we had let it go too long. I knew there was no way to measure the amount of heme and no knowledge of how much heme was necessary for "typical" body functions. I wondered about the possibility of low heme potentially contributing to Jill's physical problems and distress. I wondered if certain chemicals could "breakdown or "eat away" a body's heme supply and result in porphyric activity. Little did I know I was going in the right direction with that line of thinking—however, this time the chemical wasn't in the air—it was in Jill's body. But I had not connected that yet.

---

99 Jill's journal. March 2011.

Vanessa suggested a "med check" so I called Dr. Nyeer to make an appointment. On the way home from her session with Vanessa, Jill brought up the crying incident of the night before. "Clinton and I *didn't* have a fight. It was because I didn't want to go on anymore. He was just trying to keep me from hurting myself," she said.

I replied, "Jill, when I went to your door and you told me to go away, I figured you two had something to work out so I went away as you requested. But, Jill, *why* do you want to hurt yourself—or die?" She clamped up.

Before allowing her to return to school, KPS requested a psychiatrist's clearance. I said I would not hold her out of school until the following week when Dr. Nyeer would see her. After all she had been through with the last "school-appointed" psychiatrist, I would not subject her to a "new" psychiatrist, either. Vanessa was a licensed clinical therapist. I said they could rely on her professional opinion. So Jill returned to KPS the day after her appointment with Vanessa. Driving home, I told her we had an appointment for a med check with Dr. Nyeer coming up because I knew she wanted to feel good. I said I knew she hated the side effects she had experienced from the heme treatments, especially since she had had so many of them during eighth grade, but I was stuck. The heme had helped get her to a lengthy latency period. I had also called Dr. O'Connor but I didn't tell Jill and left a message saying Jill's mental status was deteriorating. I told him I had been in regular contact with Vanessa and had a pending appointment with Dr. Nyeer for a med check.

Jill told me she had spoken with Tori and told her she felt frustrated because she was left to independent study too much and felt she wasn't learning anything. Tori promised to provide a more appropriate teaching style. That lasted only a few days. I told Jill I would speak to Tori and Lucy* to arrange a time for me to observe a school day. Jill became agitated, "Of *COURSE* they're going to do everything perfect when you're there! They'll go right back to what was going on before you came. I've lost *TWO MONTHS* of school, Mom!"

Attempting to steer her to follow a more mature method of confronting problems, I said, "Then I'll talk to the attorney." At that Jill became verbally aggressive and screamed in my ear to the point I ordered her out of the car to walk the remaining quarter mile home.

The round-robin of updating Vanessa, Miriam, KPS and Drs. O'Connor, Alaimo and Nyeer about Jill's continual physical and mental health conditions consumed much of my time. When I had left the message for Dr. O'Connor, I had also questioned whether or not we should at least do tests again to identify ALAs/PBGs because that was considered the "definitive indicator" for AIP. Dr. O'Connor returned my call and left a message on our answering machine saying he understood about the symptoms Jill was exhibiting and when it seemed like a heme treatment was necessary, to call for an appointment. He did not answer about the lab testing.

KPS's assistant principal, Lillian, invited me to observe Jill at KPS any day and time I wanted to. When I arrived the next week I discovered a field trip had been arranged so the day's academic time would be condensed. However, during my time there, I could see how the structure of a small classroom with students ranging from ninth through twelfth grades was distracting for Jill. When Tori announced it was math time the students pulled out their individual grade level math books.

Seated in the middle of the group, Tori swiveled from one student to the next, checking the work they had done or giving each the next assignment. When it was science time, some students took out science books while others moved to areas of the room where rudimentary plant science experiments were set up. Driving home, I said to Jill, "I noticed you seemed to do the math today with no problem."

She replied, "Yeah, today's work was pretty easy, but I don't know how to do the next section and I know she won't explain it to me. We're going to be right back to where we were before you started asking them about stuff, I can see that." Jill said she was frustrated because Tori would just flip through pages, and sometimes whole chapters saying, "Don't worry about this," or "You won't need this."

"That's not teaching. I'm going to be dumb forever," she said mournfully. I told her that Ed and I would bring the issue up at the upcoming PPT.

The date of Jill's Confirmation ceremony finally arrived. She was happy about achieving this important religious sacrament. Afterward, Kevin, who was her sponsor, told us he had been worried all through the ceremony that Jill might faint. He said, "She was shaking for pretty much the whole time, especially when she was standing." Jill said that her high heeled shoes had made her legs shake. It was a logical possibility.

A new school week started. Jill woke with severe nausea and aches and pains. She went for a heme treatment where we met a new Hem/Onc physician, Dr. Winslow.* Before we left, she said the medical staff had tried to brainstorm a method to "measure heme" but it had not worked out. Nonetheless, Jill and I were heartened to hear *someone* had tried *something*. But that excitement was short lived; Dr. Winslow also said because Jill had been exhibiting so many symptoms, Dr. O'Connor recommended a second treatment for that week. Two days later we had our appointment with Dr. Nyeer who spent considerable time with Jill and me asking questions and assessing her mood. He asked if she was still cutting herself; she said she had not been "doing that as much" recently. He asked how she felt after she'd cut herself, "Not good, I don't like it." He asked about school. She talked about liking the school, the students and the adults, but was unhappy with the academic approach.

Dr. Nyeer looked at me, "What have you done about that?" I explained what I'd done so far. He ended with, "Well it's really up to the therapist, Vanessa, to continue to work with you on these matters." I said I thought we were at the maximum dosage of Celexa but it did not seem to be helping. Dr. Nyeer said the maximum dosage for Celexa was 80 mgs, and Jill could begin taking it that night. He then turned to her and told her she was at a critical point in life and she would have to "make peace" with the educational position for the remainder of the school year. He advised her to "focus on the good parts the school offers and look to the future."

On the drive home from his office, Jill announced, "I want to go back to Littleton. I'll put up with the bullies. I just want to *learn* something." I told her that was *not* going to happen. It was clear she was depressed *and* desperate. But I could not let her return to Littleton schools. I did not want an autopsy to tell me the toxins had finally killed her, or to take a chance that the bully brigade would finish her off for good. That Celexa could be the problem never entered my mind.

CHAPTER 54

Icicles

How many times can I break till I shatter...
— AS SUNG BY THE GROUP O.A.R.

Back in the infusion center, Jill relaxed and the heme treatment went well. Zofran helped ease the nausea. Being a Friday, she had the weekend to recuperate. But by Tuesday, I was called to pick her up from school *again*. This time, it was too late in the day for me to go—I had a CCD class to teach and would not be back in time to start the class so Ed went to get her. The frequency of having to pick Jill up at a school nearly an hour away had begun to work on our nerves. Ed was of the opinion because Jill was not happy with the school situation, she was "dogging it." I was worried that Celexa was not helping her depression. As I drove home after class my own irritation about having been called yet again from KPS and Jill's terrible attitude grew. Maybe Ed was right—it was time for Jill to "get her stuff together." She did not have the worry about peers bothering her. I had guessed that no homework, tests or quizzes was KPS's idea of reducing student stress. But for Jill, the lack of measurement feedback only increased her stress level. She said homebound tutoring was better because at least she had gotten feedback from Lizabeth based on the homework assignments, quizzes and tests. Jill had *always* been motivated to learn. Lizabeth's last assessment of her academic performance, behavior and attention had been positive. I could not figure out what was going on—either with Jill or KPS. If we had had a better relationship with Littleton, I would have called Bart, but I was sure doing so would somehow have resurrected the WHACK-A-Jill! game. I did not want another bout of that. My mind was so full. Was it teen angst to an extreme? Could Jill be losing her grip on reality?

By the time I got home, I was rattled and crabby. Jill was talking with Clinton on her bedroom phone. I knocked on her door and told her to hang up. "No!" she yelled. I unlocked the door. She was sitting on her bed.

I reached for the portable phone, "Give me the phone. Your conversation is over." She started screaming at the top of her lungs and stuffed the phone under the bedcovers. As I continued to grab for it, she began kicking and slapping my hands away, shrieking even louder. At last I knocked the portable phone from her hand and left the room with it. Head bells were clanging like crazy. Jill had been off heme and did really well for *months*. What had caused this awful about-face?

When Jill went to school the next day, she complained to Lucy that I had hit her, she was afraid of me and that I made her "get heme all the time that makes me sicker." It appeared she was fully in "I really hate my mother" teen mode. In the meantime, we received a notice that the PPT to set the IEP would be held at KPS. Jill had been at the school for about two months.

Jill's grounding did not include computer access and though I had told her more times than I could count to not take my computer off my desk, one day it was missing. I went to check her bedroom. The door was closed but not locked. Jill was sitting on her bed holding my work computer. I said, "I'm taking my computer because you didn't ask to use it and now you're grounded from that, too."

She said, "Sorry, let me get out of something first."

"Oh no you don't. You're grounded, remember?" I snatched the computer and took it back to my office. When I looked at the screen, I was sick. Jill had not been able to erase what was on it before I grabbed it. I had seen some of Clinton and Jill's emails and overheard snippets of phone conversations before but had not heard or seen anything like what I was looking at. This was over and above what Ed and I had set for boundaries for communication between the two. Needing Vanessa's guidance on this, I emailed her. She responded and asked to see me alone before Jill's next session. Our sessions with Vanessa usually started with me and Jill going in together, I'd give a brief update as to what had happened from my perspective since we last met then leave them to their session. This time, I told Jill that Vanessa asked to see me alone first. Jill immediately displayed an attitude. "Why?" she asked.

"Because she and I need to talk about something."

"Me?"

"Yes, you."

"Well, too bad. I'm going in with you," Jill said. "*No* you are not. You will stay here until she comes for you. Don't push it. You're already grounded for two weeks— want to make it three—or more?" I retorted and went in to meet with Vanessa who expressed concern about the Clinton/Jill inappropriate email messaging issue. "As a mandated reporter, I have to do something about this," she said and explained she had already talked to a youth officer in the town where she practiced. "I believe he's a predator," she said.

I replied, "I think you're right. Okay, what do you recommend I do? Talk to this town's youth officer? Call Littleton's local police? Call the police in the California town where Clinton allegedly lives? Call the FBI? What?"

"Start with your local police and ask them to advise you," Vanessa said. It was time for Jill to come in and I left them to their session. When I returned for Jill, I could see she had been crying. "Sorry I upset you," Vanessa offered to her. A subdued Jill and I drove home.

The next week was a repeat of so many before except Jill had really lost her spark. She was back to the pattern of attending school one day and being absent the next. She was so miserably sick and so sure she had strep throat that by the end of the week I called Dr. Alaimo's office for a strep check. A nurse swabbed Jill's throat and said she would be back shortly with the results. Jill said, "I've got strep. I just know it."

"But you don't have a fever," I said.

"Look mom, I *know* my own body." The doctor arrived to announce that Jill did not have strep but there *was* a lot of strep going around so it was good we had checked it out.

Jill missed school for the entire last week of March. I couldn't help thinking I was missing something.

CHAPTER 55

Sloppy Puddles

*Sadness is more or less like a head cold—with patience,
it passes. Depression is like a cancer.* [100]
— **BARBARA KINGSOLVER, AUTHOR**

I told Jill that Vanessa recommended police involvement to find out more about Clinton. I reminded her that none of us knew anything about him and could not be sure he was who he said he was. I said we had a responsibility to keep her safe. Jill was livid. She called Clinton and demanded his father's office phone number "so my mother can talk to him." He said no. Jill said, "Well, I just want you to know the police might come to check you out, so be ready." He then sent her an email to say he was taking his Facebook page down and hoped she would find a "good guy." She was bereft. "He promised to always be my friend. All I wanted to do was meet him." Now I was doubly sure Clinton was *not* who he said he was.

My pursuit of the Clinton issue was in the front of my mind when PPT day arrived. The school meeting had already started when Doris made a late entrance and interrupted what she apparently thought was a conversation about Jill and Clinton. She made what Ed and I felt was an inappropriate comment for a school administrator to have made, especially during a school meeting. I told her, "Jill knew the rules. Things happened and consequences followed." Tori then addressed Jill's academic performance. She said Jill had difficulty in sustaining attention, organization, a high level of anxiety and stress regarding academics and frequently underestimated her own ability. She produced an academic report of *fourteen* classes, all graded "Incomplete." Ed spoke for Jill, saying she was unhappy with the way the academics were presented, "She's continually complaining at home that she's bored

---

100 Kingsolver, B. "The Bean Trees." (New York: HarperPerennial, 1992), 173.

at school. Either the work is too easy or too hard and what's too hard is something she is unfamiliar with."

Doris exclaimed, "First I've heard of it!"

I said, "Well, Jill said she's spoken to all of you about it and I've spoken directly to Tori, Lucy and Lillian about the issue.

Ed added, "I've spent considerable time at home teaching her math, only to find it's not followed through in the classroom."

Tori replied, "She *is* very good at getting concepts. But she's missed a lot of school. It's hard to keep up with so many absences."

"Since Jill started at KPS, she's attended school only 46 percent of the days school has been in session," Bart added.

Ed responded, "Wow, I knew she's been sick a lot, but I didn't realize it was such a high percentage."

Bart said the district did not want to continue paying a substantial tuition for a student with continued absences. I was aggravated; paying for Jill to attend a private day school had to cost a whole lot more than making modifications to the school's IAQ and dealing with the bullying problem probably would have. If they had done that, there was a good chance none of the past few months' inpatient or outpatient hospitalizations, psychiatrist evaluations, alternative school interviews and paying for this school would have been needed.

As the meeting wound down, Doris said, "You know, these heme treatments aren't making Jill better; how is it determined when she should get them anyway?"

I said, "Presenting symptoms decide when treatments are needed. When symptoms appear, what usually happens is I contact Dr. O'Connor to let him know the type and frequency and whether they've been steady or are escalating. Then he calls back for more information. Sometimes this goes back and forth over a couple or a few days. If symptoms aren't getting better or are worse he may approve a treatment."

Doris was on her feet, "*That's* irresponsible!" she cried.

"Maybe you think so but that's because you don't know how unpredictable and how fast moving these symptoms can be," I replied. "Like it or not, treating Jill's illness has to be a team effort between doctors and our family."

Bart dismissively flipped his hand, "I've been dealing with this Jill thing for a few years now." Inside, I seethed, "*He* had the nerve to say he'd 'been dealing with this *Jill thing* for a few years now'? That was his *job*, one he was very well paid to do. Jill lived with 'this *Jill thing*' every day and night of her life. Our insurance company was paying for the bulk of 'this *Jill thing*.' Ed and I were going through 'this *Jill thing*' with her, constantly pulling her up, pushing her through, paying high insurance deductibles and out-of-pocket costs—all the time facing nonbelieving characters like him. Yes, as parents, it was our job to support our child, but unlike Bart, there was no paycheck for doing 'this *Jill thing*.' I calmly said, 'This *Jill thing*" had overtaken our life and consumed nearly every one of my days for over three years and a good chunk of our financial resources. *Our family* has been through so much these past few years. We fully expect Littleton to stay the education course this time."

Doris asked us, "Would you like our help? This family *needs* help; how can *we* help you?"

"Yes, of course we would appreciate help." I said, "it would be good for someone else to understand what Jill has been living with." "Would you be willing to sign releases so that we can talk to medical personnel familiar with your case?" Doris asked.

I said, "Sure, I'll get you a list of people you can talk to." Where were those damn head bells when I needed them? Doris took the wheel and our expedition took another direction.

CHAPTER 56

Raining Frogs

*Antidepressants increased the risk...of suicidal thinking
and behavior (suicidality) in children, adolescents and
young adults in short-term studies of major depressive
disorder MDD)...[101]*

In hindsight, I should have stayed in bed the next morning but went downstairs just before the school van came for Jill. She immediately started harping about the "Clinton issue" and asked when I was going to do something about it. I said, "Today." She stormed out of the house. KPS called a few hours later to say Jill had had a meltdown, threatened suicide, showed fresh cuts she had made on her arm and was on her way to Haven City Hospital. I made the drive to that hospital's ED in record time. Psychiatric APRN Brendan* spent considerable time talking with Jill, then me. He obviously knew how to work with troubled adolescents and had a good grasp on general AIP symptoms. He discussed the dangers associated with Internet online relationships, the Clinton/ Jill online connection and the fact that neither she nor her parents had actually met this person face-to-face

I said I would pursue finding out what I could about Clinton whether Jill liked it or not and whether he threatened to "cut ties" with her or not. I looked at Jill, "That in and of itself is troubling. If he said he'll always be there to support you, that doesn't sound very supportive to me!"

Brendan asked Jill if she would feel better if she could participate in my achieving my objective. Jill said yes. Then Brendan provided what turned out to be the

---

101 *Antidepressant Medications: Use in Pediatric Patients.* Center for Medicare and Medicaid Services (CMS). www.cms.gov/.../pharmacy-education-materials/downloads/ad-pediatric-factsheet.pdf. August 14, 2014.

crux of Jill's recent symptomatic behavior. "You do know, don't you that the generic name for Celexa, citalopram, is on the medication list you gave us some time ago? It's on the Possibly Porphyrinogenic list."

I was flabbergasted, "Oh noooo! I haven't used that list since the APF posted a drug database on their website and I checked that when the doctor at Mountford was looking for a safe antidepressant for Jill; Celexa had an OK! rating so I took it for granted it was safe." By then, Jill had stabilized enough to be released. I resolved to pursue the Celexa dilemma as soon as I could.

Now it was time to pursue Clinton, and Jill wanted to be involved. Once home, I dialed the police department and explained as best I could the predicament we had found ourselves in, the email messages I had discovered and Vanessa's recommendation we consult the local police department for guidance. Though I offered to go to the station, the officer said he would come out to our house. When Officer Knox* arrived, I explained what was happening, our original directive to Jill when the online communication between the two started and showed him the messages. He told Jill what he saw was inappropriate for a fourteen-year old girl to be involved with. The phone rang and caller ID indicated Clinton. I handed the phone to the officer who proceeded to ask him questions and told him that what he was looking at was not what a young girl should be involved with. The next thing we knew, Jill ran to the cupboard where her Celexa was kept and grabbed the bottle. Officer Knox was on her in a flash. She began to weep uncontrollably, saying she just wanted to die. The phone rang again. It was Clinton and he asked to speak with Officer Knox. Knox listened, then spoke about parental responsibility and expectations and said, "You sound like a really nice young man but I have to tell you, what I see is inappropriate and you need to own that. There were more exchanges and the conversation ended. He turned to Jill, "Clinton actually sounds like a nice young man. He's obviously protective of and worried about you right now. I'll do some more work and get back to your parents tomorrow with a recommendation.

Jill accused Officer Knox of "ruining my friendship with Clinton." When she could not calm down, he called for an ambulance. Jill was on her way to MedCity ED. Great. This would be the second hospitalization in one day. A few months later we discovered that my call to the Littleton Police had resulted in the arrest of fifty-something-year old "Clinton" for online child solicitation. After I had signed the requisite hospital insurance information and talked to the attending doctor who said she would be evaluated in the morning, I went home to another night of tossing and turning.

The next morning I settled in to research. Remembering the Heparin/MedCity fiasco, my stomach sunk—could Celexa contain sulfa or sulfur? I called a pharmacist to ask if Celexa/citalopram contained any trace of sulfur. After looking it up she told me it did not. I went to the computer and found what I was looking for on a National Library of Medicine (NLM)/National Institutes of Health (NIH) medication website: "Reduced hepatic function…20 mg is the recommended dose for hepatically impaired patients."[102] Ding, ding, ding, my heart skipped a beat. Jill had

---

102 *Celexa-citaprolam hydrobromide; tablet, film coated.* U.S. National Library of Medicine. DailyMed. http://dailymed.nlm.nih.gov/dailymed/search.cfm?labeltype=all&query=Celexa. April 8, 2011.

been taking well over 20 mg of Celexa daily for *months*. AIP was considered a "liver/ hepatic" disease and the information about the enzyme production problem was well-documented, but I could not find anywhere that said porphyrics were actually considered "hepatically impaired." Jill's liver tests always came out fine because the problem was with the enzyme—not the liver functioning. "Who's going to believe me now," I said to myself. I called the pharmacy again and asked for a rundown of all the dates and dosages that Celexa prescriptions had been filled for Jill. I grabbed the calendar and compared dates with the information I had just been given. The evidence was written in my own hand. "Nausea," "aches & pains," "sore throat," "stomachache," "screaming headache," "abdominal cramps?" "coming down with something," "horrible sore throat," "extreme agitation," "verbally aggressive," "cutting self" "depression" "suicidal thoughts" correlated to every boost over the original 20 mg dosage. My gut hurt. My head ached. My heart screamed. Jill had been ingesting this poison for months. *Five* doctors knew she was taking increasing dosages of Celexa and none had expressed concern. And why should they have? Even if they had known higher doses of Celexa were not recommended for hepatically impaired patients, for all any of these doctors knew, AIP patients are not considered to be hepatically impaired. This indicated to me that chemicals, which prescription medication is, could be more potent for porphyrics than the general population. Based on our unintentional Celexa experiment, when medical practitioners check blood levels for a "therapeutic dose" of certain medications, that same level could actually be considered toxic for porphyrics—especially for juvenile porphyrics.

Again, I blamed myself. I should have checked everything more thoroughly, found the information sooner and brought it to *someone's* attention. I was already considered to be over-the-top by some of the doctors I had come across, so what did I have to lose? But it was not their child living this nightmare. It was Jill and I had to make things right for her. I immediately called Drs. Nyeer, O'Connor and Alaimo and left voice messages about what I had discovered. I emailed Vanessa, Miriam and Lucy to tell them as well. I talked to Dr. Lincoln,* the MedCity doctor who was managing Jill's latest ER visit after the Clinton fiasco erupted and told him what I had discovered on the DailyMed site about Celexa/hepatic impairment connection and asked how soon the dose could safely be reduced to 20 mgs. He said, "According to her records here, she's only at 40 mgs so that's what we gave her."

"Good! So can I safely bring her down to 20 mgs within a week or so?" Dr. Lincoln said yes, that could be done. I still had not actually been told by a porphyria specialist whether porphyrics could be considered hepatically impaired, but that was how I would think of Jill from now on. After all, my kidneys work fine yet impairment of my kidney arteries had contributed to my strokes. I had long ago decided to consider myself kidney-impaired and took measures to avoid triggering symptoms.

By the time Jill returned from the hospital, she was down to 20 mgs of Celexa a day. Dr. Lincoln said she'd had "at least two seizures" while in the ED. I asked what they had done to treat her. "Nothing, she came out of them okay," he replied.

I said, "Actually, what she probably had were convulsive seizures associated with AIP and she sometimes comes out of them on her own. Simple sugars help—again,

I don't know exactly why, I just know it works. And that's why NHC's orders include D10 infusions." I signed the release papers, went to the vending machine, bought a sweetened lemonade drink and told Jill to drink it before leaving the hospital. It would have to do until she was able to get a D10 infusion.

Not only did KPS demand clearance from the hospital doctors for Jill's return to school, but they also wanted to speak to Vanessa, Dr. O'Connor *and* Dr. Nyeer before allowing her back to school. No one from KPS responded to my email update about my Celexa find and my contention that the escalating dosage of Celexa, not the heme, had likely been the culprit in Jill's latest problem. I wrote, "Because most people have no knowledge of heme or its usage, it was the obvious target, yet the fact that the top dose of an *adult-strength* antidepressant being administered daily to a juvenile was never even considered problematic." Actually, KPS's response was on the way but we would not know that for a few days. When it arrived, we would realize that Doris' offer to help was nothing more than an expansion of Littleton's GOTCHAJill! game into GOTCHAEDandJOYCE!

CHAPTER 57

Acid Rain

Judge a man [or woman] by his [her]
question rather than his [her] answer.
— VOLTAIRE

Jill had been down to 20 mgs of Celexa for a couple of days. Her agitation and physical complaints had begun to calm down noticeably. But because KPS was still waiting to hear from the doctors, she was home for the day. The doorbell rang and I opened the door to Department of Children and Families (DCF) social worker Clara.* She told me, Ed and Jill the purpose for her being there was to investigate allegations of abuse and Jill's truancy from school. The complaint had KPS stamped all over it. I had copies of diagnoses, medical records, test results, school reports and communication to and from doctors since the fall of 2007, so had plenty of tangible evidence to answer Clara's questions. The Clinton issue came up which led Clara to ask about discipline and, specifically, the incident when I had hit Jill. During my explanation of what had happened, Jill left the room. Clara asked if she could speak with her alone. Then Clara spoke with Kevin. When she asked him how Jill was disciplined Kevin said, "Losing privileges like the computer, phone, iPod, stuff like that." When she asked if there was ever any physical discipline, Kevin said, "No, but I think Jill gets away with too much."

Jill then launched into a tirade, saying she wanted to get away from "this house and these people!"

Clara said, "You really want to go? I can make that happen if you really want that."

Jill said yes, she wanted "out of this place."

Clara looked at me. I said, "If you do end up taking her, I just want you to know she really *does* have a life-threatening illness. After being stable for *months*, she got worse while at KPS. I just found out something that supports my suppositions that

Jill has been going to school 'under the influence.'" Clara looked puzzled. I continued, "She's been taking increasing prescribed doses of Celexa, a medication deemed safe by the American Porphyria Foundation—I can pull it up on the computer if you'd like—but a sharp Haven City Hospital APRN pointed out last week that it is on the potentially unsafe drug list from a different porphyria organization. I discovered an NIH medication website that says hepatically impaired people should not be taking more than 20 mg—and Jill had been taking 60, then it was increased to 80 mg a day! Obviously, her system is not fully weaned from it, so this is what we have—Jill "sort of under the influence." I continued, "There are many AIP triggers and we've found they cannot always be avoided. For Jill, stress is a big one but toxins are worse. She is extraordinarily susceptible to low level toxins, normal stuff you'd never think could harm anyone. But if she does go into attack and ultimately dies, I have to tell you that could be on your and the State's shoulders. It's up to you." I handed her the printout from the www.dailymed.nlm.nih.gov website about Celexa. "Now I just have to find out from the porphyria experts the answer to the question, "Are AIPorphyrics considered to be hepatically impaired?'"

I continued, "What concerns us is KPS has said Jill can't return to school until they've spoken to Vanessa, Dr. O'Connor *and* Dr. Nyeer. That could take some time. Dr. Nyeer is out of the country and tough to get a hold of anyway. In my opinion, KPS is withholding Jill's right to education. They are supposed to be an accredited special education school, yet their academic *and* therapeutic approaches are terribly lacking, which we've complained about. That's probably what started all this." Clara took lots of information with her and promised to get back to us. In the end, Jill ended up staying home for two weeks with no extraordinary health crises. I added Clara to the round-robin of people to update.

I had been pushing Jill to do her VLA online computer science program during the "boring' vacation," but the Jill who doggedly fulfilled schoolwork obligations was gone. She kept letting it slide. The vacation was winding down and we looked ahead to a quiet Easter. Jill had earned her landline phone privileges back when early Saturday evening, she said, "I'm going for a walk. I need some exercise and to get out of the house."

Ed's antennae picked up. "Who are you going to meet?"

"NO ONE!" she shouted and left. I busied myself but kept an eye on the clock. After an hour, it was getting dark and I began to get nervous. The phone rang. "Mom? I'm at the gas station, can you come get me?" Jill said.

"First of all, *why* are you at the gas station? You said you were going for a walk! And *why* are you calling me on *my* cell phone—you're still grounded from cell phones!" I said.

"Kandis was having a bad day; she asked me to meet her at the gas station, so I rode my bike here," she answered. I was aggravated, told her she could ride her bike back home and hung up. My head bells started jumping. It was beginning to drizzle so I drove to the gas station with Kevin. Jill and Kandis were sitting on the sidewalk in the drizzling rain. Thoroughly annoyed, I told Jill to get on her bike and to start peddling home. To Kandis I said, "You can start walking home." Jill whined, "Come on mom, can't we just put the bike in the car, you drive Kandis home then take me home?"

"No, you told your father and me you were going for a walk. You said nothing about going to the gas station or about meeting Kandis. *And* you took *my* cell phone. You rode your bike here, you can ride it back." I was determined and said I would follow her in the car with the lights on and told her to either start walking or ped-dling. Jill began walking the bike up the hill. Then my conscience got a hold of me, "She already rode her bike here; it's drizzling and starting to get dark; she got 'caught' though she *did* call me knowing she'd get in trouble, and physical *and* emotional stress can spark attacks. I'll tell her to stop at the corner—that will be enough." Just when I had gotten to that thought Jill stumbled, dropped the bike and sat on the wet ground, looking as though she might vomit. I parked, left the lights on, jumped out of the car in my socks, told Kevin to put her bike in the back of the car and said to Jill, "Get in the car, we're going home." She started hollering.

I hoped the earth would just open up and swallow me whole! A couple came out of a nearby house, "What's going on here?" the man yelled, concerned to see Jill sitting on the ground crying.

I answered, "This is my daughter. She's fourteen and snuck out of the house to meet a friend. She had been grounded from the home phone but took my cell phone and called me to come pick her up *and* wanted me to bring her friend home. I was making her walk or ride her bike home, had just decided she'd had enough punishment and was telling her to get in the car when she collapsed. She's really mad at me, and yes, I'm mad at her too."

He said the police had been called and he and his wife would wait there until "someone in authority" arrived. As community members, they were doing the right thing but I thought, "Great, *two* encounters with the PD in as many weeks." I asked Kevin to shut the car off (I'd left it running, thinking everything would be over in a matter of minutes). The officer arrived, recognized Jill and said he was familiar with her condition. By this time, Jill was repeating she wanted to die. The officer called for an ambulance. I asked Kevin to move the car so the ambulance could maneuver better. The car wouldn't start. "Surreal" doesn't begin to describe the circumstances. Kevin called Ed and asked him to come. Jill fell over in a faint and started convuls-ing. Ed arrived in the midst of the chaos. Jill came to briefly, but then fainted and resumed convulsing again. Ed used his jumper cables to start my car and move it. He gave a statement to the officer that confirmed the series of events I had just told. The ambulance arrived and surprisingly, the EMT asked which hospital Jill should be brought to! I asked why he was asking; we'd been told so many times that she *had* to be brought to MedCity. He replied, "If a medic is available, she can be brought to NHC—and a medic is on the way."

"Why hadn't anybody just told us that? It would have made things so much smoother these past few years," I said. Though she was clearly exhibiting symptoms, this time I opted for MedCity, "as long as you keep oxygen on her and remind the doctors that she has *acute intermittent porphyria*, to use Dr. O'Connor's medical plan that is in their system and if she begins convulsing again, to *please* give her Ativan. I'll be along as soon as I can. The EMT came to the car window, "What's the name of that disease Jill has?" he asked. I responded, "Acute…Intermittent…poor-FEAR-ee-ya—a, devilish affliction."

By the time I had arrived at the ED, Jill had revived. "I'm sorry, mom, I shouldn't have taken your cell and I shouldn't have sneaked out of the house to meet Kandis. But she was really upset and depressed about her boyfriend and I just wanted to help her. Actually, I didn't really want to go. But she needed me."

"Well, you made really poor choices and now your grounding is extended," I told her. A doctor asked me to step into the hallway, "Jill will be staying the night and will be evaluated by a clinician tomorrow. I have to tell you, at first blush I have concerns along the lines of a personality disorder, but from what I've seen, many times with patients who have a history of depression and self-mutilation, inpatient placement doesn't improve but worsens the condition." "Thank you for saying that," I said. "Jill's been inpatient a couple of times and I have to say only once, at the very beginning of this ordeal, did it help. I recently discovered a problem with the Celexa she had been taking and notified Dr. Lincoln from this hospital, her prescribing psychiatrist, her hematologist, her PCP and of course her therapist of that. She's now down to 20 mgs and had been doing well until this. She did a typical teenage thing in sneaking out, got caught and between the physical stress of pushing the bike up a hill and the emotional stress that went along with everything, not to mention the level of Celexa in her system may not yet be down to 20 mg, she had an episode. You know, I can't even discipline my child in a safe manner without the possibility of an attack hanging over my head!"

The doctor said that I could stay the night with Jill if I chose to. I went back into Jill's room. She was terribly pale and complaining that where the Ativan shot they had given her hurt, that she "felt horrible," was nauseous and her chest hurt. Remembering the lemonade, I offered to go to the vending machine for a sweet drink. She nodded her head. When I returned, she said, "Mom, I feel really, really bad. Would you please stay tonight? I need heme. I want to get heme tomorrow." This was the first time in a very long time that Jill had said she needed and wanted heme. She did look terrible. I was afraid to leave her in that condition and said I would stay the night so a nurse brought a reclining chair for me.

CHAPTER 58

Dense Fog

*Just because a person successfully steers
a voyage through hell doesn't mean he
ever wants to sail that route again.*
— **RICHELLE E. GOODRICH**

I watched the clock throughout the night. By six a.m. I had had enough of the hospital. Jill was sleeping and I headed home for a few hours of real sleep. When I returned, Jill was fitful, had hardly eaten any breakfast and complained her stomach hurt. I asked when the doctor might be seeing her. "Rounds end at noon, he'll be in by then," was the crisp reply. Finally Dr. Lincoln arrived. He listened carefully first to Jill and then to my story about what had happened to land her in the ED again. In the end, he reminded Jill that responsible parents "ground" kids and "after what happened yesterday, you're probably going to have to endure a longer grounding. It's something every kid I know of, my own included, have to live with." He cleared her for release. I asked if she could go back to school the next day, he said, "Absolutely." We went home, I popped the ham in the oven, prepared side dishes and we all sat down to Easter dinner.

The next morning, with Dr. Lincoln's approval and not having heard anything from KPS, Jill went to school. By noon, the phone rang. Emma at KPS said, "Jill's on her way by ambulance to Haven City Children's Hospital. You need to get there ASAP."

"Why? What happened?" I asked.

"She fainted and had a seizure," Emma replied shortly.

"Did they put oxygen on her?" I asked.

"Yes." I was on my way, head bells ringing. Jill was awake and alert when I arrived at the ED. She said brightly, Rosa's father said to say "Hi to your mom and dad," so "Hi!" I had forgotten that Jim worked in that city as an EMT.

Changing the subject I said, "So, I guess your first day back to school in a while didn't turn out so well, huh?"

Jill replied, "No, it was a weird day. First the van had some kind of problem, so they brought me to the high school to wait for another van."

I jumped to my feet, "*You went to Littleton High School? Today? Did you go into the building?*" "Yes, today and yes, I went into the building," she answered.

"Oh my Christ, please help us," I moaned.

Jill continued, "I had to go to Mr. Knight*'s office and wait for another van to come."

I was reeling, "How long were you in there?"

"Twenty minutes or so, I guess," she answered.

"Did anything at all in your body feel different while you were in there?"

"I was shaking—but I was just nervous. I don't like Mr. Knight and I was wondering what was up with the bus. After a while I got on another bus and went to KPS. I was kind of nauseous on the ride there and it got worse and worse. I got to school then I just fainted and here I am." I was sick to my stomach, too. After all my efforts to keep her out of the Littleton schools, she had been made to go into the LMS/LHS school complex, and the shaking, nausea, fainting and convulsions had returned.

"Did you have any candy or a Gatorade with you?" I asked. "No, I just thought I'd get over it." The fact that Jill's "shaking" had commenced shortly after entering the building told me that her body had reacted quickly to whatever was in there and by the time she got to KPS, her symptoms had escalated to fainting and convulsions. "I told Tori about the bus problem and being brought to LHS," she finished. I was livid. There *was* something toxic to Jill in Littleton schools, I *knew* it. And this time it'd taken less than half an hour of being in the school for Jill to end up in an ED.

During the D10 infusion, hospital social worker Myra* came in to talk about how Jill ended up in the ED this time. Myra asked if I wanted Jill to have a psych eval. I thanked her for the offer but said Jill had an LCSW therapist and they were to meet in a few days. She asked if by any chance the State was involved in Jill's case. I said, "As a matter of fact, yes. A state social worker is investigating alleged abuse and Jill's truancy from school." Myra asked how much school Jill had missed. I replied, "According to a recent PPT, 46% percent of the school days." I explained about Jill's AIP, the increasing Celexa dosage, how the Haven Hospital APRN brought the medication to my attention and how I had discovered the problem with Celexa and hepatic-impaired patients.

Myra looked at Jill, "Even though you missed a lot of school, have you been able to keep up with your make-up work?"

Jill replied, "They don't give me make-up work." Myra's eyebrows raised, "They don't?"

Jill replied, "Nope. And they don't give me homework, tests or quizzes, either. It's a very weird school that way."

"Well," Myra continued, "it's kind of hard to call a student truant when the school doesn't help by not giving make-up work."

I said, "For a State accredited special education school, I find it very disconcerting that their academic program is so lacking that they won't teach Jill in a style she requires. She's been *very* frustrated for the past few months which hasn't helped her motivation at all."

"Nonetheless, she should have been given make-up work every time she missed any session," the social worker said. "I would be better able to understand why they're making a big deal about truancy if they had been fulfilling their responsibilities."

After she left, I called Vanessa to tell her the latest and to ask her if she agreed with not having another psych eval done. "Absolutely," she said. "What can they tell us we don't already know?" Then she said she'd secured a place in St. Michael's outpatient DBT group (dialectical behavior therapy—a form of psychotherapy developed by Seattle-based author and psychologist Marsha Linehan "that helps patients address problematic behaviors such as suicidal and/or self-harming) by practicing mindfulness and distress tolerance techniques along with employing concrete strategies"[103] for Jill and an intake appointment was set for the coming Monday.

I then called Miriam to give her the same update and to ask if she would contact Bart or the school district's attorney and tell them Jill was never to be made to go into a Littleton school building again. "I understand your distress but what could they have done differently?" Miriam asked.

"I believe there is communication between transportation 'headquarters' and the bus drivers via radio and/or cell phone, right? They could have left Jill on the bus—with an adult, if necessary, and explained the situation/predicament they were in about not having a bus available to bring her to KPS right then. They could have sent another bus, called us to bring her, whatever," I said, angrily.

"You're right. Those are doable suggestions. I'll call right now," Miriam said.

Discharge papers in hand, we left the hospital. That evening, Lillian called to ask about Jill and to say they had been surprised when she had shown up at school because they had not heard from Dr. Nyeer yet. I told her no one had called to tell us that so we had sent her to school and, besides, Littleton clearly figured everything was all set because they had sent the van for her. I then told her sending Jill into LHS that morning had likely triggered the attack. Lillian ignored that and said they still needed a letter from Vanessa clearing Jill's return to school again. I asked, "In addition to you still waiting to hear from Dr. Nyeer?"

"Yes."

I was perturbed, "Wait a minute, Jill has been out of school for over two weeks—at *KPS' insistence*, a week's vacation is over, and no one from KPS notified us about not having talked to Dr. Nyeer yet so she was not allowed in school—the school that wanted her so badly in January? *Really?* And talking about school, a hospital

103 Potter, AM. *Escape from Hell, Rejecting Suicide, How Marsha Linehan's Pioneer Therapy Saved My Life.* Special to The Hartford Courant. July 27, 2011.

social worker questioned KPS's truancy claim and said it was inappropriate to have labeled a student truant yet not provided make-up work for her." I reminded her that Jill, Ed and I had each brought up the issue of deficient academics with KPS before. I added I would contact Bart and ask if he would call Dr. Nyeer and request that he please contact KPS. After that, I said, I was done. If KPS didn't want her back until someone there spoke to him, then KPS would have to deal with Littleton, the State of Connecticut and anyone else about why Jill's education was being withheld. Lillian was not happy.

The next day Jill felt well enough to help out with my final CCD class of the year and to say good-bye to the students. The mail brought notification that she was number seven on the waiting list for the coming SFTA year; there was a chance she might get in but that would not be known for sure until the end of June. I decided not to say anything to Jill about it. She had enough going on and seemed excited about the upcoming DBT group therapy program that Vanessa had arranged. Jill was stabilizing but the bizarre world in which our family existed continued to morph.

CHAPTER 59

Blue Moon

If you're going through hell, keep going.
— WINSTON CHURCHILL

At Jill's next therapy session, Vanessa said she had cleared her for return to KPS but that apparently was not in the KPS ladies' (Doris, Lillian and Lucy) game plan. She said she and they had had a lengthy, "intense" speakerphone conversation in which they claimed Jill faked all her symptoms and they did not believe she had von Willebrand, either. One said she had reached Dr. O'Connor and spoke with him about the heme treatments he had approved for Jill, and what Vanessa got out of it was that KPS pointed the finger directly at me. I said, "Well if they talked to Dr. O'Connor, *why* hadn't they asked *him* whether or not Jill had von Willebrand? He's been treating her for it for years! Furthermore, I've been accused of having Munchausen by Proxy by better trained people than them!" I was furious to hear KPS had sunk below even the repulsive level of the Littleton School District and wondered if they had used the same technique with Drs. O'Connor and Nyeer who had supported our family through AIP hell and back. Thankfully, both doctors said they had shrugged off KPS' intent.

As Jill and I were preparing to drive to the first DBT session, Clara stopped by to give me a copy of a letter she had received from KPS. In it, Lucy (and KPS) enumerated, "...concerns regarding Jill's emotional and physical wellbeing, pointed out Jill's self-injurious behavior, seizure activity and hospitalizations over a matter of weeks and that they had "...requested... Jill be psychiatrically cleared to attend school by her treating psychiatrist... [and] ...outpatient therapist...hope that this clears up any confusion or questions regarding Jill's absence from our program."[104]

---

104 KPS* social worker Lucy.* Letter to Littleton* SE director. May, 2011.

It was clear this was a CYA (cover your a##) letter, probably because I had told Lucy that the hospital social worker had challenged that no make-up work had been given to Jill, yet KPS was complaining of Jill's truancy.

In my opinion, I told Clara, AIP had been very much in control of what had been happening for at least the past month. I said it was no surprise to me that Lucy had called DCF to lodge an "abuse" complaint. But when parents are doing everything aboveboard, I said, they need not worry about being investigated. We were not. In fact, like the time Jill ended up in juvenile court, I welcomed letting the officials in on what happened in schools where inept administrators ran rampant. I explained how APRN Brendan had talked with Jill and me about the Clinton/California situation, questioned the Celexa Jill had been prescribed and that she had been discharged from the hospital less than *six hours* after her KPS-reported suicide threat. I said it was apparently okay for KPS to overlook an overdose of an antidepressant carrying clear warnings about potential adolescent suicide ideations, attempts or actual accomplishments—but they were up on their high horses about *heme*—which had been proven to be beneficial for Jill many times over.

Clara was not pleased at KPS's attempt to "try to go in a back door to get this PPT" because it wasn't a social worker's job to call a PPT, she said. Then she asked what my intentions were for writing a book (KPS had obviously expressed misgivings about my intentions). I said, "To tell Jill's story, to spread the word about acute intermittent porphyria and to hopefully help others who may find themselves in similar situations. If Jill *is* the only kid to suffer so badly from manifest AIP that she has to be treated with heme/glucose infusions, I don't think she will be the last, not with the ongoing replication of genes throughout the generations and today's toxin-overloaded society," I continued. "If we could get attention directed 1) to juvenile-onset AIP so that parents/caregivers, doctors or schools with a child, pediatric patient or student who exhibits recurrent, weird, unexplainable neurological symptoms, especially in school, might say, 'Wait a minute…could it be…porphyria?' and 2) God-willing, DNA testing might become reasonably priced and available for insurance company or individual payment, much like a blood test or other diagnostics to rule the disorder in or out, then maybe far fewer kids and their parents will have to go through this nightmare. Because that's what it's been—a nightmare," I ended. Clara understood and said KPS's "help" had turned into a big mess. Ed and I welcomed Clara's planned attendance at the PPT; I said I would fax KPS's letter to Miriam. Then I drove Jill to her DBT group therapy meeting.

A parent support group meeting was scheduled to follow the DBT program and I decided to attend. Jill agreed to wait in the car for the extra hour. As I sat in the parent group discussion, my eyes were continually drawn to the floor to ceiling, corner to corner white board covering the majority of the room. It was filled with hand written notes, goals and/or encouragements from and/or for the twenty or so adolescents in the program—all written with black dry-erase markers.

Small head bells chimed. The parent discussion was interesting and helpful. I hoped Jill would do well in the program. She finally had another "group" to be a part of. When it was time to leave, the car would not start. I called AAA roadside assistance for help. The technician responded quickly, performed a diagnostic test, provided a printout that indicated a new battery was needed and got the car started. I thanked the tech and then looked more closely at the printout and chuckled. "This is just what *you* need," I said to Jill, "a printout telling how much heme is in your liver when you need to know it. And, if we could get one that tells us the level of toxins in your system, that'd be awesome!"

That afternoon, a lengthy email with pages of makeup work attached appeared from Tori. Jill reviewed the material, then remarked, "Just like in school, no help, but *do the work, Jill!*"

She liked the DBT program but within a day or so complained of a "screaming headache" for which she took Tylenol and went to bed. The headache had tapered off the next morning. "But it feels like it could come back," she said. Dr. Mellon* called from the program the next day to report Jill had had a "pseudo-seizure." She described the seizure activity and I explained that the seizures Jill sometimes had were "sort of atypical, more like convulsions." She asked lots of questions about EEGs and neurological workups. I told her Jill had been evaluated neurologically at least five or six times, three during the past couple years alone and that she had had three or four EEGs including one in which she was required to sleep and an MRI in 2007 and everything had been found to be "in the range." I'd begun calling them "convulsive seizures," I said, because that was the best way I could describe them. At the time, to my knowledge no one had ever had an EEG machine available during any of Jill's seizures. Then I told her about Jill's possible toxin/AIP connection. As with so many before her, Dr. Mellon dismissed the notion.

She told me Jill had "come out of the pseudo-seizure" and wanted to know if I would allow her to go on the regular transportation to get home. I approved that and Jill came home complaining of a "killer headache." The first DBT week came to a close and Jill came home with yet another killer headache. She was fine on Saturday. By Sunday, I felt Jill might have had a reaction to the white boards covered with *black* dry-erase marker writing. So I faxed an explanation to Dr. Mellon:

> It occurred to me I could provide you with information that may be helpful for the remainder of Jill's DBT treatment time. The recent convulsive 'episode' Jill experienced could of course be attributed to emotional/psychiatric reasons. However, in order to make the most of the services offered to her and to minimize the potential of future disruptions for staff and patients, I offer the following suggestion based on the past four years of observing, recording and dealing with Jill's AIP. Please bear with me; I am in no way attempting to tell you how to 'run your ship,' merely sharing information in an attempt to make the time she spends there as productive for everyone as possible. As you know, Jill has been diagnosed with a genetic disorder caused by a liver enzyme deficiency. We have seen Jill react with symptoms due to certain toxin exposure/ingestion time and again. Under suspicion are the ingredients found in dry-erase markers. I ask you to make one modest accommodation to see if Jill's performance/

tolerance level improves. Simply change the color markers used on the white board and use black minimally or not at all. During her 8th grade school year I asked the same of some of her teachers. Two switched to lighter color ink markers, one continued to use black exclusively. With one exception, Jill's 'episodes' continued to happen in the class that used only black markers (the other time was in the chemistry lab which makes sense to most everyone).

Jill's body (liver) and brain are very much a 'growing' work in progress and of course there could be any number of reasons for the other day's convulsive episode. If you have any thoughts, suggestions, etc., please do not hesitate to contact me.

I faxed the message late that Sunday night. By Tuesday, Jill reported that the black markers had been put away and the teens only had access to the lighter color markers.

The next day a letter arrived from Bart, wanting to arrange tutoring for Jill. "I guess that means KPS is done," I told Ed. Lizabeth called within a day or so to arrange a tutoring time. In the meantime Tori had emailed another package of "make-up" work. "Why would Littleton pay both KPS *and* a tutor?" I wondered. Actually at that point, I really didn't care—as far as I was concerned, we were done with KPS.

Jill and I met with the allergist who had diagnosed her as being allergic to cashews, to talk about chemical testing. I was worried, though, that if he did test for certain chemicals she might have a bad reaction. In the end, I need not have worried. Dr. Shriner* said he could not do the type of testing Jill needed. He suggested I seek a tertiary facility that conducted such research and listed a few for me to check into. I checked out their websites but couldn't find anything I thought would help so decided I'd have to brainstorm another avenue.

Clara arrived for a scheduled visit and said the PPT had been scheduled at KPS and that Dr. O'Connor had agreed to be available by speakerphone. Ed exploded, "*Why* is the meeting at *KPS*? *Littleton* is in charge of Jill's education, not KPS—the school that put ridiculous conditions on us about not letting her back in until they'd harassed the doctors and Jill's therapist. And who the hell does KPS think they are, demanding the head of NHC's *Hematology* be available to talk to *them*?"

I said, "Ed's right—the meeting should be in Littleton and if KPS wants to be there, they can send someone to represent them. Why in the world Littleton would acquiesce to KPS is beyond me. I'll contact Miriam to see what can be done about this." Clara asked if we would sign a release so she could also "talk to Littleton because Bart had told her, 'Get a release; I'll tell you all about the bullying Jill Gould was responsible for.'"

The combination of KPS's malicious and meddlesome intentions and Jill's recent reactivity to both LHS's internal environment and Celexa had rekindled my determination to find out more about toxin triggers for Jill. Some dots had begun to connect, and I felt we were making progress.

CHAPTER 60

Water Spout

A society is judged by how it treats its weakest members.
— HARRY TRUMAN

"Outrageous!" Miriam said after reading KPS's letter that I had faxed to her. She told Littleton's attorney we would *not* attend a PPT at KPS but *would* attend if it was held in Littleton. She said it did not matter whether anyone from KPS attended because they were pretty much out of the picture. Bart agreed the PPT would be held in Littleton. The next day he contacted her to say KPS would not be there, but they would send a final educational report.

Clara was already at LHS when Ed and I arrived for the PPT. As we approached the meeting room, a school counselor and high school teacher who knew Kevin greeted us and asked how he was doing. They would be participating in Jill's PPT and this time, nurse Larry was on hand, too. Ed and I left a space between us for Miriam to sit in case we needed to communicate with her during the meeting. Bart started the meeting with introductions then launched into reading KPS's letter aloud. I was immediately infuriated—he had said KPS would be sending a final educational report and here he was reading Lucy's letter! It was definitely *not* an educational report. Bart concluded with, "The district feels KPS is an appropriate school setting for Jill to return to." At this point, KPS had withheld Jill from school for over a month. They had taught her virtually nothing in the four months she had spent there, made her totally frustrated and had slandered her. They had harassed and harangued three important professionals involved in Jill's care, two of whom had been with us through precarious medical phases. KPS's entire academic and therapeutic program was bogus—and the spurious *educational report* reeked of it.

I snapped, "*Jill will never walk through KPS's doors again. Ever.*" I felt the people on either side of me stiffen. "That report is garbage. I can't believe you would even *think* of reading it in this venue! Of course, nothing was said about the too high levels of Celexa Jill was expected to deal with, right?" At that, I saw Larry's brow furrow. As a nurse, he knew the problems medications could cause for Jill. Then, Bart laughed. A big, full grin accompanied the condescending laugh. My head bells screamed with rage. I demanded, *"WHY ARE YOU LAUGHING?"*

Ed yelled, "YOU THINK THIS IS FUNNY, BART? WELL IT ISN'T!" He continued, "Can anyone tell me how a school that *doesn't give homework, doesn't have tests and doesn't have quizzes* can adequately grade a student? And how about KPS claiming she's truant, but never gave her any makeup work?"

Penelope,* Littleton's attorney began, "Well, it *is* accredited by the State." Then she shrugged. Miriam tugged at Ed's sleeve, trying to get him to calm down. Clara took it all in, stone-faced. The guidance counselor and Kevin's former teacher looked stricken. Bart passed around two releases that would allow him to talk to Dr. Mellon at St. Michael's DBT program. They were blank. "Oh…no," I said firmly, "we *are not* doing this again." I filled in the date, Dr. Mellon's name and the program she was affiliated with then slashed through the remaining blank lines and sections. I gave them to Ed. "Remember last year? Don't ever sign anything this guy gives you that is blank," I said, glaring at Bart. Then I let Miriam take over. She knew what we wanted for Jill. If I had opened my mouth again, there would have been real trouble. The subject of tutoring was brought up. Jill would resume tutoring for the remainder of the school year. Bart said Lizabeth had mentioned we were also interested in summer tutoring. He said something about the summer program at LHS. I wrote Miriam a note, "Jill *cannot* be in the building!" Miriam said something about a tutorial. I was too drained to follow the discussion. Miriam took the reins and the PPT ended with plans to reconvene during the summer to make fall plans. Ed, Miriam and I gathered in the parking lot. Clara joined us saying, "I'm closing the investigation. The charges brought by KPS are unsubstantiated."

Gesturing at me and Ed, Miriam said to Clara, "They've cooperated fully with every professional or authority concerning Jill."

"Exactly. That's what I've seen," Clara said.

Ed returned Jill's books to KPS and gave them a letter indicating that all releases we had signed for them were immediately revoked. They were not to contact Dr. O'Connor, Dr. Nyeer, or Vanessa again. Then it was time to focus once again on the tutoring issue. Until it was arranged, I suggested Jill work on the online computer science program she had started in January. I was angry, but not surprised to see virtually nothing had been done beyond the first half of the first chapter. Obviously, Tori had never even looked at what Jill was doing, which had been nothing.

The DBT program manager called during the second week to tell me that Jill was on her way to the hospital. "Was she convulsing?" I asked, immediately worried and wondering which hospital I was headed to now.

"No, she didn't have an AIP attack. She couldn't handle something she was confronted with during the session. She's on her way to St. Michael's Hospital in Haven City because she threatened to hurt herself. Do you know where the hospital is located?" I sighed, said yes and went.

Jill was stable when I arrived. While the doctor completed the required physical exam, I met with the clinician and nurse assigned to Jill's case. Both Donna* and Darren* remembered us from the previous summer. They were particularly interested in the asymptomatic months Jill had had, the Celexa-induced problems and the cutting. In signing releases, one of the clinicians said something about "not needing to bother with the school" which was good, because I wouldn't have signed for them to talk with either KPS or Littleton anyway. Jill was safe for the night and had connected with a girl in the next room—a fellow DBT group member.

The next morning I spoke to Dr. Mellon and we both agreed it would do Jill good to stay at St. Michael's for a few days. Soon after ending that call, however, Dr. Frank* called to say he was nervous about Jill staying there for the long Memorial Day weekend because she had not slept well and had complained of stomach pains upon waking. Besides, he said, the clinicians would not be in during the three-day weekend to run programs and he could not guarantee that the change in weekend staff would not create a problem. I said I was reluctant to take her out because I thought she would benefit from longer term inpatient support. Then he asked if I would consider Lamictal as a medication to help Jill with her depressive tendency. "I'm sorry, but after what she's just been through with the Celexa, we just can't chance it," I said.

"It's on that list you gave us last time you were here, same as Celexa," he said, "but it's metabolized differently and doesn't seem to distress the mutant gene-affected liver enzyme." I told him I was still leery about using it because the APF drug database had no safety rating on it. He said, "Hold on a minute," then came back to the phone. He had checked an online international physician site and said, "Apparently, it's been used uneventfully by six patients with acute porphyria," and offered several other chemical/therapeutic/metabolism-related facts.

My heart in my throat, I said, "Then I guess we have to give a minimal dose a try. But I'll check the website where I found the Celexa information before I give it to her." He said he would arrange for Jill to rejoin the DBT program early in the week and asked when I planned to pick her up; the nurse shift change was scheduled for 3:00. I said I'd be there before then to bring Jill home.

CHAPTER 61

Clearing Skies

Life isn't about waiting for the storm to pass; it's about learning how to dance in the rain.
— VIVIAN GREENE

Jill's body, mind and spirit had been ravaged so much that I truly wondered if she would mend. Out of Littleton's and KPS's clutches, she began to improve. But I still worried about residual effects of all she had been through. Littleton approved summer school tutoring, largely because KPS's academic program had been so shabby. With my constant harping, she finished the online computer science program. She also successfully completed the DBT program without further incident.

We located an outpatient DBT adolescent group and Jill started there. After six weeks she expressed annoyance that "some of the kids are driving me crazy about dumb things" that I interpreted to mean she had made progress and it was time to find a school for her to start her sophomore year. Returning to Littleton was off the table; nothing had changed there as far as Jill's health impact was concerned.

I began another search for a suitable school. After the PPT blowout, Bart was more responsive and sent Jill's complete records to the potential schools I had selected. Burton Academy (B.A.) extended an invitation to attend an intake session. This time, the subject of Jill's porphyria was addressed. B.A. was receptive to not only learning about AIP, but also listened to our concerns about school toxins and readily responded to my request to eliminate black dry-erase markers throughout the school. We left with the clear understanding that Burton Academy was a therapeutic school with a population comprised of special education students, many of whom could be deemed "troubled."

Jill shrugged. "Most of the kids that were after me at Littleton were *troubled,*" she said. And she was happy to hear about the academic expectations—note-taking, homework, quizzes and tests were regular parts of school activity and though class sizes were small, grades were separated and moved from room to room. There was gym class, a lunch room, field trips and a year-end talent show. We submitted her application and Jill was accepted.

Before the start of school Jill met an LHS junior online who had noticed her Facebook page, messaged her and asked to meet her. I agreed, but only if I met him and his parent(s) too. Jeremy's* mother accompanied him to meet us at a local movie theater. As we stood talking in the parking lot, his mother gestured to Jill's neckline and asked if she had a port. Jill moved her neckline to show the mark better and acknowledged that yes, she had a port. Sarah* responded to our questioning looks by sharing that Jeremy's older brother, Derek,* had lost his battle with cancer within the year. Of course we shared condolences then explained about Jill's AIP; it was clear Jeremy and his family had had plenty of experience with NHC, too. Unfortunately, within a month or so, he and Jill had cooled. Jeremy was unable to become involved with someone who needed NHC's oncology department's regular care, which was understandable.

Thankfully, Jill quickly got into the swing of the Burton Academy school year. As promised, academics were a priority. She was relieved to see adult responses when it came to managing "problem" students. For the most part, the kids at B.A. were there because they had been removed from their home school districts because of behavioral problems. Many were rough and boorish—to everyone. Jill was regaining her sense of self and though she sometimes "smart-mouthed" her peers back, she refused to taunt anyone. Most referred to her as "Goody Two-Shoes" and more than a few tried their best to get her to act out. It was a daily struggle.

By October, we learned she had not made it into SFTA so she settled in for her sophomore year at B.A. where she appreciated the clinical support. Kandis invited Jill to "chill" with her at the Dudleytown* Fair where they met up with some of Kandis' other friends. Arnold,* a Littleton senior, liked Jill and soon they became an "item." Since she had been out of Littleton schools for so long, she had little knowledge of the student cliques. But it did not take long to figure out that Arnold did what he wanted to do when he wanted to do it with or without parental knowledge or assent. He did not like that we kept fairly close tabs on Jill and resented our parental expectations. Nonetheless, he exuberantly invited Jill to his senior prom and seemed infatuated with her—for a while. He even accompanied us on a shopping quest for a prom dress. Jill was eagerly looking forward to a chance to dress up and dance; she had missed school social functions for so long. One evening Jill was invited to join Arnold's family for dinner at a local restaurant. A few hours later, a distraught Mia* came to the front door to say, "Something's wrong with Jill. She's in the car." I went out to the driveway. The back door of their car was open; Jill was sitting in the back seat, leaning against Arnold. She was non-responsive and her arms and hands were beginning to twitch. I asked if she had been exposed to cigarette smoke, if she had drunk anything but soda or if she had been around anything that "smelled weird" like glue or smoke or something—*anything*? All heads shook no.

Ed, Kevin and I maneuvered Jill out of their car and into ours, put her seat belt on her and locked the door. I turned to Ed, "Call the doctor's office right away, tell them Jill is in attack mode and we're on our way to NHC's ED. Ask them to call ahead and give them a heads up. I turned the fresh air intake vents on full blast and headed to the hospital. Unbelievably, by the time we had arrived, Jill had revived enough to walk unaided into the reception area. While I parked the car she was put into a room. The only reason for Jill's attack I could think of was maybe Arnold's and/or Mia's school work clothing had been splashed by the cleaning fluid. Had Jill's sensitivities become so bad that fabric entrapment of toxins was cause for concern? Thankfully, a D10 infusion made her well.

When Arnold and his family left for vacation things really started unraveling. The teens kept cell phones blazing. Jill was frequently aggravated because Arnold's phone either kept losing its signal or she would hear his friend, Quincy,* in the background goading about things that were not his business to be commenting on. I advised her to stop calling Arnold and suggested she let him call *her* back if and when he wanted to talk. Jill ignored my advice and resumed calling every time his phone "died." So Arnold told Jill it was over—and to forget going to the prom. She discovered via Facebook that Arnold had already replaced her as his prom date with none other than Camerin! Jill was bereft. Dumped from the only social situation she had had to look forward to since the first dance of her eighth grade year in favor of the queen bee of the girl bully clique was devastating. Shortly thereafter, Jill was told by a prom-goer that Camerin had split well before it ended to hook up with another guy, leaving Arnold alone at his senior prom.

Life went on for Jill. She entered the SFTA lottery again and decided to participate in Burton Academy's annual talent show. She signed up for the Littleton's Parks and Recreation Department's summer camp Counselor In Training (CIT) program, hoping it would be a good experience. I was nervous because the day camps are held in and around Littleton school buildings. But I believed since school would not be in session, dry-erase markers would not be in use and doors would sometimes be left open, letting fresh air into the buildings. I prayed that Jill would be safe.

CHAPTER 62

Cloudy Spells

*Another mountain to climb. The sun burns
hot as the devil's eye. There's chaos on the rise.
The sky is raining knives. We have mistaken the
toll that it's taken on you and I.*

— **AS SUNG BY THREE DAYS GRACE**

The upcoming CIT program for the coming summer brought the Littleton school IAQ to the forefront. Jill hoped she might be able to return to regular school and so arranged a two-hour visit to LHS to see if returning there would be viable. Upon seeing her, Quincy made rude comments to her and others about her presence. Arnold ignored her completely. A few girls made catty comments and generally made her feel like she had in eighth grade. Two hours later she had left LHS and was on her way back to B.A. looking forward to that school's talent show tryouts that afternoon. The tryouts went well and Jill was comfortable with her performance. But she became nauseated on the return van trip to B.A. and, according to the school nurse's report, "Staff reported they pulled over several times because Jill felt as though she might vomit…she made it back to school…[but] I was called into the hall and saw Jill lying on the floor…unresponsive, her pulse…slightly elevated as well as her temperature and blood pressure…[she] remained unresponsive for 2 minutes and [then her] body started convulsing…[which] lasted for a little less than a minute…She was taken to [MedCity] hospital…"[105] where she received a D10 infusion. The next day she had a heme treatment. This was the second time within a six month period that Jill had ended up hospitalized with AIP reactions after having been in LHS. I was now convinced that delayed response to toxin

---

105 Burton* Academy nurse Rina.* Memo to author. May 22, 2012.

exposure was real and was doubly nervous about her participation in the summer CIT program. But I knew if I refused to let her participate in it, we would get grief from Jill who desperately *needed* to feel normal.

Based on information I had sent to the local newspaper about Jill's participation in an APF fundraiser, the editor asked if Jill would agree to be interviewed. The opportunity to let people, no matter the audience size, know about AIP could not be missed. John* wrote a front-page article that got the attention of a mother several towns away. She recognized the signs and symptoms mentioned in the article as being similar to what her daughter was experiencing, most notably the recurrent fainting episodes. She called and I briefly explained about AIP's potential for neurological, psychological and psychiatric manifestations. Melanie* said her daughter, Alyssa,* had gone through months of inconclusive testing, had been moved to home-tutoring; was ultimately diagnosed with conversion disorder (at NHC) and spent weeks institutionalized for severe depression. She mentioned that Alyssa had a tendency to cut herself and asked if, by chance, Jill suffered from "excessive sweating," too? I was intrigued and excited—might this be another case of juvenile AIP? I told her Jill had done some self-cutting, too, but did not experience the sweating she described and that I did not know if it was considered an AIP symptom (I later found some sources that in fact did list "sweating" as a symptom for AIP). I sent Melanie the list of 22 symptoms I had culled from my initial AIP research and we began to keep in touch by email.

A few weeks later, Jill sang Miley Cyrus' "The Climb" in the B.A. talent show. I sat quietly, tears welling as Jill sang. I knew how hard it was for her to climb that purple mountain facing her. The next week Jill headed into summer, excited about the CIT program. She started at the Benton School morning program that was mostly held outside on the playground, then walked to the Main Street Elementary School (MSES) to help with the next age level. During the second week, near the end of the day, the MSES site camp counselor called to say Jill had a nosebleed that would not quit and asked me to bring her nasal spray medication. I did, but by then she was feeling weak from blood loss so I took her home. She had nosebleeds on each of the next two days but since they happened early in the day, I drove to the school, administered Stimate and she was able to finish the day. The weather had been dreary, requiring more inside activities than out. Head bells chimed. Although there were no dry-erase markers in use, the janitors were using hydrogen peroxide cleaner most days. Could it be that the cleaning fluid fumes alone triggered Jill's nosebleeds? It was too much of a coincidence to ignore.

I brought AIP information when Melanie and I met for lunch. As she described Alyssa's fainting spells and other symptoms—abdominal pains, loss of speech, depression, cutting herself, temporary waist down/leg paralysis—my stomach tightened. Melanie told me about her mother's suffering from kidney failure and her own bouts of abdominal pains. She showed me page in a spiral ring notebook upon which Alyssa had written, because she had been unable to speak at the time, about her desperation and fear of what was wrong with her, and my eyes filled with tears. For their sake, I did not want to think it could be AIP, but the clues could not be dismissed. According to Melanie, Alyssa did not produce darkened urine, but

I shared with her the article about how not all porphyric children produced that symptom. I told her DNA testing was the only sure way AIP could be ruled out. Melanie was desperate to help Alyssa and decided to pursue DNA analysis.

The weather turned rainy and chilly the last week of the CIT program. Along with the rest of the staff and campers, Jill was stuck inside the middle school for the day. She looked haggard when I picked her up on Monday. Complaining of nausea, a "killer" headache, and body aches and pains, she went straight to bed. The next day she came home zombie-like and took to her bed. Incapacitated, she was not able to get up at all the next two days. When I called her supervisor, he said the janitorial staff was "getting ready for school re-opening and the smell of cleaning fluid has been very strong throughout the school." Now it made sense. Rainy outside conditions meant closed doors. The need to prepare for fall opening in a few weeks meant an increasing use of the hydrogen peroxide-based cleaner. But, little or no dry-erase markers were in use. That meant the cleaner alone produced Jill's symptoms. Why? What happened when the human body was exposed to hydrogen peroxide? Based on observations and reports from the doctor who had observed Jill's fainting/convulsive activity during the DBT program, I had figured out that marker fumes, black in particular, alone were enough to affect Jill. Now the hydrogen peroxide cleaner jumped higher on my mom radar.

By midsummer, Jill's Facebook status changed to "in a relationship," and she started hanging around with B.A. classmate, Lonny.* Jill had been drawn to him because he was not prone to bullying others and they sometimes joked around at school. Lonny and his family had issues and he began to accompany us nearly everywhere such as to Jill's monthly port flush where he wrung his hands throughout the procedure. Yet, one day at a local fair, he and Jasmine commandeered a helium balloon, sucked the majority of the helium in and quacked like ducks. He encouraged Jill to inhale the rest. She got a bad stomachache. As far as realizing the potential for toxins to harm Jill, Lonny and Jasmine just did not get it.

Jill desperately sought ways to project her budding independence and after checking ingredients in hair dyes/products, occasionally changed her hair color and/or hair tips. She had begged for a tattoo since entering her teens, inspired by Kandis who had been "inked" many times. I was adamant—her AIP was too sensitive to risk a tattoo. I held out for a long time—until after she had been so victimized by the school bullying and during her recovery had claimed the band Seether's song "Rise Above This" as her personal anthem. She desperately wanted "Rise" tattooed on one wrist and "Above" on the other so she could see the message every day and stay strong enough to stop cutting. Finally, I researched information about the tattoo process. I discovered solvents were often used as "carriers" to help move the ink through the needle and into the skin. Knowing that solvents are AIP triggers, I would not consider allowing Jill to get them injected into her skin. Next was the issue of the ink or dye made with chemicals, which seriously raised an alarm because Jill wanted her tattoo in black and those black dry-erase markers loomed large in my mind. She was heartbroken but I steeled my resolve—her health was paramount. Coincidentally, I happened upon a regional newspaper which ranked favorite retail establishments such as restaurants, pizza places, movie theaters, consignment stores—and tattoo parlors. The "favorite" regional tattoo parlor used "all natural" products. I called the owner and explained that my daughter wanted a relatively small tattoo, two words, one on each wrist. However, I said, she had a liver disorder so I needed to ask questions before I would commit to or walk away from the process. He seemed surprised that I knew what a "carrier" was but answered "we use distilled water."

"What about ink? My daughter wants a black tattoo. What chemicals do your black inks contain?"

He replied, "we don't use chemicals, especially for black. We use burnt pine nuts." Jill had eaten pine nuts in the past with no problems. I thanked him, hung up and researched pine nuts then pulled some out of the pantry and gave her a few. "Here, eat these. If you do okay, we'll try a few more in half an hour or so then more after that. If you don't have any reactions over the next couple of days, we'll make an appointment for a tattoo." She was euphoric

On Jill's sixteenth birthday, with Lonny and Jasmine in tow, we drove to the tattoo studio. I shut my eyes and prayed to God throughout the entire process that Jill would not have an episode from the pain, stress or anything else. I so hoped she would not have to be rushed to NHC. Jill was fine. "Rise" "Above" were tattooed on her left and right inside wrists—in black. It was done. She reported that tattoo pain was nothing compared to AIP pain.

CHAPTER 63

Windy

I ask not for a lighter burden but for broader shoulders.
— JEWISH PROVERB

Jill returned to Burton Academy in September, still waiting to find out if there was a chance she might get into STFA. Before that would happen, though, her wisdom teeth had to come out. The oral surgeon, Dr. Carroll,* listened to Jill's AIP history, contacted Dr. O'Connor and then made the arrangements. As we drove to the hospital the morning of the surgery, Jill was nervous. "Am I gonna die, Mom?" she asked.

"No. You're going to be fine. A little loopy, probably, but you'll be coming home with me this afternoon. Don't worry. Dr. Carroll is a conscientious doctor and Dr. O'Connor made arrangements to be here, too. You'll be home safe and sound tonight," I assured her. Just before she was whisked into the operating room, a doctor was having trouble getting the intravenous D10 line inserted. Time grew tight and he said, "I'm going to have to use a numbing agent" and plunged a syringe into Jill's arm. Within seconds, her face turned bright red, she began fanning herself and was having trouble breathing.

I ran to the doctor/nurse station, "Please come quick! Jill needs oxygen—now!" An oxygen mask was immediately put on her and she was wheeled into the operating room. I fled to the waiting area, praying fervently she would be all right. The clock ticked hospital time—15 minutes, a half hour, 45 minutes, one hour. Dr. Carroll came out and asked, "Can I see you privately?" My heart pounded. "It's done—she did fantastic," he reported. "She's in recovery and can go home in a couple of hours or so. I'll call this evening to check on her condition. Have a great afternoon."

When I saw Jill, I joked, "See? You made it! We'll be going home as soon as you get your bearings about you—so, rest up!"

STFA called during the first week in October. Jill's lottery number had been drawn and they had to know immediately if she would accept. Jill was rattled and wanted time to think it over. "Jill, they need an answer now—what do you say?" I said. Jill said yes. I called Bart's office to let them know and a few days later, his assistant called to arrange a PPT. I asked them to please make sure to invite the STFA administration to the meeting, too. Littleton called back with a date and assuming they had invited STFA, I emailed the STFA principal to say if he needed anything specific before the meeting to let me know. The day before the PPT, I received an urgent call from STFA's SE director, saying there had been a communication problem between the regional headquarters and STFA; they had no information about Jill being accepted at the school. In the meantime, Jill seemed to be getting cold feet. I called Bart to say the PPT was in jeopardy and to stay tuned. When I arrived at B.A. for the PPT, Jill confessed that she didn't feel ready for the advanced placement level class work and did not want to head into academic failure but also didn't want to disappoint *me*. I said, "Jill, I have always only wanted what *you* want. If you really don't feel comfortable right now, don't go. You can reapply for next year." I cancelled the PPT.

Thanks to Dr. O'Connor's assistance, I located a toxicologist. With fingers crossed and prayers said, I sent a package of information to Dr. Casey,* director of the Connecticut Toxicology Department,* complete with "highlights" of Jill's AIP journey and questions about the specific chemicals I suspected triggered Jill's episodes. I asked if he would *please* see us. Before long, Jill and I had an appointment scheduled with Dr. Casey.

Meanwhile, Melanie notified me that the DNA report indicated that Alyssa did not have AIP. I felt so bad that their diagnostic trials had not ended, but my heart was happy they would not have to endure the turmoil AIP could bring. The wheels in my head began turning. Alyssa's many neurological symptoms (tremors with convulsive activity, difficulty breathing, fainting, leg paralysis, sensory impairment, changes in mental status, depression) essentially mirrored the ones Jill had had in Littleton schools. Was it possible that school toxins affected other students, particularly those with underlying, perhaps undiagnosed, illnesses, too?

On the day of our appointment with Dr. Casey, Jill and I drove to the Connecticut Toxicology Department office. Dr. Casey, a gracious and gentle man said he had reviewed the information package I had sent and listened intently as Jill and I answered his questions about all that had happened since 2007. Then he turned to Jill, "Your mother has asked a lot of thought-provoking questions. Unfortunately, I cannot say with any certainty that the chemicals she has identified *do* cause your reactions. But then, neither can I say with certainty they do not." I knew he had a fine line to walk but he did it with compassion. After being brushed off for so long, I was so grateful he had not dismissed us altogether. But my hope for definitive answers had been crushed yet again, and my tears spilled over. He immediately responded with kindness and said, "There is no doubt that, in general, internal environments are known to be several times more polluted than the outside environment. If you absolutely believe these chemicals are affecting Jill, then it is your right as a parent to follow your instincts." He suggested I read scientist Rachel Carson's book, *Silent Spring*. He said our predicament was reminiscent of her identification of toxic chemicals that were affecting the earth's environment back in the 1950s or so. I thanked him for respecting us and for giving me strength and resolve to forge ahead. On the way home, I stopped at the library to borrow *Silent Spring* and read it cover to cover. Coming on the tails of learning that Alyssa's DNA test results for AIP were negative, it provided me the inspiration to finish writing *Purple Canary*.

PART V

The Aftermath

Truth goes through three stages.
First, it is ridiculed,
Second it is violently opposed.
Finally it is accepted as self-evident.

— ARTHUR SCHOPENHAUER, GERMAN PHILOSOPHER

Speak for those who cannot speak for themselves,
defend those who cannot defend themselves,
and plead the cause of those in need.

— PROVERBS 31:8-9

CHAPTER 64

Perfect Purple Storm Conditions

*We have put poisonous and biologically potent
chemicals into the hands of persons largely or
wholly ignorant of their potentials for harm.
We have subjected enormous amounts of
people to contact with these poisons without their
consent and often without their knowledge.*[106]

— RACHEL CARSON

AIP is known as a pharmacogenetic and toxicogenetic disease which means certain medications and toxins are known to adversely affect AIPorphrics; that hydra-headed, many-mouthed beast has stymied Jill, me, doctors and other medical providers many times over. The Celexa debacle that Jill endured supported the pharmacogenetics label. Having researched Heparin medication for IV locks, I found that it contained an alcohol preservative and was sure that had been the switch that triggered the whole MedCity ED problem. The NCH APRN staff agreed the notion was plausible. That opened another portal—minute amounts of alcohol. It was time to revisit all of the information I had uncovered and as I did, more dots began to connect.

As far as toxins were concerned, a favorite "Gene Reviews" article listed organic solvent, biocide, cannabis, smoking, components in wine and spirits including alcohols and congeners [substances produced during fermentation which, according to Wikipedia include acetone, acetaldehyde, esters, tannins and aldehydes][107] among precipitating AIP attack factors.[108] Porphyria Educational Service (PES)

106 Carson, Rachel. *Silent Spring*. (New York: First Mariner Books edition 2002). 12
107 *Congener*. Wikipedia. https://en.wikipedia.org/wiki/Congener_(alcohol).
108 Thunell, S. *Hydroxymethylbilane Synthase (HMBS) Deficiency; Porphobilinogen Deaminase Deficiency, HMBS Deficiency. Includes: Acute Intermittent Porphyria (AIP)*. http://www.ncbi.nlm.nih.gov/books/NBK1193/. Initial posting September 27, 2005. Last Update March 23, 2010. Author note: the con-

newsletters strongly recommended that porphyrics avoid the inhalation of chemical fumes...and noted, "[m]any porphyria patients have found themselves with a high degree of sensitivity to a large variety of chemical toxins. [109]" Interestingly, I also learned that the CNS is a common target of solvent distribution.[110] Having observed the results toxins had on Jill's system, I studied the logs I had developed about her AIP/school activity; watched the CEDSA machine's green light appear and heard the technician say what troubled Jill at school came through the HVAC system; received input from other AIPorphyrics; researched AIP and toxic exposure in-depth; spoke to numerous doctors, then toxicologist Dr. Casey and felt I was on an "it makes sense to my gut" track.

As a child, I developed skin reactions when the household laundry detergent was changed so the school's cleaning product came to mind when Jill developed recurrent symptoms. But I had been assured over and over that the cleaner was "green," "safe" and approved by the EPA so I had backed off. And the large quantity of dry-erase markers used in the schools was the only thing I could think of that was different between the schools' internal environments and other public access buildings where Jill had not experienced symptoms so I dug in.

The majority of my research came from MSDSs; government agencies like OSHA, NIOSH, EPA; and universities' and states' toxicological department websites though I was not above checking out Wikipedia. I started with solvents used in paints, varnishes, pharmaceuticals, adhesives, printing inks, pesticides, cosmetics and household cleaners—and as it turned out, dry-erase markers and quickly learned that "...different solvents are often used simultaneously."[111] Such was the case with the brands of dry-erase markers chiefly used in Littleton schools. The ingredients included a combination of solvents: Special Industrial Solvent 200 Proof, Ethanol, Isopropyl, Alcohol, N-Proposal, 2-Propanol, all known as "industrial alcohols." Alcohol is a known poison of the liver and appears on most AIP trigger lists although I had always assumed it meant consumable alcohol. So I was intrigued as I scrutinized the individual ingredients contained in the "safe, harmless," government approved dry-erase markers that had replaced chalk in so many modern schoolrooms and learned that they contained "alcohol" which is, when used in that respect, a *solvent*. And when I discovered that solvents can cross the blood-brain barrier and dissolve in neural tissue, leading to nervous system diseases and that metabolic conversion of solvents into other substances may cause heart and liver diseases,[112] my head bells really started ringing. I scrutinized each ingredient:

tent of this URL was apparently changed to *Acute Intermittent Porphyria; Synonyms: PBGD Deficiency, Porphobilinogen Deaminase Deficiency* by Sharon D. Whatley, PhD and Michael N. Badminton, PhD, FRCPath. Last Update: February 7, 2013. This latest version does not contain the quoted statement.

109 Sommerfield PhD, J Professor of Biochemistry. *Porphyrinogenic chemicals and pharmaceuticals*, PES Bulletin. http://porphbook.tripod.com/vol2_43.html. October 29, 2000.

110 Rutchik, JS MD, MPH. *Organic Solvents Clinical Presentation*. http://emedicine.medscape.com/article/1174981-clinical. Published online by Medscape. Updated April 4, 2012.

111 Chen, Seaton. *A meta-analysis of mortality among workers exposed to organic solvents,* citeseerx.ist. psu.edu/viewdoc/download?doi=10.1.1.559.3724&rep=rep1&type=pdf, downloaded from http://occmed.oxfordjournals.org/. April 28, 2013.

112 Ibid.

According to the <u>Special Industrial Solvent 200 Proof</u> MSDS, its "shipping name" indicated Alcohols, Flammable, Toxic, N.O.S. (Ethanol); *Chemical Name(s)* are Ethanol, Methanol, Methyl Isobutyl Ketone, Ethyl Acetate; and *Chemical Family* includes alcohols, ketones, acetates. The *Emergency and First Aid Procedure* section of that MSDS offered guidelines for inhalation reactions: Remove victim to fresh air. Artificial respiration should be given if breathing has stopped and cardiopulmonary resuscitation if heart has stopped. Oxygen may be given. The *Health Hazard Data* noted: May cause dizziness, fainting, drowsiness, decreased awareness and responsiveness, euphoria, abdominal discomfort, nausea, vomiting, staggering gait, lack of coordination and coma. Irritation of the nose, throat and eyes will begin at ~200 ppm MIBK [methyl isobutyl ketone]. Inhalation of high concentrations can produce dizziness, fainting, drowsiness, nausea and vomiting. Symptoms depend on the level and duration of exposure... [and] ...may exacerbate liver injury..."[113]

Ethanol...known as grain alcohol or <u>Ethyl Alcohol</u>. "[E]xposure health effects can include eye, nose, skin irritation, headache, fatigue, narcosis, cough, liver damage, teratogenic and reproductive effects [malformation of embryo or fetus]...Affected organs: eyes, skin, respiratory system, CNS, liver, blood, reproductive system. Among other things, the MSDS's *Emergency Overview* stated, May cause central nervous system depression... [and] ...respiratory tract...irritation. *Warning!* May cause liver, kidney and heart damage. Target Organs: Kidneys, heart, central nervous system, liver...vapors may cause dizziness or suffocation. *First Aid Measures:* Inhalation: Remove from exposure and move to fresh air immediately. If not breathing, give artificial respiration."[114] I further learned that acetaldehyde [a congener, which is an AIP trigger as noted above] is "the toxic byproduct of ethanol metabolism in the liver... [and] ...alter[s] liver function and structure and may be responsible for ethanol's actions in the CNS..."[115] [which, remember, readily distributes solvents]. Lastly, according to OSHA, "contact between isopropyl alcohol and air may result in the formation of dangerous peroxides."[116] A toxicologist noted that ethanol is among "the worse of the toxins."[117] A head bell clanged as I remembered Dr. Plapp's detailed explanation about hypotheses for what might cause AIPorphyric neurovisceral complaints, and the word "peroxidation" had been noted.

Isopropyl Alcohol aka <u>rubbing alcohol</u> is a synonym for <u>Isopropanol</u>. OSHA's health guidelines noted permissible exposure limit (PEL) for isopropyl alcohol to be 400 ppm, at which "three to five minutes resulted in mild irritation of the eyes,

---

113 *MSDS No. SISC190, Special Industrial Solvent General Use.* Commercial Alcohols/The Industrial & Beverage Alcohol Division of GreenField Ethanol Inc., February 11, 2011. Note: This information no longer directs to the MSDS in question.

114 North American Fire Arts Association. *Material Safety Data Sheet. Ethyl Alcohol, 70%m ACC#91791.* http://www.nafaa.org/ethanol.pdf. April 17, 2001 and Occupational Safety & Health Administration. *Chemical Sampling Information, Ethyl Alcohol.* http://www.osha.gov/dts/chemicalsampling/data/CH_239700.html.

115 Deitrich, Zimakin, Pronko. *Oxydation of Ethanol in the Brain and Its Consequences.* Alcohol Research and Health, http://ncbi.nlm. nih.gov/pubmed/3181606.

116 Occupational Safety & Health Administration. *Occupational Safety and Health Guidelines for Isopropyl Alcohol.* http://www.osha.gov/dts/chemicalsampling/data/CH_239700.html. Based on 1992, 1993 and 1996 NIOSH, OSHA and DOE sources.

117 Jones, Dr. L. Toxicology & Cell Biology. *Focus: Toxicology.* Porphyria Educational Services (PES) Weekly Bulletin. http://porphbook.tripod.com/vol2_49.html. December 10, 2000.

nose and throat,"[118] that exposure to high concentrations has narcotic effects producing symptoms of dizziness, drowsiness, headache, staggering, unconsciousness and possibly death."[119]

2-Propanol is yet another synonym for Isopropyl Alcohol and Isopropanol. A manufacturer's MSDS warned that "inhalation of high concentrations may cause central nervous system effects characterized by nausea, headache, dizziness, unconsciousness and coma. May cause narcotic effects...causes upper respiratory tract irritation."[120] OSHA identified health factors as "eye, nose, throat and skin irritation; cough, sore throat, bronchitis; headache, nausea, dizziness, drowsiness, incoordination; vomiting, diarrhea [and noted that] affected organs include the eyes, skin, respiratory system, CNS."[121] Additionally, another MSDS stated that the chemical can aggravate pre-existing conditions: "Persons with pre-existing skin disorders or impaired liver, kidney, or pulmonary function may be more susceptible to the effects of this agent."[122]

n-Propanol aka 1-Propanol is a solvent of which "vapours may cause drowsiness and dizziness....[and] should not be released into the environment."[123] NIOSH (National Institute for Occupational Safety and Health) reports that 1-Proponal may produce ataxia, confusion, dizziness, drowsiness, headache, nausea, weakness, dry skin, eye redness, pain and blurred vision.[124]

My concerns about solvent/alcohol fumes intensified when I came across, "Most organic solvents affect the central nervous system, primarily the brain."[125] That and the fact that a manufacturer of n-propanol (synonym for most of the "industrial alcohols") stated that the chemical should not be released into the environment added to the concern that molecules associated with all of these chemicals are released into Littleton school buildings where they "mix" (or don't) with molecules released with myriad other products. Both alcohol and solvents are known AIP triggers.

Whether directly ingested in liquid form, inhaled or entering through the skin, like everything that enters the human body, alcohol is metabolized in the liver at the cellular level. Jill's reactions when exposed to industrial alcohol-loaded dry-marker fumes was beginning to make sense to me.

Carbon Black is a coloring ingredient used in many products—including dry-erase markers. I located specific information about the chemical's ingredients on

---

118 Occupational Safety & Health Administration. *Occupational Safety and Health Guideline for Isopropyl Alcohol.* http://www.gov/SLTC/healthguidelines/isoprophylalcohol/recognition.html. pg. 2
119 www.unil.ch/.../files/live/sites/cig/files/FAQ/Safety/PDF/MSDS/isopropanol_MSDS.pdf
120 Manufacturer Avogadro. *Material Safety Data Sheet for 2-Propanol, 99-100%, ACC#12090.* http://avogadro.chem.iastate.edu/MSDS/2-propanol.htm. Creation date: July 23,1999, Revision date: October 12, 2001.
121 Occupational Safety & Health Administration. *Chemical Sampling Information, 1-Methoxy-2-propanol.* http://www.osha.gov/dts/chemicalsampling/data/CH_250962.html. Date last revised: March 4, 2005.
122 Manufacturer JT Baker. *Material Safety Data Sheet for 2-Propanol Number P6401.* http://www.jt-baker.com/msds/englishtml/P6401.htm. September 16, 2009.
123 Sasol Chemical Industries. *MSDS n-Propanol Version 1.11.* Revision date July 16, .2007.
124 CDC. NIOSH. *International Chemical Safety Card, 1-Propanol.* www.cdc.gov/niosh/ipcsneng/neng0553.html.
125 No identified author. SixWise.com. *The Toxic Chemicals Most Linked to Depression.* www.sixwise.com/newsletters/05/06/15/the_toxic_chemicals_most_linked_to_depression. Undated.

the Artline Whiteboard Marker MSDS. Varying amounts of Ethanol, 2-Propanol and 1-Propanol are used in manufacturing the black, blue, red, and green markers:

"Chemical	Black	Blue,Red,Green
Ethanol	20~30	35~45
2-Propanol	30~40	30~40
1-Propanol	20~30	5~15
Carbon Black	1~10"[126]	

I noted that carbon black is used *only* in the black dry-erase markers, which I had already identified as being problematic for Jill. Information about carbon black was not abundant but I was eventually able to determine that exposure to carbon black echoed the effects of other dry-erase ingredients including recommendations to move an affected person to fresh air, administer oxygen if breathing is difficult, to give artificial respiration or cardiopulmonary resuscitation (CPR) and to immediately call a physician if not breathing or no heartbeat occurred. In spite of the miniscule amount of Carbon Black used in the black markers, it seemed reasonable that I try to keep Jill away from the black marker fumes permeating Littleton's schools.

Early on, a CT DPH representative had told me that the amount of dry-erase vapors found in schools was not enough to send a child into fainting or convulsive fits. I now thought, "Maybe not *individual* markers, but what about the cumulative vapor volume from hundreds of dry-erase markers used every day, all day, five days a week?" Not being a scientist, I surmised (correctly or not) that molecules emitted from open markers combined with those released from the friction of frequently used erasers became air-borne and either entered school occupants' bodies via inhalation, eyes, mouths, skin; settled on objects such as pens, pencils, food, fingers, arms; and/or were swept into the HVAC system where they were returned to the supply of internal building air to start the process all over again. I remembered the Littleton school district's decision one summer to use an industrial-strength solvent to clean the schools' HVAC systems and shuddered.

Leaders and participants in Jill's former DBT group could attest to her fainting/convulsive episode when only black markers had been used, and once the administrators had switched to using only lighter colors, she had had no neurological symptoms for the remainder of the summer. Comparing the similarities among symptoms Jill suffered in Littleton schools, those presented by product manufacturers and the warnings about CNS and/or liver impact, it seemed like I was on the right track in suspecting solvent-laden markers affected Jill at the cellular level.

Noting "biocide" on the list of triggers, I looked up the word—destroys microorganisms—and switched my attention to the "green" cleaner slathered on virtually every surface throughout Littleton's school buildings. I emailed the manufacturer to ask whether EnvirOxH2 Orange 2 was considered to be a biocide, and if so, why the product was considered to be safe if hydrogen peroxide itself was termed harmless? A customer service representative replied, "[The product] ... is considered a pesticide

---

126 Shachihata, Inc. *Artline Whiteboard Marker, EK-577, EK-579, MSDS No. AA1007A-9401.* May 6, 2011.

per EPA requirements since we have the sanitizer/viricide/HBV kill claims with this chemical...Hydrogen peroxide is listed as a hazardous ingredient on the MSDS because it is the 'active' ingredient in our chemical. The EPA requires that all 'active' ingredients are listed as hazardous ingredients because of their 'active' nature...." [127]

I checked out OSHA's guidelines for hydrogen peroxide (HP). One of the first things I learned was that "[h]ydrogen peroxide released to the atmosphere will react very rapidly with other compounds found in the air." [128] And that HP is incompatible with certain agents and when "[m]ixed with "alcohols, acetone [isopropanol metabolizes into acetone and/or]...aldehydes [129]...can cause 'spontaneous combustion.'" Because I was investigating molecular amounts, I certainly was not envisioning explosions of major proportions! However, I remembered that acetone and aldehyde were among the fermentation substances which can precipitate AIP attacks and wondered what, if any interaction happened when these incompatible compounds "met?" Dry-erase markers are solvent- (aka alcohol) laden products. Swedish experts warn, "Jobs involving the use of solvents are not suitable for AIP carriers. All exposure to solvents should be avoided." [130] I supposed that microscopic metabolites could wreak life-threatening havoc on Jill's internal system and my thoughts went wild, "It *must* be possible for hydrogen peroxide and alcohol molecules like ethanol (an 'incompatible substance') from the dry-erase markers to individually or collectively bind/cleave somehow and get into Jill's system." I envisioned infinitesimal alcohol/solvent- and hydrogen peroxide-laden molecules circulating through the air in Littleton school buildings, entering bodies and making their way to the livers of occupants who were able to metabolize them—except for Jill. In her case, I visualized miniscule detonations along her metabolic pathway where they became obstructions in her deficient metabolic process. I became convinced that Jill's porphyria caused her to be *poisoned* by the combination of toxins in the "safe, green" school environment and the proof was in the number of times she had been transported from school to ER rooms for treatment of acute attacks.

Next I was determined to find out what affect HP had on the human body. Internet articles talked about its oxidizing abilities for sterilizing medical implements, teeth whitening capacity and wound irrigation. Regarding the latter, while the impressive "bubbling action makes it look like it is doing its job by loosening damaged material and cleaning out bad bacteria, the problem is that hydrogen peroxide not only does this but also damages the healthy cells trying to heal the wound." [131] Understandably, medical guidelines no longer support HP's use as an antiseptic.

OSHA guidelines for HP state, "exposure...can occur through inhalation of the vapor or mist, ingestion, and eye or skin contact...Vapors are...[a] poison hazard

---

127 EnvirOxinfo. Email reply from customer service representative regarding EnvirOx. August 13, 2010.
128 ATSDR. *ToxFAQS™ for Hydrogen Peroxide*. http://www.atsdr.cdc.gov/tfacts174.html. April 2002.
129 Occupational Safety & Health Administration. *Occupational Safety and Health Guideline for Hydrogen Peroxide*. http://www.osha.gov/SLTC/healthguidelines/hydrogenperoxide/recognition. html.
130 Socialstyrelen. *Acute Intermittent Porphyria, ICD 10 Code, E80.2A*, http://www.socialstyrelsen.se/rarediseases/acuteintermittentporphyria. 2010.
131 The Survival Doctor, Hydrogen Peroxide for Wound Cleaning: Water's better! http://thesurvivaldoctor.com/2013/02.20/hydrogen-peroxide-for-wounds-is-it-better-than-water. Original article appeared in Sept/Oct 2009 issue of "My Family Doctor."

indoors...[s]evere systemic poisoning may cause headache, dizziness, vomiting, diarrhea, tremors, numbness, convulsions, pulmonary edema, unconsciousness ..."[132] —symptoms Jill had experienced in Littleton schools so many times. I had wondered if it was possible for her to be tested for HP exposure and, if so, how that could be accomplished. But OSHA had something to say about that too, "No signs or symptoms of chronic exposure to hydrogen peroxide have been reported in humans...Biological monitoring involves sampling and analyzing body tissues or fluids to provide an index of exposure to a toxic substance or metabolite. No biological monitoring acceptable for routine use has yet been developed for hydrogen peroxide."[133] So, apparently, no information existed about how "safe" hydrogen peroxide is for *anyone*, children or adults, especially when used in quantity. More information bombarded my brain, "[HP]...has caused DNA damage in vitro [in glass] human test systems...The Prescribed Exposure Limit (PEL) is 1 ppm (parts per million); inhalation of 7 ppm causes lung irritation." [134]

Then I found, "Hydrogen Peroxide has a weak potential to cause or promote cancers. The way it acts is unclear, but could involve direct damage to DNA...[and] hydrogen peroxide can lead to the production of hydroxyl radicals." [135] While it was important to know EnvirOxH2 Orange 2 "kill[ed] 99.9% of common bacteria [and] specified viruses,"[136] the reference to DNA damage concerned me greatly. Feeling like "The Magic School Bus'" Ms. Frizzle, I dug further and learned that HP "is produced by all cells of the body for many different physiological reasons... it is involved in many metabolic pathways"[137] and ultimately becomes an oxygen-derived radical which essentially means it is a by-product of oxidative metabolism. To that end, if left unchecked, HP accumulation can be a potentially dangerous side effect of oxygen metabolism as it would quickly endanger the organism.[138] I found that HP is known as one of the major reactive oxygen species (ROS) and has both beneficial effects in that it helps in cell creation and elimination of pathogens and/ or negative effects as the source of oxidative stress, cell death. This dual capability, a sort of Jekyll/Hyde role, is reflected in a medical hypothesis I found in the article, *Hydrogen Peroxide Has Been Shown to be a Potent Cytotoxic Agent in Causing Cellular Damage and Used in the Possible Treatment for Certain Tumors.*[139] It was good to know HP has the potential to fight cancer *and* kill germ cells but free radicals and oxidative stress can damage healthy, non-cancerous cells that could in turn possibly run

132 Occupational Safety & Health Administration. *Occupational Safety and Health Guideline for Isopropyl Alcohol.* http://www.gov/SLTC/healthguidelines/isoprophylalcohol/recognition.html.
133 Ibid.
134 Ibid.
135 GreenFacts. *Tooth Whiteners & Oral Hygiene Products Containing Hydrogen Peroxide; 2.4 Can hydrogen peroxide cause cancer or harm reproduction?* http://copublications.greenfacts.org/en/tooth-whiteners/. 2007.
136 EnvirOx. Online advertisement, *H2Orange2 Concentrate 117.* http://www.enviroxclean.com/safe-cleaning-products/h2orange2-cleaning-system/
137 Farr, Dr. CH. *The Truth About Food Grade Hydrogen Peroxide.* http://www.foodgrade-hydrogen-peroxide.com/id43.html. 1986.
138 No author identified. wiseGeek. *What are catalase enzymes?* www.wisegeek.org/what-are-catalase-enzymes.htm
139 Symons, MC. *Hydrogen peroxide: a potent cytotoxic agent effective in causing cellular damage and used in the possible treatment for certain tumors.* http://www.ncbi.nih.gov/pubmed/11421625. Published online in "Science Direct" via PubMed. July 2001.

full circle to illnesses. I also discovered that during the metabolic process, alcohol is oxidized by organelles that contain oxidative enzymes called peroxisomes into hydrogen peroxide and results in acetaldehyde as the metabolic processes' end product.[140] And that closed a loop—I was back at the beginning when I had started researching the ingredients of dry-erase white board markers. Adding molecular amounts of HP released by the cleaner—on top of whatever Jill's body metabolized on its own *and* the marker solvent emissions—surely seemed to be another dot connection.

As I continued to research I learned about the different grades of hydrogen peroxide, from the drug or grocery store variety to food grades that are regulated by the Food and Drug Administration (FDA). Researching "food grade" hydrogen peroxide, I found articles that touted peroxide as a cure for various medical conditions, although AIP was not one of them. Methods of administering HP to patients ranged from inhalation of a hydrogen peroxide/water vapor mixture to intravenous administration. The late Dr. Charles H. Farr (1927-1998, first president of the American Board of Chelation Therapy) advocated the use of intravenous hydrogen peroxide therapy to treat various ailments. An article written by him helped me understand hydrogen peroxide's effects within the body: "hydrogen peroxide stimulates enzyme systems throughout the body. This triggers an increase in the metabolic rate, causes small arteries to dilate and increase blood flow, enhances the body's distribution and consumption of oxygen and raises body temperature."[141] Head bells grew louder and my hope soared. I now knew that HP is produced in the human body and that the enzyme peroxidase helps break it down *and* that metabolic rate increases with the introduction of HP. I wondered if the amount that Jill was exposed to daily and cumulatively throughout her entire school career in the Littleton school buildings, combined with what her body produced had become too much for her porphyric-affected metabolic pathway. If the miniscule amount of HP used in Dr. Farr's bio-oxidative therapy was enough to increase metabolic rate, cause small arteries to dilate, increase blood flow, enhance the body's distribution and consumption of oxygen and raise body temperature in non-porphyric *adult* patients, therefore, it made sense to me the school's HP vapors that gained entry to AIPorphyric Jill's metabolism produced the very symptoms that Dr. Farr reported. The memory of her "increased temperature" recorded by the B.A. school nurse following Jill's visit to LHS made for another "dot" connection.

I went back to my research on alcohol and found, "Alcohol-induced oxygen deficiency (i.e. hypoxia) in tissues, especially in certain areas of the liver…required extra oxygen to metabolize the alcohol."[142] HP's effect of increasing blood flow, enhancing the body's distribution and consumption of oxygen *and* raising body temperature clearly meant a need for increased heme production. Adding the

140   Britain Society for Cell Biography. *Peroxisome.* http://bscb.org/learning-resources/softcell-e-learning/peroxisome and Wikipedia. *Peroxisome.* http://en.wikipedia.org/wiki/Peroxisome.

141   Williams, Dr. DG. *Hydrogen Peroxide—Curse or Cure?* PureHealth Systems website; http://pure-healthsystems.com/hydrogen-peroxide-2.html, 2012

142 Defung PhD and Cederbaum PhD. *Alcohol, Oxidative Stress, and Free Radical Damage, from National Institute on Alcohol Abuse and Alcoholism* website. pubs.niaaa.nih.gov/publications/arh27-4/277-278.htm. October 2004.

effects of the dry-erase marker ingredients known to affect the CNS resulted in a wide range of potential symptoms: abdominal pain, cough, convulsions, diarrhea, dizziness, death, drowsiness, eye irritation, fatigue, headache, incoordination, irregular heartbeat, narcosis, nausea, nose irritation, throat irritation, unconsciousness, weakness, and vomiting. It could not be simply repeating coincidences. Jill's liver *must* be ultra-sensitive to every one of the elements, individually and collectively, floating around in the schools' IAQ fumes. I deduced that, for Jill, H2Orange was the fire and dry-erase markers the gasoline. Add alcohol-induced oxygen deficiency, the haranguing peers and punitive, insensitive adults in the Littleton schools and perfect AIP storm conditions had materialized for AIPorphyric Jill.

Now that I had more knowledge, I rescrutinized the State of Connecticut Department of Labor Division of OSHA (CONN-OSHA) Benton School 2008 IAQ report I had filed away. When I read, "Monitoring of several substances commonly evaluated to assess indoor air quality was conducted,"[143] I noted that HP was not mentioned—and probably had not even been considered for evaluation—because it was deemed *safe*. And as I read the *Summary of Monitoring Data*, I understood that "[t]he sampling strategy utilized included carbon dioxide, carbon monoxide, temperature, and relative humidity. None of the substances evaluated resulted in concentrations exceeding limits found in CONN-OSHA regulations."[144] They had been ably set up to evaluate only those specific factors that might result in what had been found and legislated in previous IAQ incidents such as mold, dust, radon, "bus fumes," a similarly known toxins. They had concluded, "The overall results of monitoring did not reveal elevated or excessive levels for any of the contaminants monitored as described here and in the Monitoring Data section of this report."[145] There was nothing about testing for ambient chemical fumes released by "benign" products approved by the government because—they are "safe." CONN-OSHA had touched all the bases they had been trained to touch, but had gone no further.

Reading with better knowledge this time, I noted clues on the *Monitoring Report* that on been there all along—I had actually highlighted them but did not know enough then to challenge them. Now I did. The dry-erase marker ingredients had not been flagged for testing, yet had registered alarming results. The report stated, "On the day of the consultation, the most prominent compounds detected were isopropanol and ethanol...Most substances detected could be attributed to cleaning agents, personal fragrances, and fugitive emissions from the laboratory. All levels were well below any regulatory limits found in CONN-OSHA permissible exposure limits [PEL]."[146]

The substances isopropanol and ethanol, both of which registered "Exceeds Calibration Range" *are not* ingredients of the EnvirOx agent used by the school system, but they *are* ingredients in dry-erase markers. Coincidentally, Jill suffered

---

143 Connecticut Department of Labor, Division of Occupational Safety and Health. *Benton School* initial industrial hygiene report #504610155. April 17, 2008.
144 Ibid.
145 Ibid.
146 Ibid, pg. C-7 of 20

fainting and convulsive spells in the two locations, principal's office and cafeteria, where the chemicals—not meant to be measured—had been identified as exceeding calibration range.

My theory about ambient exogenous HP being too much for Jill's metabolism to handle was validated when I saw the effect the HP cleaner alone had on her during the summer CIT program. Add what I found in a National Institute on Alcohol Abuse and Alcoholism (NIAAA) article, "…ethanol metabolism tends to increase the hepatocytes' oxygen uptake from the blood"[147] meant to me that the combined alcohol/solvents and HP molecules Jill had been exposed to in Littleton schools made her metabolism speed up. This required more and more oxygen, reaching right down to the base of Jill's AIP heme/oxygen binding problem and the spewing of precursors in order to keep up with the demand for more blood cell production.

By this time I was aware there was "little question that individuals who are genetically predisposed to a porphyria can have clinical [neurological] manifestations of porphyria triggered by exogenous [outside the body] chemicals…."[148] But I still wanted to know *why* and then I found, "[a] number of chemicals… are known to be porphyrinogenic, that is, they are capable of inducing changes in heme synthesis…."[149]

Regarding chemical poisons, Rachel Carson noted, "One part in a million sounds like a very small amount—and so it is. But such substances are so potent that a minute quantity can bring about vast changes in the body."[150] Like any other substance that enters the body, toxins are sent to the liver, where enzymes are found, to be metabolized. She continued, "When [an] enzyme is destroyed or weakened [because of chemicals], the cycle of oxidation within the cell comes to a halt… [this is] potentially capable of the whole process of energy production and depriving the cells of utilizing oxygen. This [has] disastrous consequences…[151] Regarding chemical exposure and children, Ms. Carson reminds us that while the quantities may be small "they are not unimportant because children are more susceptible to poisoning than adults."[152]

I understood that Jill has an illness that can present with physical, neurological and psychological symptoms because "[t]he CNS, rich in both blood supply and lipid content, is a common trigger of solvent distribution."[153] Now knowing what I did about the AIP metabolic process and vapors associated with the "safe" OSHA-approved products, it was realistic for me to think the solvent-based cleaner and markers' "incompatible" ingredients triggered AIPorphyric Jill's intermittent irritability, moodiness, tremors, fainting, tachycardia, increased body temp, convulsions

147 Zakhari PhD. *Overview: How is Alcohol Metabolized by the Body?* From National Institute on Alcohol Abuse and Alcoholism website. http://pubs.niaaa.nih.gov/publications/arh294/245-255.htm. pg. 6
148 Daniell et al. *Environmental Chemical Exposures and Distribution of Heme Synthesis.* http://www.ncbi.nlm.nih.gov/pmc/articles/PMC1470308. Published online in "Environmental Health Perspectives." August 1996.
149 Ibid.
150 Carson, R. *Silent Spring.* (New York: First Mariner Books edition 2002), 22.
151 Carson, R. *Silent Spring.* (New York: First Mariner Books edition 2002), 204
152 Carson, R. *Silent Spring.* (New York: First Mariner Books edition 2001), 23.
153 Rutchik, Dr. JS. *Organic Solvents Clinical Presentation.* http://emedicine.medscape.com/article/1174981-clinical. Published online via "Medscape." May 2, 2012.

and other AIP manifestations. The Swedish Porphyria Foundation's warning that all exposure to solvents should be avoided made complete sense to me. I'd found the connection between Jill's AIP flare ups and Littleton schools' IAQ. Between the HP toxins with the ability to gobble oxygen cells, the chronic toxic solvent/alcohol molecules that poisoned those same oxygen cells, and her mutant gene, it was *no wonder* Jill fainted and collapsed in Littleton schools. Perhaps that was why her red blood cells were misshapen that time when Dr. O'Connor did not know why.

Whereas experts have for years had a good handle on outdoor pollution issues that affect air, land and water, it seems that indoor pollution (IAQ) issues have been recognized, but progress on setting regulations for internal school environments remains elusive.

Throughout Jill's school career, I had ascribed most of the periodic concerns about her irritability and mood swings to not having slept well, having been hungry or personality quirks. As time went on, the realization came that maybe she *did* have an emerging personality disorder or mental illness, which is how and why we ended up at Dr. Bludonowitz's office in the first place. But with research comes knowledge and with time comes wisdom. I had done plenty of research and the years brought wisdom. I was able to challenge the CONN-OSHA statement, "all levels were well below any regulatory limits found in… permissible exposure limits…" because those guidelines, PELs and standards are set for *adults*–not children. And I found no studies about low-level, long-term effects of these school-used and government endorsed chemical fumes.

Just because a short-term exposure to a single dry-erase marker does not pose an immediate threat to "typical' humans (adults—children don't count) or the fumes from a gallon of EnvirOxH2 cleaner are largely imperceptible to the nose of typical humans (again, adult) doesn't mean the aggregate fumes from hundreds of markers and gallons of HP-based cleaner used every day in school buildings and held captive in HVAC systems then recirculated throughout school buildings day in and day out are "safe." One can only wonder what effects such toxins actually have on occupants—especially children and fetuses of pregnant women—short- *and* long-term because who would be willing to purposely subject children to clinical trials to prove exactly what happens when toxins are inhaled, ingested or otherwise introduced to their systems? Yet for *years* that has been done every day in schools throughout the country.

My concerns were not welcomed by the Littleton school district so no help was forthcoming. As a taxpayer, it was not logical that in tough economic times Littleton school district had shelled out thousands of dollars to ship Jill out of the district when a simple solution could have involved maximizing fresh air intake and switching to water-based brands and quantity of dry-erase markers. In her book, *Is This Your Child's World? How You Can Fix the Schools and Homes That Are Making Your Children Sick*, author Dr. Doris Rapp tackled the prickly issues of children's sensitivities and school environments. She urged parents, teachers and school administrators to "be aware that minute odors from many commonly used items like chalk, freshly printed paper, marking pens, ordinary crayons can cause symptoms."[154] She goes on to say that schools should use water-based markers and reminds parents to "insist that only safe markers be used in schools and that our government protect its citizens more fully from harmful chemicals."[155] Several companies have already heeded the call for water-based coloring agents; PPG Industries has even developed a water-based car paint with proven durability.

As a parent, I could not comprehend why school leaders who are supposed to keep children safe, would not. I theorized that if the school IAQ could be made safe for Jill, chances are it would be that much healthier for all occupants. Yet the Littleton school district chose to ignore the information I asked to present. Other medical cases in the Littleton school district came to my attention. With all that I had learned about school-used toxic products and their effects on humans, and Alyssa who had fainted and experienced sensory impairments in her school, too, I wondered if it was possible for these toxic agents to have an adverse effect on school occupants with underlying, perhaps unknown, medical conditions that depend on oxygen intake, for example, asthma, allergies and cancer. Actually, some cancers *thrive* in low oxygen levels. I contacted a Connecticut Department of Public Health specialist about what I had discovered. I suggested that testing for such agents as hydrogen peroxide and dry-erase marker solvents, in schools that use them, be included along with the "standard" school IAQ testing for mold and radon. He responded that the amount of chemicals used in schools was not enough to cause problems and thanked me for my "well documented explanation." I then contacted the state hygienist who had prepared the 2008 Benton School report. I told him what I had discovered about the HP-based cleaner, the dry-erase markers and that none of those chemicals had been included for evaluation, yet the marker ingredients had registered at concerning levels. He was pleasant and listened to what I had to say. Then he said the PELs, set for healthy, adult males, had been lowered since that report had been prepared. Several organizations have already recommended that schools replace solvent-based markers with water-based markers and pay particular attention to cleaning products used in internal environments.

I have been belittled and scoffed at many times about my concerns for the "safe" and "harmless" toxic chemical products used in Littleton schools. However, given what Jill and I have been through, I believe that Jill *is* a canary with the ability to warn of toxic harm and the potential identification of more juvenile AIPorphyrics. In response to my concerns about school IAQ, an AIPorphyric adult male with knowledge of air quality issues offered, "It seems it is the little things that can cause the biggest problems. Regarding your concerns about the air quality at school… older HVAC systems recycle the same air over and over again. I highly recommend a fresh air exchange system. Check your local building code and ask your school board. It's good for all."[156]

154 Rapp, Dr. D. "Is This Your Child's World? How You Can Fix the Schools and Homes That Are Making Your Children Sick." (New York: Bantam Books). 1996, 518.
155 Ibid. 190.
156 Contributor requests anonymity. Letter to author. May 28, 2012

Thank you, Mr. B, I concur. Optimal fresh air intake and extreme reduction, or better yet, elimination of toxins would make schools everywhere safer for *all* occupants—even purple canaries.

CHAPTER 65

Purple Dayz

Leo* Generous, Faithful, Caring, Original, Outgoing
— *JILL'S ASTROLOGICAL SIGN; MESSAGE ON A FAVORITE T-SHIRT

*Life is a game that can be hard. It's a roller coaster ride. Both the good and bad memories stay with you. You will laugh and cry, learn and sometimes get burned, love and hate and that's what I had to learn. Life is **not** fair. A regular day for me can be getting up first thing in the morning, having to worry about whether or not I will make it through the day without an attack, what will the kids be like and staying focused on the school work and not the drama. Unfortunately something always happens to me. My mom says that trouble just seems to find me. I don't know why.*[157]

Sadly, too many children carry heavy crosses and too many adults respond to those burdens with talk of childhood resiliency, "He's/she's young—he/she will get over it" and if "character building" is not said, it is implied. The theory is routinely intoned by parents, psychiatrists, psychologists, medical doctors, educational professionals and others. There is no doubt some children often can and do rebound after setbacks. But setbacks are one thing; crosses and lifelong burdens another. Being human, children *do* have resiliency—but also fragility. And while children are often resilient, as humans we are also *residual* beings. Those physical, emotional, medical and/or social crosses can surreptitiously reappear in the future, impacting individuals *and* society, sometimes for better, sometimes for worse.

Manifest acute intermittent porphyria has been Jill's cross to bear since sixth grade. For her, it is not a static disorder. MAIP gouged a hole in her 'tween and teen years and took over our family's life as we struggled to help her cope with its various forces. She lost the better part of three full school years. She was then shunted to

---

157 Jill's journal. March 2010.

schools for troubled students largely because the school district used the SE-OHI designation with malevolent intent so it would not have to deal with the bullying issue and the problematic school IAQ/Jill connection. What I had hoped would be her educational salvation turned out to be anything but.

With society's "expected child resiliency," Jill dealt outwardly with a gargantuan medical condition as nothing more than an inconvenience to everything she hoped to achieve in life. Only once do I remember her initiating a conversation about why she "got" AIP. It was during eighth grade and she had left school early again; we were on our way to another heme treatment. Mrs. Podurski told me that Jill had become teary-eyed while preparing her backpack to leave. As we approached NHS, she softly murmured, "Why do you suppose I got AIP?"

I answered, "A lot of kids get rare diseases—no one ever expects to get that kind of news." She replied passionately, "Well, *no one* should have to get this disease. *No one.* I don't care if they are twenty, thirty or sixty years old. No one should have to live with the pain and scariness that porphyria makes. No one."

Sometimes I'll be in my room wondering, why me? Every now and then my disease will get to me and I don't understand. Other times I'll be in school and start to feel side effects from the medicine or symptoms of the AIP and I just break down. But I've also realized that I am who I am and this was what God wanted for me. I've learned to cope with it as best I can and always try to rise above the times when I wish I didn't have AIP because in the end I know that's just not going to happen. So many people have said to me that middle school is one of the hardest times to get through and when you live in a small town it can be harder to deal with the drama. Sometimes the drama will cause me to have an attack because I get so overwhelmed. Every morning so many questions run through my head and I just want to know everything will be okay, but see I am an extrovert and tend to open my mouth way too much. I get caught up in the moment and don't care who you are. If you're giving me trouble I will stand up for what I believe in. And unfortunately because of that I am labeled as a troublemaker. But a lot of people don't understand what I've been through and so they don't know what to think or just don't care so they give drama.[158]

It helped considerably that Jill's MAIP activity calmed down once she entered Burton Academy, allowing her to keep porphyria from the forefront for months at a time. But the ridicule and scorn from LMS peers and adults had made indelible impressions on her psyche and feelings of fear and depression often came back, especially when actions and words from B.A. students were directed at her.

I happened upon a stack of papers in Jill's bedroom, with a title page of *"My Name is Jill Gould. I am a survivor of bullying."* When I asked about them, she said they had been part of a planned script for a YouTube message to "help victims of bullying." It was clear the school bullying she had experienced had been more to process for her than AIP.

During her lengthy latent porphyria period, Jill enjoyed a break from heme treatments. The notion that heme could be considered a preventative measure as far as exposure to certain toxins was concerned kept niggling at me. After everything Jill had been through, I did not necessarily think it was so. Then, almost to prove it,

---

158 Jill's journal. April 2010.

a sequence of events beginning in late fall 2012 launched a round of MAIP activity and ushered in a return of Purple Days.

An odorous smell was in Jill's bedroom one morning. She felt "yucky" but went to school where she promptly collapsed and was transferred to NHC's ED. Even after infusion of the first round of D10 followed by heme, Jill's head, back, leg and abdominal pain and mental status changes escalated. In addition to mounting pain, she complained about blurry vision, dizziness and an icy pain shooting through her hands to her fingertips, "My hands feel like they're going to fall off!" She insisted I stop shaking her bed. I was standing a foot away from it. She begged for morphine which she had always tried to forego because, "I hate how it makes my head feel!" She was having difficulty breathing and asked for oxygen. She said, "My life sucks, Mom." She asked if she was going to die.

Although I firmly answered, "No," I *was* nervous. The ED doctor and I agreed to stay with the protocol and go ahead with the heme then the post-hydration D10 infusion. Having just read the *Silent Spring* chapter concerning cell respiration, I asked him if he would increase the oxygen level while infusing heme. He did. Within twenty minutes, Jill "came back," brightened considerably and wanted to go home.

Her new beau, Aaron, and his family members were heavy cigarette smokers. Jill often came home from visits there feeling nauseous, achy and saying, "My nose is stuffy—maybe I'm coming down with something." One day their home furnace malfunctioned and filled the house with fumes. She called to be picked up. We immediately opened all the car windows, even though it was January with below freezing temperatures, for fresh air. She went directly to bed when we arrived home. The next day she complained of nausea, headache, aches and pains. She did not go to school. By the next morning abdominal and back pains came screeching in and she ended up in the ED for a heme treatment. It took longer than usual for her to recover following that treatment, too. A few days after that incident, the B.A. school nurse called to say a staff person had been spray painting in a storage area and indicated that Jill was not feeling well because of the paint fumes. She asked permission to give Jill her inhaler. I suggested she take Jill outside *then* give her the inhaler so she could breathe clean, fresh air. I said I would be right there to pick her up and asked the nurse not to allow her back inside until the building had been fully aired out.

Thankfully, B.A. staff members remained vigilant about keeping identified toxins such as black dry-erase markers, which they had banned, away from Jill. Also, they did not use the same cleaning products as Littleton school district did. Then, in mid-March, 2013, Jill was ill for more than a week with an unusually bad cold and a heavy menstrual period combination. Following that, she remained fatigued, irritated and anxious. She could not sleep, grew nauseous, had aches and pains and complained on and off about headaches. After attempting a few days of home remedies such as rest, plenty of fluid intake and eating a high-carb, multi-grain diet with simple sugar snacks in between, I arranged for a heme treatment. However, before we would get to the appointment Jill begged to be taken immediately to the ED. Asked to describe her pain, she rated it eight on the scale of one to ten. She said it felt like her back, leg and stomach were on fire and asked for morphine that hospital staff quickly administered. By the time the heme arrived from the hospital pharmacy, the pain level in her back had decreased only to a "two or three." Then, midway through the heme infusion, her back pain ramped up to a "seven." The doctor ordered more morphine. In a few minutes, the abdominal and leg pain disappeared but the back pain leveled off only at "two" which lasted until about one-third of the way through the post-hydration glucose infusion. By the end of the infusion, Jill complained her back pain was up to about a seven again and reiterated her "My life really sucks, Mom!" refrain. But the infusion was finished—and, accordingly, so was the emergency. It was time to go and hope the heme would work. We had an appointment to see Dr. O'Connor in less than two days, and we could always call him if the pain did not relent. As Jill and I drove home, I tried to think what the genesis of this recent attack could have been. Suddenly, an illustration from a favorite AIP article [http://www.art.com/products/p14441601075-sa-i6715325/ nucleus-medical-art-illustration-of-red-blood-cells-rbcs-transporting-oxygen-molecules-bonded-with-hemoglobin.htm] showing hemoglobin transporting oxygen flashed into my head. A head bell chimed and I had a forehead-smacking thought, "*Oxygen!* Problematic heme/oxygen binding is involved with MAIP activity. We need to add oxygen *during* the heme treatments! Oxygen had worked well in January—and it had worked from day one back in 2007. In fact, she had improved every time supplemental oxygen had been administered or fresh air brought in when she was in AIP distress. *WHY hadn't I thought of it before?*" I said to Jill, "I just thought of something that might help you next time. Remember in January when you had that attack and I asked for oxygen and you got better within twenty minutes or so?" She nodded. "I'm going to ask Dr. O'Connor about adding oxygen to your heme protocol from now on. It's worth a shot. Dr. Piersen told us a long time ago if oxygen helped you, then you should have it." She nodded again. She was exhausted—and still in pain.

She *really* railed at porphyria and what it had done and was doing to her. I tried to comfort her, but she was in immense pain and scared. "My life *really* sucks!! I can't do this anymore. I just can't. I don't want to go on," she sobbed. Many, many porphyrics have confessed they thought that their lives were over or prayed for death to deliver them from the onslaught of the horrific pain and terrifying symptoms. Admittedly, there *were* times, especially before the Panhematin infusions had been figured out when I wondered whether or not Jill would make it through certain attacks.

At our next appointment, we updated APRN Kym and Dr. O'Connor about the toxin exposures she had had during the past few weeks and the very concerning recent decreasing effect of heme/D10 treatments. I showed them Ovation's (previous Panhematin manufacturer) MSDS specifications that stated, "If breathing is difficult, give oxygen."[159] Then I suggested the idea of adding oxygen to Jill's AIP treatment protocol. They agreed to try it.

All in all, Burton Academy's use of dry-erase markers was minimal which I was convinced helped in keeping Jill's episodes to a minimum. The combined DBT,

---

159 Ovation Pharmaceuticals. *Material Safety Data Sheet for Panhematin*. March 10, 2008.

ongoing individual counseling sessions with Vanessa and B.A.'s clinical staff had helped strengthen her sense of self. It was time for Jill to move on to her senior year. She toyed briefly with returning to Littleton to finish her education with the class she had started preschool with. But because she had ended up in the ED following the two brief times she had been in LHS while attending Burton Academy, the CIT experience and the DBT black dry-marker experience, I was against her return to Littleton schools.

Summer was looming. Jill received and accepted an invitation to participate in the Hole in the Wall Gang's teen camp for a week. She was nervous when I dropped her off because it meant a full week away from Aaron. But Jill being Jill, she soon made friends with the campers and counselors and began to settle in. Eight and a half hours later she was on her way to NHC ED with severe abdominal, back and chest pains. As I drove to the hospital, I thought that stress had triggered the problem. But, when I arrived at her room, Jill reeked of smoke and told me how they had been sharing stories around the campfire when the symptoms started. I wondered aloud if the wood smoke might have had something to do with it. Jill snapped, "Oh come on, mom—it was just the stress." A few days later, I Googled and Bing-ed wood fire/AIP connection?" and found possible clues in World Health Organization (WHO) and PES articles warning porphyrics to avoid dioxin exposure. Dioxins are omnipresent environmental pollutants[160] [that] ... can present as unintended byproducts of natural events such as ... forest fire."[161] Given Jill's heightened sensitivity to toxins, stress *and* the chemicals from the campfire's smoke could have caused her reaction.

Three years after she let the SFTA opportunity go, Jill ended up with Littleton-provided tutoring for the morning hours and afternoons at SFTA for her senior high school year. A creative writing class assignment was to write about an incident that "all of us have had." Jill wrote about scars. In the essay she told of her trials with illness and the vicious bullying she endured at Littleton. She explained how the tattoos on her wrists and arm had come to be. Those were the places she had once chosen for self-cutting. Reading her words brought pride in the young woman that Jill had become:

I went to school every day with a smile on my face but by sixth grade I started realizing I was an outsider. I tried so hard to fit it, because let's face it when you're that young, that's the only thing you care about. If you look closer at my wrists, you'll see the marks of my struggles from schools, bullying and my health issues. These words on my wrist tell a story. They mean something to me. It's a promise to my friends and family—but most of all a promise to myself that I wouldn't self-inflict wounds on my body just because I have them inside. It's a promise to always RISE ABOVE the hurt, anger, pain, heartache, and struggles in life. And although my skin is still pale, my bones still ache and my heart is still bruised, it's a reminder of what I went through as a victim of bullying. The tattoos remind me that I

160 World Health Organization (WHO) Fact Sheet N°224. *Dioxins and their effect on human health*; http://www.who.int/mediacentre/factsheets/fs225/en/. June 2014.
161 Neis, P MNS, NP. *Dioxin Exposure to Be Avoided by Porphyrics*. Published online at Porphyria Educational Services (PES) Monthly Newsletter, *Metabolic Disorders*. http://porphbook.tripod.com/Autumn2006.html. Autumn, 2006.

was able to get through one of the most traumatizing times in my life. It's been over a year since I've cut and I feel so much better about myself. I'm not gonna lie and say the thought hasn't come up since then, but I've accomplished so many goals in my life, including this one, and the person I've become, is a strong, beautiful, smart, young lady. I love who I am despite what anyone says."[162]

My beautiful daughter, with a purple canary badge of courage newly tattooed on her upper arm, was on her way back to life.

---

162 Jill. Creative writing assignment. June 2014.

CHAPTER 66

Fog Covered Purple Mountains

Once you go purple, you never go back.
— COMIC/VENTRILOQUIST JEFF DUNHAM'S PEANUT CHARACTER

Stories can conquer fear, you know.
— BEN OKRI

My interest in porphyria started the moment the word slipped off the tongue of the neurologist Jill and I met in 2008. Matthew 7:7 says, "Ask and it will be given you ...."

I asked and "...something called porphyria ..." came out of the doctor's mouth. I searched, and thanks to the Internet, information about the porphyrias flooded my computer screen from online sources. My fascination with AIP was cemented once DNA testing confirmed that Jill had the acute porphyria. I was particularly fascinated with the molecular aspect of AIP and the chain of events that started at the cellular level, different from blood levels, I assumed, and culminated in a convulsive, fainting, breathing with difficulty, over-the-top-pain-filled and sometimes psychotic patient—my daughter. That's where I started and found a plethora of resources to learn from. The concept of heme being the key element of metabolism and its fundamental purpose wholly dependent on its ability to bind oxygen in order to move oxygen and energy throughout the body intrigued me.

A 2010 Swedish National Board of Health and Welfare Agency article describes what happens. "Because the third step [of an eight-step blood building process] is regulated by the deficient [HMBS also known as the] PBGD enzyme, it functions at only fifty percent of normal. However, that's enough in most circumstances to ensure an uninterrupted flow of heme. [But] sometimes the cells need to accelerate production of heme to such an extent that the defective third step of the process just cannot meet the [demand]. The result is that two enzymes, PBG (porphobilinogen) and ALA (aminolaevulinic acid), which PBGD usually helps to convert [into usable blood products], start to accumulate"[163]"…in tissues and are excreted in excess in urine…."[164] This was the explanation for the darkened urine (purple, red, rust, brown or other in that spectrum) color that AIP is noted for. For years, several sources identified ALAs and PBGs as being potentially toxic and the basis for acute symptoms. However, a relatively recent study provided "convincing evidence that delta-aminolevulinic acid (ALA) is the cause of pain in the acute porphyrias."[165] Also, Dr. Bylesjö noted that ALA most likely increases the effects of heme deficiency.[166]

When I first learned about the AIP/heme building process, an "I Love Lucy" episode came to mind. Working in a chocolate factory with her best friend, Ethel, Lucy's job was to pick individual chocolates off a conveyor belt, individually wrap each in paper and return it to the moving conveyor belt for packaging. As the conveyor belt sped up, the women began to have trouble keeping up with the process. Things became funny when the line moved faster and faster and the women could not keep up; they resorted to stuffing chocolates into their mouths and then hats and clothing. "The girls" got stomachaches from eating so much chocolate and being so stressed. The "Lucy" episode is hilarious, but when AIP trigger conditions call for an AIPorphyric liver to rapidly produce more and more blood cells and results in neurotoxic precursor/porphyrin overflow, the result is anything *but* funny.

In real life, the process negatively impacts the CNS that in turn affects the peripheral and autonomic nervous systems (PNS) and can result in physical, neurological and/or psychiatric AIP manifestations. And because individual body makeup varies, the symptoms may present individually or collectively in varying intensities.

Claims that AIP is under-diagnosed in the United States are becoming more common. One source noted, "[p]orphyrias are relatively uncommon conditions but probably under recognized…and prevalence underestimated in the general population because…studies have focused on family members of affected individuals and less on the general population."[167] Years later, that is still the case as far as Jill, with no documented family history of AIP available, goes. How the AIP gene found its way to my adopted daughter will forevermore remain a mystery. Discovering that notable people of the past like England's King George III; Mary, Queen of Scots; Vincent Van Gogh; Edgar Allen Poe; Paula Frias Allende and more recently, Kurt Cobain of Nirvana fame were suspected of having or known to have an acute porphyria did not alleviate the pain of knowing that Jill has it.

163 Socialstyrelsen. *Acute intermittent porphyria.* http://www.socialstyrelsen.se/rarediseases/acuteintermittentporphyria. website article ICD 10 code. E80.2A. Publication date: 2010-2011.
164 Sassa, S. *Modern diagnosis and management of the porphyrias.* http://onlinelibrary.wiley.com/doi/10.1111/j.1365-2141.2006.06289.x/full. Published online via British Journal of Haematology. September 4, 2006.
165 Bissell, DM. et al. *Role of delta-aminolevulinic acid in the symptoms of acute porphyria.* http://www.ncbi.nlm.nih.gov/pubmed/25446301. Published online in "American Journal of Medicine" via PubMed. March 2015.
166 Bylesjö, I. *Epidemiological, Clinical and Pathogenetic Studies of Acute Intermittent Porphyria.* Medical dissertation, Umea University. www.diva-portal.org/smash/get/ diva2:141227; FULLTEXT01.pdf. 2008, 17.
167 Daniell, William E. et al. *Environmental Chemical Exposures and Disturbances of Heme.* www.ncbi.nlm.nih.gov/pmc/articles/PMC1470308/pdf/envhper00326-044.pdf. Published online via Environmental Health Perspectives. August 29, 1996.

After Jill's positive DNA test results came back in 2008, I revisited the APF web-site's member stories and found that sixty percent of them mentioned childhood MAIP symptoms. Those accounts supported my theory that MAIP *can* produce clues in early life. Of the nearly 100 letters I sent to AIP patients requesting informa-tion about their early recollections, approximately thirty percent were men. Many shared tormented accounts of pain- and fear-filled suffering throughout childhood and into adult life. The average age of diagnosis based on symptom presentation was thirty-seven.

Along with the memories received via U.S. Mail, telephone communications and emails, Jill and I collected porphyria-management tips from the AIPorphyric patients, some of whom have managed the affliction for many years. Learning that older people struggle with AIP let Jill know that in spite of acute intermittent por-phyria, she has a future, too. We are grateful to the following anecdotes shared by AIP patients.

AIPorphyric women remember:

- A woman shared that she felt sick most of the time as she grew. She explained it as a sickness she couldn't describe even to herself. She remembered being a young teen and telling herself that someday she would know why she was "very, very sick." Eventually diagnosed with AIP, she said everything began to make sense. She explained because children have nothing to use as a comparison, she thought everyone experienced her symptoms at one time or another.

- "I [grew up] in the south where fruit and vegetables were the main foods eaten and mostly homegrown. I was basically healthy [but] had belly aches, bowel problems, and sometimes severe depression. I did struggle in school because I found it hard to concentrate. I remember at age 8 I became ill and was in a coma for about 2 weeks. When I awakened I had trouble walking and the doctor [told] my parents I needed to be in an emotion-ally safe environment. I had the pain as always, vomiting, etc. but learned early to keep to myself as much as [I] could. Your description of symp-toms [matched] what I tried to describe to many doctors to no avail."[168]

- "I was always a sickly child with constant sore throats, sinus/ear infections and respiratory infections. They removed my tonsils (a big cure for sore throats in those days) when I was only 18 months old. I continued to catch every[thing], measles, mumps, chicken pox and strep throat, numerous times. When I started my menstrual cycle at age 11 is when I experienced my first acute AIP attack. My abdomen swelled so I looked 9 months pregnant. This was accompanied by severe abdominal pain and nausea. The doctors believed the pain and the swelling were gynecological. I have always suffered muscle weakness and general fatigue. I never played sports or ran around like the other children. I remember having insomnia even as a child.

---

168 Bruno, R.D. Email to author. October 29, 2009

I think I realized that stress (physical or emotional) made me feel "bad" so I avoided it whenever possible. When I was 15 our high school made every child take the President['s] Fitness Test. One of these tests was to time us running ¼ mile. I got 1/3 of the way around the track and doubled over with chest pains. My [P.E.] teacher screamed obscenities at me in disgust. When I got home, my mother took me to our GP who diagnosed growing pains. When I was 16, I had my first acute AIP attack that was not associated with my menstrual cycle. I was taking my preliminary college boards and doubled over with abdominal pain. Afterwards, my parents took me to our doctor who admitted me to the hospital with 'appendicitis.' The surgeon was unsure of the diagnosis and put me on glucose IV and bed rest. After three days, the pain and swelling disappeared and I was sent home. When I was 17 and tried to learn tennis, I blacked out on the tennis court. They decided it was "the heat." I never tried sports again. Between 16 and 25, I had numerous "appendicitis" attacks (in addition to the pain associated with my menstrual cycle): abdominal swelling, diarrhea, severe abdominal pain, fever, fluctuating pulse and blood pressure and nausea."[169]

- "I remember having stomach problems my whole life and suffered frequently with abdominal pains and vomiting especially with periods. [I] do not remember having darkened urine until age 28."[170]

- "While growing up I was around all kinds of pesticides. Also the main drugs were sulfas and barbiturates. When I began school I also began bouts of repeated pneumonia. Those, coupled with the drug [reactions] were my earliest indicators of AIP. When I began teaching, [my] classroom was a storeroom for the biology and chemistry departments, I would often get nauseous but would think I was pregnant or maybe had the flu. [After years of illnesses too numerous to mention (including spontaneous abortion/late-term miscarriages); medical visits, testing, etc.] the big breakthrough came when my new husband and I [travelled] to New England. I was very tired but had trouble sleeping. Insomnia, restlessness, sweating, gut pain, a slight nausea. The next morning I was shocked to see a toilet bowl full of red urine. I knew it could not be what it appeared to be because I'd had a hysterectomy." [Note: this person has AIP and acquired PCT.]"[171]

AIPorphyric men shared memories:

- One man said he developed whooping cough and measles at age twelve that led to frequent episodes of vomiting, pain and hallucinations. AIP was diagnosed when a urine sample left to stand turned color.

169 Sadowniczak, S. Letter to author. November, 2009
170 Williams Dr. J. Telephone communication. November, 2009
171 Deats-O'Reilly, D. *My Porphyria Story.* http://porphbook.tripod.com/153a.html. As published on-line via Porphyria Educational Services.

- Another indicated he was often susceptible to prolonged illness and had more than his share of injuries and broken bones. When he was not yet ten, he said he was "studied" medically because of a tendency to develop multiple boils and carbuncles. Around the time of high school graduation he recalls being in the hospital for several weeks with ailments he feels were misdiagnosed as Mono and/or Hepatitis.

- A third man's severe pain in his side at eleven or twelve years of age stumped the family doctor. Incidents of extreme abdominal pain persisted for the next several years. When he complained during his time in the military service, he noted that MALINGERER had been written in large, red letters on his file. Finally, at the age of twenty-four, a doctor told him to urinate in a clear glass jar, put it on a sunny windowsill and to call him the next day. The urine had turned purple, he says, one of the very few times that his urine had ever been purple.

AIPorphyric juveniles:
As adults, who among us has not attributed a child's complaint of aches, pain (especially abdominal), occasional shakiness or being dizzy to growing pains, coming down with something, wanting attention, a "phase," or something to "get over?" Like adults, perhaps even more so, children are at risk of being written off as complainers or attention seekers. But with minds and bodies still developing, children may be at an even greater disadvantage than adults when AIP surreptitiously harbors in their liver.

A 1974 article about childhood diseases where AIP was concerned asked, "Is it the disease or merely the diagnosis that is so rare in childhood?" and noted, "37 cases were found…A port-wine coloured urine was not always noticed in proven cases that have been published; possibly because the urine was not left standing long enough [a theme in more current diagnoses also.] Though this disease is thought to be very rare in childhood, mild cases presenting merely with abdominal pain may escape diagnosis."[172] The article gives fair warning, "This a disease in children which is potentially fatal and can present with minimal symptomology but may not be diagnosed until the final attack…thus a high degree of suspicion among both pediatricians and pediatric surgeons appears to be the only way to improve the diagnosis rate."[173]

An abstract from the "Journal of the American Academy of Child & Adolescent Psychiatry" titled "Acute Intermittent Porphyria in a Children's Psychiatric Hospital" described "…bizarre behaviors…seen in cases of organic mental dysfunction and toxic psychotic states. The author reports on two cases of AIP in children who were initially diagnosed as atypical psychosis in an inpatient children over a 3-year period."[174] Unfortunately, attempts to obtain more information from hos-

---

172 Barclay, N. *Acute Intermittent Porphyria in Childhood. A neglected disease?* http://adc.bmj.com. Published online by group.bmj.com. (Archives of Disease in Childhood). British Medical Journal. 1974. 404.
173 Ibid. 405.
174 Boon, Franklin, Ellis. Abstract: *Acute Intermittent Porphyria in a Children's Psychiatric Hospital*; www.sciencedirect.com/science/article/pii/S0890856709654848. February 9, 1989.

pital contacts were not successful but the following anecdotes about AIP children are revelatory:

- A mom reported that two of her three children have struggled with active acute porphyria for years. All three siblings underwent DNA testing; two received positive results. However, she said, "We were told by the doctor that it was impossible for my daughter to have symptoms as children do not have acute attacks. It obviously stems from the fact that [some] children don't produce urine porphyrins (she does not but my son had elevated urine levels at age 7). He still wasn't treated for it as this specialist considers porphyria attacks not important to treat!"[175] Note: And there was a time when infants were operated on without anesthesia because the medical community believed they could not feel pain.

- A mother whose adult son has AIP said her grandson (her son's nephew) was about to undergo testing and was interested to find out about Jill's testing protocol because "his psychiatrist diagnosed him with a mood disorder (juvenile bipolar). I don't think the prescribed medicine is helping at all. The pediatrician is working with us to find out [how to determine whether or not he has AIP and is] going to do the 24-hour urine test first. [She needs to] try to see how much blood needs to be drawn, what [tubes] to put them in, etc."[176] Note: This communication about another child labeled with a mood disorder/bi-polar diagnosis with plans to medicate him for behavioral issues, struck to the heart of why this book is needed.

- Another female respondent, herself struggling with recurrent AIP episodes expressed concern about a nephew who had developed AIP symptoms as a pre-teen following a severe bacterial infection. His main symptom was abdominal pain in his lower right side and no appetite. The symptoms significantly impacted him during school. She said that according to the doctor they had consulted, AIP biochemical confirmation is virtually impossible at the boy's age.

Relatively early in this writing, a U.S. nationally recognized porphyria expert provided answers to several questions Jill and I had. They are included throughout the remainder of this book. You will note them in the sequence: Q# (question from Jill and/or me) followed by A# (the doctor's answer). Along with his responses, information obtained from other expert sources is also included:

Q1: I recognize doctors must be skeptical when it comes to diagnosing disorders, never mind rare/orphan ones, but are you aware of *any* other cases of juvenile-onset MAIP requiring D10/ Panhematin treatment?

A1: AIP symptoms before puberty are very rare, and it would always be important to be sure that some other condition is not present, and that porphobilinogen

---

175 Hanna, A. Email to author. Fall 2015.
176 Shelor, J. Emails to author. October 2009

is elevated. I don't know of any patients with onset of symptoms before puberty. Your daughter will probably need repeated evaluation later as she matures.

Dr. Sassa, writing in the "British Journal of Haematology" confirmed that hepatic porphyrias are rarely seen before puberty but noted they are quite common at puberty or after.[177] Jill had entered puberty about six months before the strange neurological symptoms appeared. Her DNA report stated the splice-site mutation in one of her HMBS alleles was consistent with AIP. Since fall, 2007, even before those test results came back, Jill had presented with AIP clinical symptoms with the exception of heightened U-PBG and U-ALA measurements, coma and death.

We have been stymied time and again when it comes to Jill's urinary PBG production not being "up to snuff." Based on what we have discovered, we are not ready to give up yet as Swedish experts contend, "The urine of the patient may turn red from a surplus of PBG … [but t]he absence of red-coloured urine does not in itself exclude the presence of acute intermittent porphyria."[178] Jill connected with other AIPorphyrics who indicated that their urine discoloration was variable during attacks, acknowledging the *intermittent* symptom presentation of AIP. This is confirmed by a Japanese medical team that conducted a four-year study and concluded, "…an abnormal urinary profile of ALA, PBG, UP…shows wide variations from status to status in the same subject."[179]

The issue would not go away. Jill has had debilitating neurological attacks for years, set off by known AIP triggers, yet only once had her urine been discolored. Unfortunately, hospital staff did not analyze it.

I came across an article that reported, "An important feature of the intermediates in heme biosynthesis, as well as in heme degradation, is their chromophorphic character, some are colored while others are not. An easy way to distinguish which will have a color and which will not is to look at the suffix of the compound name. All heme intermediates and degradation products that end in –ogen (e.g. phorphobilinongen [sic]) will be colorless and those that end in –in (e.g. bilirubin) will be colored.[180] This seemed in conflict with the "colored urine can confirm AIP diagnoses" mandate.

My interest was piqued a few years ago when I began to notice a theme running through some of the articles I read. That is the subject of measuring PBGD (porphobilinogen deaminase) erythrocyte (blood) levels during attacks. Most, if not all, articles stated that *increased* urinary biochemical marker (ALA/PBG) excretion is required to diagnose AIP. But some also mentioned that *decreased* PBGD could play a part in that diagnosis.

---

177 Sassa, S. *Modern diagnosis and management of the porphyrias.* http://onlinelibrary.wiley.com/doi/10.1111/j.1365-2141.2006.06289.x/full. Published online by British Journal of Haematology. September 4, 2006.

178 Socialstyrelen. *Acute Intermittent Porphyria, ICD 10 Code, E80.2A.* http://www.socialstyrelsen.se/rarediseases/acuteintermittentporphyria. 2014.

179 Tanaka, H. et al. *Long Term Follow-up of Erythrocyte Porphobilinogen Deaminase Activity in a Patient with Acute Intermittent Porphyria: The Relationship Between the Enzyme Activity and Abdominal Pain Attacks*; www.osaka.med.ac.jp/deps/b-omc/articles/533/533tanaka.pdf. Published online by Bulletin of the Osaka Medical College. June 18, 2007.

180 King, PhD, MW. *Porphyrin and Heme Metabolism, Biology Research Reagents.* http://themedicalbiochemistrypage.org/heme-porphyrin.php. Last modified: April 4, 2015.

"The author of a 1986 "Clinical Chemistry" article states, "occasionally the amount of PBG in the urine is normal. If this is so and the clinical story is convincing...I proceed to measure erythrocyte PBG deaminase...."[181] A "PubMed" abstract confirms, "97 of 107 patients with AIP had enzyme activity below normal range [which] underscores the utility of this test [measuring PBGD in red blood cells] in confirming the diagnostic of acute intermittent porphyria."[182] Furthermore, the authors of "Behavioral Aspects of Acute Intermittent Porphyria" (mentioned in Chapter 18) contributed to a 2009 "PubMed" abstract explaining how a 15-year-old female patient's [previously diagnosed with autism] "normal urinary [ALA] and [PBG] findings... [were] not compatible with symptomatic porphyria according to well established criteria...could have led to a missed diagnosis of neuroporphyria. But the diagnosis of AIP was established on the basis of a 64% reduction in erythrocyte HMBS activity...and the finding of a known causative AIP mutation."[183]

Another article noted that reduced porphobilinogen deaminase measurement "...provides excellent laboratory aid in the diagnosis of acute intermittent porphyria particularly in those patients who are asymptomatic or in whom the disease is not biochemically manifested by porphyrin precursor excretion."[184] Not finished yet, a relatively recent article stated, "In anuric [absence of urine formation] patients, diagnosis of AIP can be established by measuring serum PBG."[185]

That became a niggling notion and I began to pay better attention to it. I pulled together the PBGD blood test results Jill had had. There weren't too many. But, in comparing the results to Jill's AIP activity log that I relied on, there was a definite trend. Her first PBGD test had been done prior to the DNA test. It registered 6.1 (of an expected 7 "normal"). She had been ill enough for me and doctors to be concerned. Within a matter of weeks her condition deteriorated. When she ended up in the hospital with breathing difficulty, severe nosebleeds and "sleep apnea>64 seconds," Dr. Wade's handwritten notes indicated her PBGD was 5.3.

Still, according to U.S. experts, Jill's urine test results have not produced a high enough level of PBGs to be considered MAIP.

As Jill philosophically has said, "Only time will tell. We'll wait."

181 Hindmarsh, JT; *The Porphyrias: Recent Advances* from Clinical Chemistry www.clinchem.org/content/32/7/1255.full.pdf. 1986
182 Pierach, CA et al. *Red blood porphobilinogen deaminase in the evaluation of acute intermittent porphyria.* http/www.ncbi.nlm.nih.gov/pubmed/3783903. Published online by JAMA. March 15, 1987.
183 Luder, AS et al. *Awareness is the name of the game: clinical and biochemical evaluation of a case of a girl diagnosed with acute intermittent porphyria with autism.* http://www.ncbi.nlm.nih.gov/pubmed/19267997. Published online by Cellular and Molecular Biology. February 16, 2009.
184 Peterson, LA et al. *Erythrocyte Uroporphyrinogen 1 Synthase Activity in Diagnosis of Acute Intermittent Porphyria.* www.clinchem.org/content/22/11/1835.abstract?sid=67edodd6-dacc-4ae9-925c-53d2f2bc72fa. Published online by from The American Association for Clinical Chemistry.1976.
185 Besur, Hou, Schmeltzer, Bonkovsky. www.mdpi.com/2218-1989/4/4/977/htm. *Metabolites.* 2014

CHAPTER 67

Potential for Squalls

*My precious child, during your times of trial and
suffering, when you see only one set of footprints,
it was then that I carried you.*

— FOOTPRINTS

Even with known familial AIP connections, I have heard of "next generation-ers"
or "not direct-line blood relatives" who have been run through multiple testing
cycles and were still left without a definitive diagnosis. There is no universal con-
sensus of what defines an AIP attack. Many experts acknowledge, and AIPorphyrics
confirm, that symptoms can develop over several hours or days. For some, attacks
begin with ambiguous complaints such as lethargy or depressive feelings. Many cite
pre-flu-like symptoms. For others, AIP acute symptoms are sudden and harsh and
the person and those in his/her proximity instantly know that AIP is afoot. Some
porphyrics have reported ongoing or recurrent attacks lasting for months, a year, or
in at least one case I heard of, over a year's time.

Once unleashed, MAIP can wreak havoc on the CNS, the systemic structure
that allows us to keep upright, moving and thinking and the PNS, attached to the
CNS that coordinates the organs, glands and muscles that we use to see, smell, feel,
touch, taste and hear. Dr. Ingemar Bylesjö describes what can happen when AIP
activity impacts the CNS: "Psychiatric disturbances, aphasia, apraxia, disturbed
consciousness and epileptic seizures…Motor neuropathy (movement of arms/legs)
is the most common involvement of the PNS and may involve the cranial nerves
[which control swallowing, talking, movement of tongue and lips and sometimes
respiratory paralysis] …myalgia, paresis, ascending flaccid paralysis of the limbs…

can lead to severe complications such as motor paralysis."[186] [Note: PNS dysfunction is known as *neuropathy*.]

In addition to the list of symptoms created during my initial research phase, AIPorphyrics responding to our query/survey letter provided others:

- abdominal distention

- anxiety

- appetite loss

- bladder dysfunction: urinary retention or painful urination

- blood labs: electrolyte imbalance; low potassium; low oxygen

- blood pressure fluctuations. (Normal systolic <120; normal diastolic <80; crisis stage systolic >180; crisis stage diastolic >110.)[187]

- delirium

- fatigue, moderate to extreme

- fever/temperature fluctuations

- heart: pain, elevated heart enzymes

- flu-like symptoms

- hypotranemia, low serum sodium, mental status changes

- insomnia (may precede actual attack)

- malaise

- muscle pain, cramping and/or muscle weakness including fainting

- pain: head, back, chest, shoulders, arms and/or legs, skin, kidney, liver

- restlessness

- sensory symptoms

- skin coloration (change to a putty or reddish/ruddy tint)

- social withdrawal

---

186 Bylesjö, I. *Epidemiological, Clinical and Pathogenetic Studies of Acute Intermittent Porphyria.* Medical dissertation, Umea University. www.diva-portal.org/smash/get/ diva2:141227; FULLTEXT01.pdf. 2008, 9.
187 American Heart Association, *Understanding Blood Pressure Readings*; www.heart.org/.../understanding-Blood-Readings_UCM_301764_Article.jsp. Last reviewed August 4, 2014.

Combined with the list from Chapter 12, it is easy to understand why some would question the legitimacy of what is going on. It takes another porphyric or caregiver to porphyric(s) to understand the frustrating disparity of symptoms. AIP has been mistaken for somatization disorders, Guillian Barre Syndrome, growing pains, epilepsy, depression, acute appendicitis, gall bladder distress, chronic fatigue, Parkinson's, irritable bowel syndrome (IBS), and many, many other conditions. Porphyria diagnostic entities consider family history to be the first clue of MAIP presence. But even without known familial connections, medical providers have laundry lists of differential diagnoses to consider. Figuring out MAIP can be a long, drawn-out challenge.

Of all the symptoms listed, three garnered the most mention from respondents: sensory effects, severe pain and mental status changes.

Sensory effects

Because of nervous systems' involvement, symptoms reported included: coordination impairment involving vestibular or balance affect; optic muscle movements; sight vision impairment such as blurred, foggy; double vision; living in a mist, slowly turning into fog, gray, visual distortions; "weak eyes," temporary total or partial loss of vision (known as cortical blindness); smell, a distorted sense of smell, "can't stand the smell of food," many things "smell bad," a heighted sense of smell to one's own body odors; taste, "food tastes awful" or doesn't taste "right;" touch including pain; burning, tingling like pins and needles, "freezing" fingertips, loss of sensation or paralysis; hearing—partial or complete loss; high pitched whine/hum; fluctuations in hearing--overly loud or "too" soft, ringing in ears; speech—garbled, halting, slurred, stuttering and aphasia ranging from an inability to speak at all to forgetting and/or mixing up words, ideas); movement problems with arm or hands and/or legs or feet ranging from twitching, a decreased feeling or muscle weakness; diminished reflexes; difficulty using the arms or hands or legs or feet; "arms wouldn't cooperate" to difficulty walking and/or bouts of paralysis.

Pain

By far, severe abdominal pain, sometimes called "colicky," is the most commonly recognized AIP symptom. For some porphyrics it may begin as a stomachache or cramping and may include the belly button area, which is why so many porphyrics lost their appendix to surgery—increasing, unrelenting pain surrounding the navel can be an early indication of appendicitis. Others are shocked by a sudden, overwhelmingly brutal pain concentrated in the lower right quadrant of the abdomen, the proximity of the liver.

AIP abdominal pain, which begins with irritation to the intestinal lining, has been described as horrific—but to the observer, it can seem out of proportion to physical signs, leading to great skepticism about what is really happening. An AIPorphyric woman reported that multiple bouts of labor and deliveries did not come anywhere near the pain of porphyria. Although severe abdominal pain did not appear for the first eight or nine months of Jill's manifestation, she has since experienced both types of pain development. Asked to describe her abdominal pain during an acute attack when she was younger, she said, "*It feels like the huge-est cramp ever that someone sets on fire.*"

It is well-established that AIP pain can become intractable or chronic and is not confined to the abdomen. When under AIP siege, Jill has complained about head-ache to migraine level; chest; lower, middle and upper back and neck; shoulder; arm, leg and hand/finger; ankle, foot and even toe pain. Jill has described the pains as "breathtaking," a "raging burn" or shooting "icicles." Whether met with weeping howls or silent tears, the feeling of helplessness smothers us all when AIP pain holds her hostage.

In short, it is a pain OTC medications cannot touch. It responds best to opioids, often in large quantities, containing chemicals that bind to opioid receptors found in the gastrointestinal tract.

Changeable mental status

The AIP changeable mental status connection is well-documented. AIP is known to mimic a number of psychiatric conditions and in fact, it has been documented that psychosis can be the *only* symptom of AIP:[188] "psychiatric findings include insom-nia, agitation, hysteria, anxiety, apathy or depression, phobias, psychosis, organic disorders, delirium, somnolence, or coma."[189] A National Coalition for Health Professional Education in Genetics (NCHPEG) article expanded on the above: "...25-80% of [AIP] cases [may present with psychiatric characteristics includ-ing] anxiety, depression, schizophrenia symptoms, social withdrawal, delusions, catatonia, disruptive behavior, hysteria, insomnia, restlessness, violence, delirium. Common presentation includes brief psychotic episodes often indistinguishable from schizophrenia or bipolar disorder...." It also noted, "[o]ccasional port wine color in urine."[190] Interestingly, the American Psychological Association released an abstract about a report it conducted on schizophrenia which identified a "... polymorphic...site....within the [AIP] gene that showed a significant association with the presence of illness...Data suggests that either the PBGD gene itself or an unknown gene linked to and/or in linkage disequilibrium with the PBGD locus predisposes some individuals to schizophrenia."[191] Could this be the reason why some AIPorphyrics present with schizophrenic-type symptoms?

---

188 Ellencsweig, Scoenfeld, Zemishlany. *Acute Intermittent Porphyria: Psychosis as the only clinical manifestation.* http://www.nlm.nih.gov/pubmed/16910386. Published online by The Israel Journal of Psychiatry and Related Sciences. 2006.
189 Thunell, S. *Hydroxymethylbilane Synthase (HMBS) Deficiency: Porphobilinogen Deaminase De-ficiency, HMBS Deficiency. Includes Acute Intermittent Porphyria (AIP).* Posted on GeneReviews-NCBI Bookshelf ID: NBK1193 PMID: 20301372. Initial posting: September 27, 2005; Last update: March 23, 2010. [Note: this article appeared at url http://www.ncbi.nlm.nih.gov/books/NBK113/ for years; it was sub-sequently moved to url www.researchgate.net/publication/221964097_Hydroxymethylbilane_Syn-thase_Deficiency but is only available to scientific subscribers to the researchgate.net forum.]
190 National Coalition for Health Professional Education in Genetics (NCHPEG). *Acute Intermittent Porphyria.* http://www.nchpeg.org/index.php?option=com_content&view=article&id=132&Item id=118. Undated.
191 Sanders, AR et al. American Psychological Association. PsycINFO journal article. *Association between genetic variation at the porphobilinogen deaminase gene and schizophrenia.* Schizophrenia Research, Vol 8(3) at http://psycnet.apa.org/psycinfo/1993-33649-001. January 1993.

The psychosis/AIP mimicry has been decried by many medical professionals as a "diagnostic quagmire." I cringed when I saw of the ten disorders listed in a "Karger Psychotherapy and Psychosomatics" article that Jill had presented with nine of them at different times. While the presence of porphyrins/ALAs and PBGs was discussed, the definitive test was to "measure monopyrrole porphobilinogen deaminase (PBGD) in red blood cells." The AIP diagnosis, it said, should be considered in seven situations: a) unexplained leukocytosis (as when Dr. O'Connor said Jill's blood cells were "misshapen?"), b) unexplained neuropathy [like being able to hear while experiencing full body paralysis?], c) etiologically obscure neurosis or psychosis [like Jill's sporadic hallucinations?], d) "idiopathic" seizure disorder [like the convulsions that do not present as typical seizures?], e) unexplained abdominal pain [like the *huge-est cramps ever that someone sets on fire?*), f) conversion hysteria [or conversion *disorder?*], and g) susceptibility to stress[192] [like when NHC staff refused oxygen, or told her she was to be discharged from the hospital with a mental illness diagnosis, or when Beatrice or Shirley or Camerin or Shana or Geoffrey or Geraldine or Angelica or Miranda or Tammy or Tony or Bart or Yvette and so many others did or said whatever?]. If so, then yes, AIP should really have been "entertained."

A few years ago, a newspaper story told about a young Connecticut adult female psychiatric patient who had suffered severe suicidal tendencies for years and no longer responded to treatment. She was transferred to a prestigious out-of-state psychiatric facility. Less than six months later, twenty-four-year-old Madeline* was found "unresponsive" in her bed despite the presence of two twenty-four-hour staff members assigned to watch her even as she slept. According to a news reports, the medical examiner listed her death as "natural causes—sudden death/ventricular arrhythmia due to schizophrenia."[193] My Mom antenna shot up. I wondered, *"What if this was a MAIP case gone wrong?"* AIP *can* present solely with psychiatric symptoms—often described as schizophrenic in nature. The young woman had been treated for schizophrenia and likely ingested medication(s) at levels deemed safe for schizophrenics, but *if* she was porphyric (or comorbid porphyric/schizophrenic), while testing within "therapeutic levels," the medication might have actually caused an untenable toxic situation for her, much as escalating amounts of Celexa had done to Jill, but with more severe consequences. It is well-documented that respiratory insufficiency can result in MAIP death. As Madeline slept, could it have been possible the young woman's lung muscles ultimately stopped working because of typical, "therapeutic" levels of antipsychotic/sleep or antidepressant medications that were, in reality, toxic? Had the differential diagnosis of acute porphyria ever been considered? And/or was she ever tested for an acute porphyria (before *or* after death)? I will never know, but the story lit a fire in my heart of major proportions, and I was truly afraid for Jill's future. Would she, too, possibly be shuttled off to some facility that would, as the Littleton School System, MedCity Hospital and

---

192 Burgoyne, Swartz, Ananth. Porphyria: Reexamination of Psychiatric Implications.
http://karger.com/Article/Abstract/289001. Published online by Psychotherapy and Psychosomatics, Vol 64, No 3-4, 1995.
193 Kovner, J. *Family Still Seeks Answers in Psychiatric Death*. "The Hartford Courant." April 02, 2011.

medical professionals did, ignore her physical symptoms, tolerate her neurological symptoms and amplify the psychiatric aspect of MAIP?

AIPorphyics will generally do all they can to avoid the aforementioned presentations. Some offered tips for consideration when walking the MAIP line:

- When doctors prescribe medications, *always* check trusted "safe-drug" lists.

- Get food down you right away when you start shaking or feeling "weird."

- One man says when he feels something coming on he takes two tablespoons of sugar. He reports that usually helps.

- "My diet is kept simple...anything with garlic, onion powder, artificial sweeteners, preservatives...is not going to be good...[and] no diet anything!"[194]

- I avoid soft drinks, sugar substitutes and processed food as much as possible...I try to always carry a supply of "emergency food" (bottled water, bananas, grapes) with me. I became a doctor of nutrition and developed "Dr. Janie's Eating in the Zone" so I could live.[195]

- "A dietician helped me design a diet on www.myfitnesspal.com that allows me to lose/maintain weight while satisfying an AIPorphyric's calorie/carbohydrate requirements. Mine is a 60% carbs, 15% protein, 25% fat formula. I followed these guidelines for several months, lost 23 lbs and haven't had an acute attack."[196]

- "Cleaning supplies with strong smell or fragrance are of no use to me. Products that are OK for me include Febreeze, Colgate Cavity Protection toothpaste, Suave unscented shampoo and Ivory soap. Be careful with deodorants because of long term alcohol contact. Perfume is not my friend."[197]

- One AIPorphyric figured out that attacks can be triggered by aerosol bug sprays. Since the advent of Jill's AIP, we haven't had the opportunity to use aerosol bug spray, but even before that, when needed, it was applied sparingly only to her clothing (pant legs, socks), shoes/sneakers, hat and jackets, etc. Many reported problems with outdoor "yard bug bombs" and/or when aerosol insect repellents such as Off are used on or in their proximity. A PES newsletter stated "insecticides can induce heme synthesis... Symptoms include general body weakness. Sweating, convulsions, difficulty in breathing, urinary problems, irritation of the nose, eyes and throat, and skin discoloration may present...Life-threatening paralysis and death can occur very quickly especially in AIP patients who are all ready [sic] sensitive

---

194 Contributor requests anonymity. Letter to author. May 28, 2012
195 Williams, Dr. Janie. Telephone conversation/interview with author, October, 24, 2009
196 Sadowniczak, C. Email to author, 2015
197 Contributor requests anonymity. Letter to author. May 28, 2012

to chemical toxins."[198]

- "Any chemicals, herbicides, weed or bug spray should be left to the professionals. Always wear protective clothing and a respirator. Do not use insecticide or spray anything on your skin.[199] Living near a forest keeps us on perpetual insect-alert. We rely on a homemade boric acid and sugar brew as an effective lure when the ants march into our living quarters. We have switched to using inexpensive brands of shampoo—sometimes mixed with baking soda, to get shower stalls, bathtubs and bathroom sinks and bowls sparking clean thereby eliminating the need for toxic bathroom cleaners.

- I use sunscreen in moderation. What you put on skin is absorbed by the skin." [200]

- A woman noted that secondhand smoke put her into porphyria attack mode and warned porphyrics to avoid being around smokers that indulge. One good reason is because "tobacco contains polycyclic aromatic hydrocarbons, which induce cytochromes and increase heme synthesis."[201] The Swedes have found a definite "association between smoking and a high frequency of AIP attacks."[202]

- One man told how the familiar abdominal pains come a day or so after his wife has done her nails.

- Regarding solvents: a man reported that he had to leave employment in an auto painting business. Jill's system could not tolerate the combination of cleaner/dry-marker vapors wafting throughout Littleton's school buildings. One woman respondent noted that her AIP symptoms crop up in stores' detergent aisles. Other AIPorphyrics cited sensitivities to carpet and paint stores, ordinary cleaners, perfumes, nail polish and similar products.

- Several porphyrics have shared that an over-the-counter medicine, Tagamet, helped diminish and/or resolve their episodic symptoms. It has offered relief for Jill on several occasions. [Note: Dr. Janie Williams' program notes that Tagamet depletes nutrients Vitamin B12, Folic Acid, Vitamin D, Calcium, Iron and Zinc.][203]

- In short, maintaining a stable metabolism is the key to living with AIP. Many factors can affect the metabolic rate: body mass, body composition, age, gender, hormones, nutritional supplements, nicotine, pharmaceuticals,

198 Pfeiffer, P. *Avoiding Pesticides in Porphyria*. http://porphbook.tripod.com/Apr2005.html. Published online by PES Monthly Newsletter. April 2005.
199 Contributor requests anonymity. Letter to author, May 28, 2012.
200 Ibid.
201 Cojocaru, I et al. *Acute Intermittent Porphyria—Diagnostic and Treatment Traps*. www.intmed.ro/attach/rjim/2012/rjim112/art06.pdf. Published online by Romanian Journal of Internal Medicine. 2012.
202 Bylesjö, I. *Epidemiological, Clinical and Pathogenetic Studies of Acute Intermittent Porphyria*. Medical dissertation, Umea University. www.diva-portal.org/smash/get/ diva2:141227; FULLTEXT01.pdf. 2008, 43.
203 Williams, Dr. J. Email to author. October 24, 2009

fever and/or infection, stress/emotional excitement, exercise, weight loss and caloric restriction.[204] Weight loss and caloric restriction, also known as fasting (even skipping meals) has been known to induce AIP attacks because it increases the level of a protein that helps to create glucose in the liver. When this happens, ALA production is increased, which may lead to acute attacks.[205]

204 Unidentified author. *Factors that affect your metabolic rate*. www.bodyfi.com/s/factorsthataffect-metabolism.pdf. published online by "What's your Metabolic Fingerprint?" Microlife, Inc. 2006.
205 Secko, D. *Link between porphyria and fasting uncovered*. http://www.cmaj.ca/content/173/8/864.2.full. Published online by Canadian Medical Association Journal. October 11, 2005.

CHAPTER 68

Silver Linings, Rainbows & Fogbows

You are not alone…if we ask anything
according to His will, He hears us.
— 1 JOHN 5:14

The "knowledge is power" adage got additional meaning when American columnist Marilyn vos Savant said, "To acquire knowledge, one must study, but to acquire wisdom one must observe." [206] Through study, observation and experience, the Swedes gained knowledge, wisdom and considerable power over the dreaded AIP and continue to be recognized and respected the world over for their knowledge and management of it.

While it originated in the Nordic region of the world, AIP can now be found throughout the globe. Regardless of when it arrived in America where, for the most part it remained hidden and largely unknown to the general public and most doctors, the earliest mention for this country I could find was a relatively recent report of a 1949 University of Minnesota Hospital case study, featured in "Psychosomatic Medicine" journal.[207] For generations, the vast majority of U.S. doctors had no knowledge of the disease and no inkling why some patients presented with a variety of peculiar, seemingly unrelated symptoms for which there seemed no reason to "connect the dots." That began to change when the not-for-profit APF was established and the founders set out to increase awareness about the genetically-generated porphyrias. Unfortunately, there are still too many doctors who do not

---

206 Vos Savant, Marilyn. "Goodreads." www.goodreads.com/author/quotes/44295.Marilyn_Vos_Savant
207 Visher MD and Aldrich MD. *Acute Intermittent Porphyria: A Case Study.* www.psychosomaticmedicine.org/content/16/12/163.full.pdf. 1954. [Note this url no longer carries this document; subscribers can access it at: http://journals.lww.com/psychosomaticmedicine/Citation/1954/0300/American_Intermittent_Porphryia

know anything about AIP—and even more who either do not understand it, do not want to know anything about it or just do not accept a diagnosis of the disease. I recently spoke with a Midwestern patient who, upon having finally located a doctor who said he was treating several AIPorphyrics, asked him about his testing and treatment strategy. His reply? "I keep them medicated with psyche drugs." Another told her he did not believe porphyria was real and refused to entertain questions or concerns about it.

On the other hand, during the 1990s, Dr. Morton, a U.S. west coast doctor diagnosed a significant number of cases of porphyria that he claimed were caused by exposure to environmental toxins. He presented about ninety symptoms[208] and argued that his diagnosis of porphyria was virtually synonymous with multiple chemical sensitivity syndrome [MCS], a condition with varied symptoms, many similar to AIP, "that appears following a person's exposure to any of a wide range of chemicals. Such exposure may occur as a major event [such as a chemical spill] or from long-term contact with low-levels of chemicals. As a result of exposure, people with MCS develop sensitivity and have reactions to the chemicals even at levels [tolerated by most people]."[209] Legal action was taken against Dr. Morton. Trial records from that case indicate that the root issue was whether or not "exposure to chemicals in ambient air causes porphyria." Peer-reviewed medical literature essentially dismissed the theory that short-term ambient exposure to chemicals causes porphyria.[210] Dr. Morton ultimately surrendered his medical license in lieu of further investigation. But information presented during the trial was troubling— even from a lay mom's perspective. First, to my knowledge, none of Dr. Morton's patients' DNA had been porphyria-tested to see if any were predisposed to *any* form of genetic porphyria (though there *is* a type of porphyria that can be "acquired" and that is porphyria cutanea tarda (PCT)). And since at least 1993, urinary or bio-chemical testing for the acute porphyrias has been known to be "problematic"[211] by U.S. experts. Fifteen years ago, "…two porphryia experts at UMass Medical Center …warned [then] that the test was not reliable, had not been validated, and should not be used."[212] Yet still today, U.S. "experts" insist high-level biochemical measure-ment is the "be all to end all" in diagnosing AIP.

Knowing what Jill has been through since the fall of 2008 when DNA tested positive for AIP and after researching myriad chemicals, observing her numerous AIP bouts connected to toxin exposures, *and* re-examining the Benton School chemical evaluation results, as a non-scientist, non-medical mom, I think the AIP/MCS connection has some merit. As I found out about conversion disorder being an AIP symptom, I believe MCS must be considered as a possible *symptom* of AIP

208 Morton, Dr. W. *Porphyria-Liver Problems via Poison Dioxin* mirrored from Geocities. www.oocities. org/fltaxpayer/endocrine/13porphy.html.October 2009.

209 WebMD. *Allergies Health Center, Multiple Chemical Sensitivity;* http://www.webmd.com/allergies/multiple-chemical-sensitivity

210 FindLaw. Court of Appeals of Washington, Division 1. www.caselaw.findlaw.com/wa-court-of-appeals/1368600.hmtl. May 21, 2001.

211 Astrink, Desnick. *Molecular basis of acute intermittent porphyria: mutations and polymorphisms in the human hydroxylmethylbilane synthase gene.* http://www.ncbi.nlm.nih.gov/pubmed/7866402. 1994.

212 "MCS" and Porphyria." http://www.quackwatch.com.search/webglimpse. cgi?ID=1&query=Porphyria.

and recognized that while toxins do not *cause* AIP, they can aggravate the heme biopathways and *trigger* porphyric symptoms.

One of the most important things we have been able to figure out from Jill's many experiences with various chemical exposures was that she has to be extraordinarily careful regarding medications, too. In today's world, medication generally means chemicals and too many times, when acute porphyria and certain chemicals mix, the result can be adverse reactions to "safe" medications. Fortunately, several acute porphyria-related drug databases have become available for doctors and AIPorphyrics to refer to. My favorite is the Canadian Porphyria Foundation/Sweden Porphyria Center's (CPF/SPC) collaborative safe drug list, "Patient's and Doctor's guide to medication in acute porphyria," written by Swedish Dr. Stig Thunell and published by the CPF in 2005. Jill and I still keep copies readily available. The CPF is now called the Alberta Porphyria Society (APS) which favors the South African drug list which happens to be the Nordic Drug Database (NAPOS) list. Fortunately, the SPC list is incorporated into the NAPOS list. However, the individual CPF/SPC list is still available through the APS at http://albertaporphyriasociety.weebly.com/patients-and-doctors-guide-to-medication-in-acute-porphyria.html for a nominal fee. As a base, it is well worth the price.

A short history of porphyria drug lists can be found at http://www.drugs-porphyria.org/epnet.php that includes EPNET (European Porphyria Network) and NAPOS (Nordic Drug Database).

As medications come and go with unbelievable rapidity, I have learned to look to and compare several sources before Jill ingests any med she has no experience with. Some online sources to consider:

- http://www.porphbook.tripod.com/2.html (PES Unsafe Drug List—however, somewhat dated);

- www.porphyria-europe.org/03-Drugs/selecting-drug-safe-theme.asp European Porphyria Initiative (EPNET) primarily tracks medications available in Europe.

- www.drugs-porphyria.org is Norwegian Porphyria Center (NAPOS), offers language choice (select UK for English) and tracks medications available in Sweden, Norway, United Kingdom.

- www.porphyriafoundation.com tracks meds available in USA. However, this list provided an "OK!" rating for Heparin yet we learned the preservative in Heparin for IV locks sent Jill into severe attacks—twice. It gave OK? ratings for Celexa and Lidocaine, both of which turned out to be problematic—as we discovered when Celexa sent Jill into frightening neurological, physical and psychiatric symptoms and, while she relies on "surface" Lidocaine for port access, one dose of *injectable* Lidocaine launched her into red-faced respiratory distress. However, my trusty CPF/SPC list had rated Celexa (citalopram) as possibly porphrinogenic and warns its use should be only when no safer alternative is available. It rated injectable lidocaine as probably porphrinogenic, to be used only on strong or urgent indication.[213] I was impressed when NCH's surgeon and anesthesiologist asked to review this list prior to Jill's port replacement surgery in 2014.

If there is a disparity between lists, if a med cannot be found, or if a med is suggested for Jill that she has not yet used, I turn to www.dailymed.nlm.nih.gov and www.rxlist.com, and/or scrutinize MSDS sheet(s) for more complete information about contraindications, precautions and warnings, interactions and side effects. I purposely search for mentions about liver-impairment. If I still come up short of information, a visit to our pharmacist for clarification usually helps.

Clinical treatment of AIP attacks

Oxygen

In an emergency MAIP situation, many things happen simultaneously but first and foremost, the airway, breathing and circulation must be stabilized because without a constant supply of oxygen, the brain can sustain irreversible damage. Jill's acute symptoms were improved many times when supplemental oxygen was administered. And once the decision was made for her to receive oxygen (level 2-4) during heme infusion, breathing problems and chest pains that sometimes had developed were essentially eliminated.

Early in our AIP odyssey, I wondered whether hyberbaric oxygen therapy (HBOT), which involves treating patients with high levels of oxygen for injuries relating to stroke, cerebral palsy, multiple sclerosis and other neurological problems including metabolic syndrome, might be helpful for porphyrics. I have since discovered that HBOT works by stimulating blood flow, metabolism and tissue growth. After learning so much about agents that stimulate metabolism/heme synthesis that can be harmful to porphyrics, I am no longer interested in HBOT as a possible treatment for Jill.

Glucose/carbs

Glucose, which is a brain food, is not generally a recommended snack of choice, but it has been proven many times to ameliorate AIP symptoms. This is because the body converts carbs into sugar which is stored in the liver and muscles as an energy source known as glycogen. Many sources explain that glucose helps to level the porphyria metabolic imbalance. One in particular describes how that is accomplished: "glucose suppress[es] the activity of aminolaevulinic acid synthesis, thereby reducing the overproduction of porphyrins and precursors—this can lead to remission [of the particular attack.]" [214]Another offers, "[the] underlying mechanism of the "glucose effect" has recently been explained: the glucose down-regulates...a

---

213 Thunell, S. *Sweden Porphyria Centre/Canadian Porphyria Foundation Patient's and Doctor's guide to medication in acute porphyria.* Published by The Canadian Porphyria Foundation. 2005.
214 Wright, Michelle Dr., original author; Tidy, Colin Dr., current version. *Porphyrias.* http://patient.info/doctor/porphyrias. Published online in "Patient." August 17, 2015.

protein which directly induces the transcription of ALAS1."[215] An AIPorphyric woman reported that different frequencies of intravenous dextrose treatments were tried before settling on weekly infusions to keep her symptoms in check. She stressed that paying attention to dietary intake and avoiding other triggers helped, too. Of particular interest is a statement Dr. Sassa made in the British "Journal of Hematology," "Glucose and insulin together might...be more effective than glucose alone, as insulin blunts the PBC-1α effect."[216] I wondered if that is so, why would not glucose/insulin be considered standard practice in AIP treatment? Is insulin too expensive, too hard to acquire? Is it not known what ratio works best? What is the reason?

Pain Relief

It has been well established that AIPorphyria pain responds best to opioids because they contain chemicals that bind to opioid receptors found in the CNS system and the gastrointestinal tract. The danger of these medications, however, is that they can be highly addictive and must be used judiciously under medical guidance. As was mentioned previously, several acute porphyrics, with physician endorsements, shared that an OTC medication, Tagamet (generic: cimetidine) provided cost-effective relief for their symptoms so I researched it further. It turns out "cimetidine can decrease ALAS activity [because] through inhibiting cytochrome P450 medicated drug metabolism, it reduces heme oxygenase activity."[217] In fact, "administering cimetidine orally decreases ALA and PBG excretion rapidly to the normal stage."[218] Another source noted the medication's value, but warned it should not be used instead of hemin or glucose.[219] This made sense to me because, in my view, cimetidine has served as an effective bandage for Jill. But it does not replace heme.

Porphyria experts in China recently found that out when a porphyric patient with recurrent attacks was treated with high concentrations of glucose which proved to be minimally effective so intravenous cimetidine treatments were given. The patient was discharged but unfortunately could not tolerate oral cimetidine daily at home and another attack started. Ten days later, the patient died after being brought back to the hospital, unconscious.[220]

---

215 Bylesjö, I. *Epidemiological, Clinical and Pathogenetic Studies of Acute Intermittent Porphyria.* Medical dissertation. Umea University, New series No. 1150 ISSN 0346-66-12. www.diva-portal.org/smash/get/diva2:141227; FULLTEXT01.pdf. 2008, p12.

216 Sassa, S. *Modern diagnosis and management of the porphyrias.* http://onlinelibrary.wiley.com/doi/10.111/j.1365-2141.2006,06289.x/epdf. September 4, 2006.

217 Xanyan Zia et al. *Cimetidine in the Treatment of Acute Intermittent Porphyria from Onset to Death.* www.omicsonline.org/...ermittent-porphyria-from-onset-to-death-2155-9864-1000331.pdf. Published online in "Journal of Blood Disorders and Transfusions." 2015. p1.
See also: Rogers, PD. *Cimetidine in the treatment of acute intermittent porphyria.* http://www.ncbi.nih.gov/pubmed/9066947. Published online in "Annals of Pharmacotherapy." 1997.

218 Ibid, p2.

219 Epocrates. *Acute Intermittent Porphyria: Emerging Therapies.* http://online.epocrates.com/u/2943235. 2016.

220 Xanyan Zia et al. *Cimetidine in the Treatment of Acute Intermittent Porphyria from Onset to Death.* www.omicsonline.org/...ermittent-porphyria-from-onset-to-death-2155-9864-1000331.pdf. Published online in "Journal of Blood Disorders and Transfusions." 2015.

Another source reported that cimetidine has been used for hematin-resistant AIP.[221] Oddly, while a U.S. porphyria drug lists cimetidine as safe, mention as to its success in ameliorating acute porphyric symptoms has yet to be found in the group's literature.

[Note: The question and answer format between me and a U.S. porphyria expert, introduced in Chapter 66, resumes here and continues into the next chapter. Reminder, information from other sources is also included.]

Panhematin (aka "Hematin" or "Heme")

Q2: Does Panhematin have a restorative and/or preventative effect on the liver? That is, does the administration of Panhematin strengthen the liver in any way against trigger exposure? For example, if a patient has been infused with Panhematin and soon thereafter is exposed to an AIP trigger such as a toxin—external exposure or ingested, physical and/or emotional stress, is the newly infused liver able to resist trigger exposure any more or less than if it would have without the Panhematin application?

A2: *Hemin repletes the regulatory heme pool in liver cells, and therefore ALA synthase decreases. Its effects last for only a matter of days, since the liver rapidly degrades hemin.*

Panhematin is an enzyme inhibitor derived from processed red blood cells[222] (human blood) currently manufactured in the United States by Recordati Rare Diseases Inc. Considered to be an "orphan drug," that is, a medication or biologic approved specifically to treat a certain rare medical condition,[223] Panhematin is a biologic, meaning it is made from natural, not chemical, sources. It was developed specifically to correct heme deficiency in AIPorphyrics' attack-mode livers by returning porphyrin and porphyrin precursor levels to a more normal state. A 2011 Brazilian case report describes how that happens. "[H]ematin...inhibits the action of the first enzyme involved in the heme synthetic pathway, thereby blocking porphyrin production and accumulation."[224] And by repressing, or limiting, the dreaded ALAs, Panhematin has been proven to help minimize or eliminate certain neurological deficits from improving cognition to regaining mobility, associated with MAIP attacks. It has worked for Jill—many times.

Panhematin arrives from the manufacturer in powder form with instructions to reconstitute it just prior to use. However, the biologic agent contains no preservatives and begins to deteriorate immediately when mixed with liquid and has no means to stop bacteria growth. So, in order to maintain its potency and hygienic property, it needs to be used immediately upon reconstitution. For these reasons, experts recommend covering the dosing vial with an amber bag to protect it from light during reconstitution through infusion. Though manufacturer Recordati's MSDS says Panhematin should be reconstituted with sterile water, many experts

221 Shah, Remoroza, Aziz. *Acute Intermittent Porphyria. Case Report.* www.turner-white.com/pdf/ hp_feb02_acute.pdf. Published online in "Hospital Physician." 2002.
222 *Panhematin.* http://www.rxlist.com/panhematin-drug/html. Published online at RxList. September 18, 2013
223 Wikipedia. *Orphan drug.* https://en.wikipedia.org/wiki/Orphan_drug.
224 Goncalves Menegueti, M et al. *Case report: Acute Intermittent Porphyria Associated with Respiratory Failure: A Multidisciplinary Approach;* http://www.ncbi.nlm.nih.gov/pmc/articles/PMC3113262/. March 16, 2011.

instead recommend using human albumin, a protein manufactured by the liver, because it is more stable than water and it reduces the possibility of vein inflammation, or phlebitis, occurring. It is also strongly recommended that Panhematin be administered into a large peripheral vein such as in the arm, or central venous vein (as in the chest or neck).

Jill's Panhematin mixed with albumin treatments were timed to arrive directly from the hospital pharmacy upon completion of the pre-hydration D10 infusion. It is essential that patients and doctors communicate throughout each Panhematin treatment period to establish what works best for the patient.

As far as dosing goes, Recordati's Panhematin MSDS recommends "…a dose of 1-4/mg/kg/day given over a period of 10-15 minutes for 3-14 days based on the clinical signs. In more severe cases, this dose may be repeated no earlier than every 12 hours. No more than 6 mg/kg…should be given in any 24-hour period. The company also recommends that Panhematin be administered through a sterile 0.45 micron or smaller filter.[225] Rxlist.com offers, "The dosage is based on your weight, medical conditions, and response to therapy."[226] This was the first time I had seen in print anything near "customizing" Panhematin treatment(s) to the patient's response and condition. I encourage U.S. experts to develop a better method of Panhematin dosing and frequency. As Jill and I have learned, when she is severely heme deficient, she needs heme "until." It seems ludicrous that one size fits all is the current U.S. method of dosing.

When heme therapy was first introduced, the practice was to infuse heme only after several days of glucose therapy. Nowadays, in order to get Panhematin's maximum benefit, experts recommend "the therapy should be started without delay in moderate and severe attacks."[227]

As wonderful as it is, Panhematin is not without potential side effects. As mentioned previously, its use can cause phlebitis, particularly when given by small veins; coagulopathy, or reduced blood clotting ability, and used in excess can cause renal failure, perhaps because "excess free-heme is highly toxic due to its ability to promote oxidative stress and lipid peroxidation, thus leading to membrane injury and, ultimately, apoptosis [cell death]."[228] Dr. Bylesjö explained that "excess porphyrins or their precursors may be nephrotoxic (poisonous to kidneys)," possibly resulting in blood pressure problems.[229] Renal failure has been known to happen when heme is given in excess, however, it is said to be reversible.[230]

225 *Panhematin. U.S. Prescribing Information.* recordatirarediseases.com/products. Published online at Recordati Rare Diseases, Inc.

226 *Panhematin.* Patient Info. htttp://www.rxlist.com/panhematin-drug/consumer-uses.htm. Published online at RxList.

227 Bylesjö, I. *Epidemiological, Clinical and Studies of Acute Intermittent Porphyria.* Medical dissertation, Umea University. www.diva-portal.org/smash/get/ diva2:141227; FULLTEXT01.pdf. 2008, p12.

228 Chiabrando, D et al. *Heme in pathophysiology: a matter of scavenging, metabolism and trafficking across cell membranes.* http://www.ncbi.nlm.nih.gov/pmc/articles/PMC3986552. Publisher: Frontiers in Pharmacology. April 8, 2014.

229 Bylesjö, I. *Epidemiological, Clinical and Pathogenetic Studies of Acute Intermittent Porphyria.* Medical dissertation, Umea University. www.diva-portal.org/smash/get/ diva2:141227; FULLTEXT01.pdf. 2008, 10.

230 www.rxlist.com/panhematin-drug/overdosage-contraindications.htm

After observing Jill's response to 140 Panhematin maintenance and attack treatments over the years, we can say it *does* have a certain restorative affect. But the quality of that restorative affect depends on any number of details, one of the most important being the type of trigger(s) and intensities. While it has been noted that heme "correct[s] the oxidative metabolism of drugs [and, I am assuming, environmental toxins] in AIP,"[230] my observation is that for Jill, certain types of medications and environmental toxins have produced the most severe and most difficult attacks to remedy.

As said earlier, adding supplemental oxygen during the actual infusing of heme significantly enhanced her treatment experiences.

Many AIPorphyrics laud Panhematin's life-saving properties and if Dr. Piersen had not provided guidance about the quantity and frequency of administering it to Jill when she did, this book might have been a tribute to her short life. Instead, though Jill swears it "tastes like car oil," and looks like it, too, we are grateful supporters of Panhematin and know the importance it has had in Jill's life.

Yet, we have heard from patients whose systems cannot tolerate Panhematin and are left on the outside looking in—as if having MAIP were not enough. Some have endured severe allergic reactions such as developing a rash or hives, difficulty breathing, dizziness, swelling of the face, lips, tongue or throat, others cannot tolerate the side effects sometimes associated with it: fever, achiness, malaise, easy bruising, urinating less than usual or not at all, pain, or irritation around the IV needle[231] and yes, phlebitis, but in most, if not all, phlebitis cases I have heard of, the patient had received the Panhematin in "any available vein," not a large or central vein as recommended.

Manufacturer Recordati states that each vial of Panhematin" contains 313 mg hemin, 215 mg sodium carbonate and 300 mg of sorbitol.[232] One has to wonder if perhaps some of the aforementioned patients' systems rejected the blood product because of excess free-heme toxicity or if they reacted to the sodium carbonate and/ or sorbitol. Or maybe insufficient oxygen was the problem? Reality is that every patient's treatment experience can vary because endogenous and exogenous circumstances are not static. What works good one time may not the next.

Recordati Rare Diseases and other sources have noted that Panhematin is contraindicated in patients with known hypersensitivity to the drug. But as with any drug, that is tough to know before it is tried! And because 100 mg of Panhematin contains 8 mg of iron, monitoring iron and serum ferritin concentration is strongly endorsed, particularly when patients are receiving multiple administrations of Panhematin.[233]

---

230 Ibid, p15.
231 *Panhematin. U.S. Prescribing Information*.www.recordatirarediseases.com/products. Published online at Recordati Rare Diseases, Inc.
232 Chiabrando, D et al. *Heme in pathophysiology: a matter of scavenging, metabolism and trafficking across cell membranes*. http://www.ncbi.nlm.nih.gov/pmc/articles/PMC3986552/. Published online by Frontiers in Pharmacology. April 8, 2014.
233 Whatley, S and Badminton, M. *Acute Intermittent Porphyria, Synonyms: PBGD Deficiency, Porphobilinogen Deaminase Deficiency*. http://www.ncbi.nlm.nih.gov/books/NBK1193. Published online by GeneReviews [Internet]. Last update: February 7, 2013.

The manufacturer also advises that anticoagulants be avoided during Panhematin therapy. Jill has von Willibrand, a bleeding disorder that can act as a "natural" anticoagulant. She never experienced excessive bleeding episodes during or after Panhematin infusions. Her Panhematin treatments were always filtered appropriately. Blood levels (including iron, serum ferritin, electrolytes and, at minimum, basic CBC stats) were monitored before, sometimes during and following every infusion. We were lucky to have caring and interested doctors to treat her.

Though not a cure, Panhematin has long been recognized as the greatest development made for treating MAIP activity. Heme arginate, or Normosang, a similar blood product is considered more stable than Panhematin with fewer side effects, is used for AIP attacks outside the United States, but it is not approved for use in this country. It should be.

A new drug that may be more universally AIPorphyric palatable is said to be on the horizon. As of this writing, this drug is in the clinical trial stage and questions remain about patient suitability, potential side effects and cost. It sounds great, but like cimetidine, will not replace heme and will likely be needed again once an AIP trigger strong enough to flare an attack is encountered.

Life can be full of extraordinary challenges and grave crises for AIPorphyrics. Any day can become a roller coaster of physical and emotional challenges often dismissed or minimized by others, leaving the porphyric to feel very much alone. Many porphyrics told of spouses, friends, parents and children who stayed by their side through good, bad, ugly and horrific AIP days. A mother's love creates a particularly unique connection and AIPorphyrics shared heartfelt memories of the maternal connection:

- An AIPorphyric woman has memories of her mother telling her about when she was a baby and people advised her to put the infant in the sun as she was very fair. Her mother tried it but the child passed out every time and her mother refused to do it anymore. The patient relates how her mother, never having known what was wrong with her child, suffered with guilt for the rest of her life. The woman was not diagnosed with AIP until she was twenty-three.

- An acute porphryic man recalled that his mother was often sick and very tired, so much so that many people thought she was a hypochondriac. He regrets that she passed away before he was diagnosed with AIP and is sure now that she also had AIP. He remembers her with deep love and affection as his true friend and inspiration.

- *It's true when they say your life is a story with many different chapters. Through the years I've been put through challenging obstacles. The fact that my biological mother did different kinds of drugs didn't help my situation. But through all these obstacles my mom has been with me each step of the way. With blood, sweat, tears, pain and anger she fought for my life. Although my story only covers a certain time period of my life, I still continue to battle a life-threatening disease. My mom was always there and still is with me.*[234]

- The mother of a now grown AIPorphyric son noted, "It's almost like you live from attack to attack. As I've read from others who care for a porphyric, my son is such a good, sweet, and loving person, it breaks my heart that he has to go through this. [AIP] is an illness that takes over your life when it involves your child. It is pretty scary when you realize that your child is so sick and even the medical professionals know nothing about this."[235]

- Another mom, who happens to be a nurse and AIPorphyric, lovingly describes how after a particularly horrific death defying AIP experience, "My oldest son quit his job, brought me home and became my 24 hr. 7 day a week nurse. My husband and youngest son were there to help but my oldest learned how to care for my track [tracheostomy opening] and puree food, etc. AIP is not something I would wish on anyone but it has taught me so much and I have the BEST NURSES EVER, my husband and sons. They learned a lot from my nurses training, I practiced on them when I was a student and they studied me as little children and then years later as big strong men they took over my care. Carried me, taught me to walk again, dressed me, and prayed for me, read to me and so much more. "[236]

More than a few respondents said they were blessed and/or grateful for people that porphyria brought into their lives. Some mentioned receiving professional therapeutic support, which Jill and I champion. Several referred to connections made with other AIPorphyrics because it helps the heart to talk with someone who has walked or is walking the same road as you. Internet porphyria support groups have sprung up around the world with information, patient stories and support being only a few keystrokes away.

It is not surprising that many people rely on their faith, especially when illness attacks their or love ones' bodies and/or psyches. *Many* AIPorphyrics rely on faith and prayers, not only during difficult attack times, but also as a major theme in their everyday lives:

- "Ultimately, I have found spiritual peace within myself. May you be blessed with the knowledge and understanding you seek." [237]

- An AIPorphyric woman reported that she does lots of praying and that her faith has helped her through many attacks and hospitalizations.

- *"I hope that God likes me the day that we meet ... if only a chance, to sit at His feet and be by His side year after year while all of the bad things just disappear. So when*

---

234 Jill. Fall 2015
235 Shelor, J. Emails to author. October 25, 2009
236 Bruno, R.D. *Why and How I became a Nurse.* Originally appeared on APF website; permission granted by R.D. Bruno to publish here, February 2006.
237 Contributor requests anonymity. Letter to author. October 28, 2008.

life gets tough and it's hard to be strong, I'll never forget Heaven is where I belong."[238]

Caring cannot be taught in medical school. It comes from the heart, so finding a doctor willing to team with the porphyric patient and his/her family is a God-sent gift and can mean so much to maintaining the emotional and physical strength needed for an AIP diagnosis. Nurses and medical staff, too, play an important role in helping AIPorphyrics manage what can become a medical minefield. Jill and I are forever grateful that Dr. O'Connor agreed to take Jill's case—and that serendipity connected us to Dr. Piersen when it did. In addition to being top-notch hematologists, both are wonderfully caring clinicians and *good* people.

Despite a U.S. surge in the expansion and building of new medical schools, the Association of American Medical Colleges predicts a shortage of physicians by 2020. There is also evidence that medications developed for certain diseases may be able to be re-purposed for use against rare diseases. To that end, large pharmaceutical companies have begun to show interest in rare diseases primarily because funding for common diseases is dwindling. How this all will play out as it affects future U.S. AIP identification, treatment and potential cures is uncertain.

---

238 Poster on Jill's bedroom wall

CHAPTER 69

Overcast, Possible Lightning Strikes

*When you have knowledge, let others
light their candle on it.*

— MARGARET FULLER

AIP is a complex disorder but as we found clues, clarification and corroboration in others' documentations, we hope this chapter will do the same for others.

Heme Deficiency
Noted Rockefeller University Biochemist Dr. Shigeru Sassa stated, "Mice with PBGD [heme] deficiency...display some of the symptoms observed in patients with AIP such as impaired motor function, ataxia....and decreased haem [heme] saturation of liver tryptophan pyrrolase. This model should be useful to further define the mechanisms of neurological damage in acute porphyrias."[239] After learning more about the heme pool, I wondered if Jill's heme supply somehow eked out little by little, if that was even possible, and whether the resulting decreased level of heme might contribute to AIP attacks. Then I found, "A critical deficiency of heme could lead to reduced levels of key heme proteins...resulting in direct or indirect effects on the nervous system...,"[240] and further, "[a]cute attacks of AIP may be accompanied by heme deficiency...."[241]

---

239 Sassa, Shigeru. *Modern diagnosis and management of the porphyrias.* http://onlinelibrary.wiley. com/doi/10.1111/j.1365-2141.2006.06289.x/full. September 4, 2006.
240 Bylesjö, I. *Epidemiological, Clinical and Pathogenetic Studies of Acute Intermittent Porphyria.* Medical dissertation. Umea University, New series No. 1150 ISSN 0346-66-12. www.diva-portal.org/smash/get/ diva2:141227; FULLTEXT01.pdf. 2008, 14.
241 Ibid, 35.

Before we had a handle on what AIP or heme even was, Jill had been fainting repeatedly—just like Paula's father, Michael, in Ms. Allende's memoir. And like her family, ours became accustomed to it. I ultimately discovered that heme deficiency or heme degradation, which *leads* to heme deficiency, was directly related to Jill's fainting and convulsive spells as well as a host of neurological problems. That was proven many times when Panhematin coursed through her liver and ameliorated attacks or increased the amount of time between infusions when she was pummeled by low-level toxins and emotional stress.

I pestered one doctor after another by asking if the "heme pool" was measurable, reasoning that if Jill and other AIPorphyrics could get an idea of what her or their level of heme was at any given point (much like diabetics are able to do with glucometers) then perhaps measures could be taken to manage or avoid crises:

Q3: Is there a method for measuring heme levels in the human body? If so, how is that accomplished? Perhaps through the liver or maybe blood cells that carry heme throughout the body?

A3: *There is not a way to measure heme in the whole body. Heme deficiency in AIP is primarily in the "regulatory heme pool" which is a small pool of heme in liver cells that regulates the enzyme ALA synthase. Otherwise, there is little indication that heme is deficient in other tissues, such as the nervous system or red blood cells.*

Q4: Over time, is it known whether heme can deplete naturally in AIP patients to a dangerously low level, potentially prompting attacks? Obviously, this could be different for each case?

A4: *Heme does not become generally depleted in all tissues in AIP.*

This assertion was countered by Dr. Sassa's 2000 scientific explanation of Type III AIP in which he explained, "The same PBGD defect is found in all tissues."* Knowing that the PBGD (also known as the HMBS) gene is wholly responsible for heme production, it only made sense to me that heme could indeed become deficient in all tissues. I had no idea how to go about getting Jill's tissues tested for PBGD deficiency and no medical practitioner we approached would entertain my hope of confirming that Jill's AIP was of Dr. Sassa's Type III.

Still interested in heme depletion, I found, "heme is produced rapidly in response to metabolic needs draining the free cellular heme pool"[242] and that "[t]he concentration of heme generated within the mitochondrion [part of cell responsible for producing energy] is insufficient to inhibit the enzyme and ALAS (ALA synthase) control is therefore "thought to be exerted by a putative [supposed to exist] free heme pool" in the cytosol [liquid found in cells where cell metabolism occurs].[243]

---

242 Ibid, p5.
243 Ibid, p8.

In addition to the regulatory heme pool in the liver, cells carry heme in a "free range" kind of arrangement throughout the body. Dr. Bylesjö stated that the "…pathogenesis of symptoms in AIP relates to heme deficiency in nerve cells, linking the disorder's biochemical, clinical and neuropathological findings." [244] Then I found, "neurologic manifestations result from porphyrin precursor toxicity rather than heme deficiency and suggest that porphyrin precursor toxicity is primarily responsible for the acute neurologic attacks in…AIP and other porphyrias."[245] But I still wondered if the heme supply could be adequately sustained, would that better insure ALAs would be kept in check?

Regardless of what makes heme levels diminish, "Heme administered intravenously is taken up well by hepatocytes and can replete heme pools rapidly and correct the defects caused by HMBS [hydroxymethylbilane synthase] and other synthetic enzyme deficiencies."[246] Not being a scientist, I stand by my personal long-term theory that when Jill's heme level is deficient, the door is open for marauding AIP symptoms to creep or slam in. I continue to hope that someday AIPorphyrics will be able to pull out their own personal "heme-ometer" to check heme levels and therefore possibly reduce or intercept acute porphyric activity.

That may well be in the future as medical researchers find that heme deficiency may be connected to many more ailments than the acute porphyrias.

Seizures/convulsions

Q5: Seizure(s) during AIP attacks are not unheard of. What physically happens to the body and/or brain during such convulsive activity? Why do some consider them to be psychogenic, or somatic, or pseudo-seizures that are able to be stopped at will?

A5: *Seizures may occur during acute attacks due to hyponatremia or from AIP itself. Sometimes patients with AIP also have epilepsy or some other cause of seizures that is not the AIP. Whether a patient has seizures or pseudo-seizures is determined by a neurologist on an individual basis.*

Seizure is included in the symptomology of many different illnesses and conditions. MedicineNet.com defines seizure as "Uncontrolled electrical activity in the brain, which may produce a physical convulsion, minor physical signs, thought disturbances, or a combination of symptoms."[247] Virtually every medical person who saw Jill in attack mode remarked that her seizures were not "true" or "real" seizures [that

244 Ibid, p17.
245 Solis, Martinez-Bermejo, Naidich, Kaufmann, Astrin, Bishop, Desnick. *Acute Intermittent Porphyria; Studies of the Severe Homozygous Dominant Disease Provides Insight Into the Neurologic Attacks in Acute Porphyrias.* http://www.ncbi.nlm.nih.gov/pubmed/15534187. Published online in "Archives of Neurology" via PubMed. November 2004.
246 Besur, Hou, Schmeltzer, Bonkovsky. *Clinically Important Features of Porphyrins and Heme Metabolism and the Porphyrias.* www.mdpi.com/2218-1989/4/4/977/htm. published online by "Metabolites." November 2014.
247 *Seizure.* www.Medline.net

is, trademark tonic-clonic or grand mal activity] as seen in patients with epilepsy where muscles stiffen; air, forced past the vocal cords, causes a cry or groan; the person is rendered unconscious, may bite his/her tongue or inner cheek and his/her face may turn blue and is followed by arms and legs jerking rapidly and rhythmically, bending at the elbows, hips and knees; with uncontrolled bladder and/or bowel results. Of her many "events," no one had ever reported that she made any sound just prior to or during the episode or that her face turned blue. I have witnessed her lapse into convulsions many times and can say with certainty that she never uttered a sound beforehand or during them. Additionally, there was no evidence she bit her tongue or the inside of her cheek, nor has she ever lost bladder or bowel control during any of her episodes. When at school, reports were that she simply fell to the floor or ground where her body was racked with convulsive tics—sometimes more forceful than others. There did not seem to be a noticeable start point or sequence for the tics. And while some patients with fainting disorders have reported auras or other warnings before seizing, Jill reported tingling or tremors in her arm, hand, leg, and/or torso, blurry or fuzzy vision, a blinding headache, nausea or vomiting prior to blacking out at school. For the most part, having fallen into a nonresponsive state (with the few exceptions when she was able to hear, and remember what was going on around her), she recalled nothing of them. And she nearly always returned to consciousness drowsy, confused, agitated, scared and/or depressed.

Though seizure is not among the highest symptom prevalence of AIP attacks, it can and does occur. A "PES" bulletin noted, "When a porphyric loses their electrolyte balance, small electric shocks sent through the nervous system signal changes ahead...[and] [t]hey are also thought to contribute to seizure activity and muscle spasms.[248] Some studies suggest that AIP seizures or convulsions are either a direct neurologic manifestation of the condition, or are precipitated by hyponatremia (low serum sodium), "During an acute attack, including those with seizures, hyponatremia and hypomagnesemia can be present and contribute to symptomatology."[249] Sources recommend that plasma osmolality (the blood's electrolyte/water balance) and electrolyte values should always be checked when AIP seizure is suspected.

Since the 1980s, it has been acknowledged that the "electroencephalogram (EEG) is often abnormal during an acute attack, and in some patients, this persists during remission."[250] But it seems that EEG is an underutilized diagnostic tool when patients are *in* actual seizure or convulsion mode. While Jill underwent several EEG tests, none happened to be conducted while she was exhibiting seizure or convulsive activity. So many opportunities were lost.

Some sources refer to AIP seizures as epileptic in nature (epilepsy being a general term used for seizure tendency). The issue of epilepsy/AIP comorbidity (having more than one health condition simultaneously) is intriguing. Interestingly,

248 Reuter. *Electrolyte Balance Essential in Acute Porphyrias.* http://porphbooktripod.com/Summer2006.html. Published online in "Porphyria Educational Newsletter." Summer 2006.
249 Bylesjö et al. *Epidemiology and Pathogenetic Clinical Characteristics of Seizures in Patients with Acute Intermittent Porphyria.* www.ncbi.nlm.nih.gov/pubmed/8598180. Published in "Epilepsia." March 1996.
250 Laiwah, Goldberg, Moore. *Pathogenesis and treatment of acute intermittent porphyria: discussion paper.* http://ncbi.nlm.nih.gov/pmc/articles/PMC1430194/?page=2. Published online in "Journal of the Royal Society of Medicine." May, 1983.

an Epilepsy Foundation report about epileptic seizures discusses coexisting epilepsy and metabolic disorders, "[A]lthough all patients with epilepsy have seizures, the converse is not necessarily true, particularly for patients with seizures from metabolic disturbances… Intracellular accumulation of toxic substances is one way that metabolic disorder cause seizures… [However], seizures due to metabolic disorders present diagnostic as well as therapeutic challenges. Close collaboration between the neurologist and the medical specialist is essential in caring for patients with seizures with metabolic origin… acute metabolic derangements can be fatal if left untreated, neurologists must consider this group of disorders when patients present with new-onset seizures or when patients with epilepsy have an unexplained worsening of seizure frequency or severity."[251]

Respiratory Distress
Q6: What actually happens to cause the respiratory distress that AIP patients can quickly ratchet up to during an attack? I have heard doctors tell Jill to "breathe," then say, "Her brain can breathe if she wants to." Yet her lips were gray, she was squeaking because she couldn't talk or breathe and collapsed into severe convulsions. When oxygen is finally administered, she resumes breathing and eventually comes around.

A6: *Porphyria can impair respiratory muscle strength.*

"But how does that happen?" I wondered. The topic of respiratory distress brought me back to the subject of hypoxia which had captured my interest from the beginnings of Jill's AIP ordeal. I pursued the question:

Q7: What is the connection between AIP and hypoxia? Some AIP sufferers have reported problems with flying and/or when they are at high altitudes.

A7: *AIP causes hypoxia if there is weakness of the respiratory muscles. Hemoglobin, which carries oxygen in blood is not impaired.*

I went to the Federal Aviation (FAA) website and refocused on oxygen deprivation and found: "*hypoxic hypoxia* occurs at the lung level and is caused by decreased oxygen in the air; *hypemic hypoxia*, which, though there is adequate supply of oxygen to the brain, the blood's capacity to carry oxygen is impaired; *stagnant hypoxia* occurs at the circulatory level; oxygen cannot get to the body's tissues, and *histotoxic hypoxia* happens at the cellular level; cells cannot use oxygen to support metabolism."[252]

251 Schachter S and Lopez M. *Metabolic Disorders*. http://www.epilepsy.com/information/professionals/co-existing-disorders/metabolic-disorders, published online in "Epilepsy Foundation." April 2004.
252 Boshers, L. *Beware of Hypoxia*. http://www.faa.gov/pilots/training/airman_education/topics_of_interest/hypoxia. Published online by Federal Aviation Administration, Airman Education Programs.

The heme connection is paramount to breathing. Since at least 1993, it has been known that "...heme is an essential component of respiratory proteins."[253]Aware of the potential for inferior binding of heme/oxygen at the cellular level in AIP, I quickly connected the FAA-identified effects of hypoxia to the symptoms Jill had frequently suffered in the Littleton schools.

I also researched brain connections to bulbar paresis (also known as bulbar palsy). Bulbar means the muscles of the throat and mouth, of which the brain stem is "in charge" of operating. The respiratory muscles are similarly controlled by the medulla, or lower brain stem, and wondered if perhaps what I had seen that day when Jill's mouth and throat had been working so oddly at Benton School in 2007 had been related to bulbar activity.

An AIPorphyric woman who responded to my 2009 query/survey letter sent me a copy of a 1995 *Discover* magazine article titled, "The Girl Who Mewed," a story about a nine-year-old girl who was ultimately diagnosed with AIP. As I read the article, I found similarities between the little girl who suffered odd attacks and Jill's odd presentations. The article described a strange mewing sound the child some-times made. It caught my attention because by the time Jill was in middle school, she sometimes made squeaking sounds that I had come to identify as early attack symptoms. In fact, "[In] ...severe cases (of AIP attacks) respiratory tract muscu-lature is affected, complicating breathing and weakening the voice...."[254] Indeed when Jill's voice begins to weaken noticeably, it often indicates that AIP activity is brewing. Still, it was the first time I had actually heard of someone else besides Jill making such sounds. Between the article and what I had learned about connections between autonomic movements of the mouth, throat and brain, I came to better understand why porphyria can impair respiratory muscle strength. Oxygen is nec-essary to keep lung muscle cells, which keep us able to breathe and functioning.

The importance of what I had learned could not be dismissed. One AIPorphyric woman reported that she sobbed uncontrollably when she went up into the moun-tains of Ecuador. She said she stopped crying after boarding the plane and it pres-surized. She told of another woman with porphyria who experienced uncontrol-lable crying while visiting Lake Tahoe and attributed these problems to the lack of oxygen at the high altitude.

Why would that be so? Because the air at high altitudes causes, "...an increase in breathing and heart rate to as much as double, even while resting. Pulse rate and blood pressure go up sharply as our hearts pump harder to get more oxygen to the cells."[255]And for AIPorphyrics, that means the heme biosynthetic pathway is required to jump into overdrive in order to produce new blood cells.

The brain is a high consumer of oxygen.[256] In his book, *Proof of Heaven*, neuro-surgeon and author Dr. Eben Alexander discussed what happens when the brain

---

253 Elder, GH. *Molecular genetics of disorders of haem biosynthesis.* http://www.ncbi.nlm.nih.gov/pmc/articles/PMC501676/?page=1. Published online at "Journal of Clinical Pathology." November 1993.
254 Socialstyrelen. *Acute Intermittent Porphyria, ICD 10 Code, E80.2A.* http://www.socialstyrelsen.se/rarediseases/acuteintermittentporphyria. 2010, 2014.
255 No author identified. *Adapting to High Altitude.* http://anthro.palomar.edu/adapt/adapt_3.htm
256 Chernova T, Nicotera P, Smith AG. *Heme Deficiency is Associated with Senescence and Causes Suppression of   N-Methyl-D-aspartate Receptor Subunits Expression in Primary Cortical Neurons.*

is deprived of oxygen: "lessen the degree of oxygen it gets by a few toor (a unit of pressure) and the owner of that brain is going to experience an alteration in [his or her] reality."[257] Because the livers of AIPorphyrics have difficulty binding heme and oxygen cells, it stands to reason that "brain dysfunction" can occur.

The connection between high altitude and hypoxia made sense too, but I wondered if a hypoxic situation could occur *without* the high-altitude factor. I checked the online dictionary for the definition of histotoxic hypoxia: "a deficiency of oxygen reaching the bodily tissues due to impairment of cellular respiration especially by a toxic agent (as...alcohol)."[258] This definition instantly brought Littleton schools' markers to mind. My mind whirred when I read about low oxygen and the danger of carbon dioxide retention. Apparently, when the lungs expand by taking in air, the body exchanges the oxygen for carbon dioxide that can lead to a carbon dioxide buildup in the lungs. A pulse oximeter measures oxygenation, not *ventilation*—the primary problem in neuromuscular dysfunction.[259] I concluded that measuring the level of carbon dioxide was an indicator of whether a patient was in danger. My intuition told me that insufficient oxygen had been involved with Jill's Littleton school problems. Had I known this earlier, I would have pressed the doctors harder for arterial gas measurements every time she ended up on school floors.

I interpreted the information about hemoglobin not being impaired when hypoxia was afoot and weakening respiratory muscles as meaning oxygen in blood carried to the finger attached to a pulse oximeter was not significantly impaired until a severe deficiency had been reached and by then, mechanical resuscitation would probably be necessary. [Note: For information purposes, a normal pulse-ox stat is 95%-100%[260] and stats of <92% during attack in air is considered life threatening.][261] I shared all of this with APRN Kym who immediately recommended pulmonary functions tests to establish a baseline for lung function. The tests exhausted Jill and she became dizzy and anxious afterward, but a baseline had been set for comparison's sake in the event of future respiratory difficulty.

The opportunity to ask that Jill's blood be tested when exposed to the inside of any of the local school buildings, particularly if or when she began presenting with AIP signals never materialized because she was moved to out-of-district schools.

Immune System
Q8: Could AIP patients be considered to have an impaired, compromised or otherwise affected immune system?

A8: *As far as I know, there is no good evidence that AIP affects the immune system. Nutritional deficiencies might do that, as in any chronic illness.*

---

http://molpharm.aspetjournals.org/content/69/3/697.full. Published online at "Molecular Pharmacology," November 23. 2005.
257 Alexander, Dr. E. "Proof of Heaven" (New York: Simon & Schuster), 138.
258 www.merriam-webster.com/medical
259 http://curecmd.org/cmd-care/in-depth-tutorial
260 www.copd.about.com/od/glosssaryofcopdterms/g/pulseox.htm
261 www.patient.co.uk/doctor/pulse-oximetry

For much of her life, Jill battled one cold, flu, upper respiratory or lower gastric bout after another. As she grew, illnesses were often followed by unrecognized (at the time) AIP activity. Once she left Littleton's school system, colds and other upper respiratory ailments and the frequency and number of AIP attacks retreated to manageable levels.

The liver
Everything that enters the body passes through the liver and is transformed into biochemical products to either be used or disposed of. The liver makes proteins, aids in digestion, helps fight infection by cleaning the blood, neutralizes toxins and is unique in that it is the only internal organ with the ability to regenerate itself.

Q9: Jill's liver function tests, for the most part, are always within the acceptable range yet she often reacts to chemicals, even at low, acceptable OHSA levels, especially solvents, including safe, green U.S. approved products and others within the pesticide category. Upon further research of those products' ingredients, virtually all indicated something to the effect of "not safe for hepatic impaired individuals" and sure enough, AIP symptoms rear up when she is exposed to them.

A9: *There may be mild abnormalities in what are called "liver function tests." This reflects mild damage to liver cells but overall liver function is not impaired as it is in cirrhosis or acute hepatitis, for example. The main concern in AIP is risk of liver cancer later in life.*

Dr. Bylesjö reported that "[i]n AIP, structural and functional alternations in the liver are generally slight."[262] Enzyme panel testing or liver workups help determine the general status of a liver's functioning but won't point to AIP except perhaps when it is too late. For the most part, many patient stories indicated pre-AIP and post-diagnosis, that their liver enzymes showed little or no abnormalities. However, liver cancer is a very real threat so it is important for physicians with AIPorphyric patients to regularly monitor an AIPorphyric patient's liver health.

A direct connection between the gut, which includes the liver, and the brain has been medically accepted. In fact, a "Psychology Today" article, *Your Backup Brain* described how within days of conception, precursor cells destined to become neurons in the gut come together in the embryonic neural crest (where brain and spinal cord develop) then migrate to the gut. The gut's brain is technically known as the enteric nervous system (ENS), though some consider it to be a branch of the autonomic nervous system. Scientists have come to know more about intestinal intelligence and now understand that the cross talk between the gut biome and the brain is continual.[263] It is almost a certainty that more will be known about gut-brain illnesses, including AIPorphyria, in the not too distant medical future.

---

262 Bylesjö, I. *Epidemiological, Clinical and Pathogenetic Studies of Acute Intermittent Porphyria.* Medical dissertation, Umea University. www.diva-portal.org/smash/get/ diva2:141227; FULLTEXT01.pdf. 2008, p11.
263 Hurley D. *Your Backup Brain.* Published in "Psychology Today." November/December, p82.

Perhaps that imagined "heme-ometer" would end up proving helpful for *many* future illnesses.

In fact, where AIP is concerned, it has already begun. A medical team at the Osaka Medical College undertook a four year study that followed the relationship between onset episodes of AIP abdominal pain and the activity of urinary enzymes (ALA, PBG, UP) *and* blood PBG-D. They discovered a definite connection between increased abdominal pain and *decreased* PBG-D levels. They concluded, "Presently PBG-D testing is performed for the diagnosis of chronic or acute intermittent porphyria. We propose that monthly range PBG-D monitoring is crucial for using the negative deviation of PBG-D from the mean value as a clinical benchmark to predict and prevent AIP attacks. Physicians treating porphyric patients should use monthly testing schedules to estimate the potential rise of an AIP attack and to establish opportune heme therapy."[264] Dr. Bylesjö stated that AIP is diagnosed based on genealogical data, clinical symptoms, standard biochemical [urinary] criteria, erythrocyte PBGD and confirmed by DNA mutations in the PBGD gene.[265] He also noted that the PBGD deficiency resulted in the "accumulation of its substrate PBG...during attacks of AIP."[266]

Interestingly, "[i]ncreased levels of ALA and PBG have been reported in the cerebrospinal fluid (CSF) during an acute attack...however, it is doubtful that the increased amounts of ALA and PBG in the CSF are sufficient to cause neurological dysfunction."[267] More than ever, this information supported my belief that erythrocyte PBG-D measurement *must* play a more definitive role in AIP diagnosis, maintenance and treatment. It should be noted, however, that there is a non-erythroid form of AIP in which PBGD may not change, which adds to diagnostic complexity. All of this points to AIP neurological problems such as headaches, abdominal pains, vision problems, mental status changes and others not originating in a porphyric's brain, but rather, in his or her *liver*.

---

264 Tanaka, Usuda, Tanida, Imanishi, Kono. *Long-Term Follow-up of Erythrocyte Porphobilinogen Deaminase Activity in a Patient With Acute Intermittent Porphyria: The Relationship between the Enzyme Activity and Abdominal Pain Attacks.* www.osaka-med-ac.jp/deps/b-omc/articles/533/533tanaka.pdf. Published online by Bulletin of the Osaka Medical College. June 18, 2007.
265 Bylesjö, I. *Epidemiological, Clinical and Pathogenetic Studies of Acute Intermittent Porphyria.* Medical dissertation, Umea University. www.diva-portal.org/smash/get/ diva2:141227; FULLTEXT01.pdf. 2008, 7.
266 Ibid, 9.
267 Ibid, 13.

EPILOGUE

Cloudy Future with Chances for Clearing

The race is not to the swift, nor the battle
to the strong but to the one that endures.
— TRUISM BASED ON COMBINED SCRIPTURE (ECC 9:11; MATT 24.13)

As a parent, watching one's child suffer with a chronic illness is grueling. When that illness is dismissed by highly educated adults who are supposed to know better, grueling is not strong enough to describe the feeling. Shunting a sick child to schools where academics are dumbed down when the child really wants to learn is gutless and heartless. Fortunately, decades ago, the U.S. government had the foresight to recognize that children with disabilities and/or special needs have the right to be educated—and to not be mishandled. Adding bullying students and persecuting taxpayer-paid school adults to that equation is despicable—and illegal. Schools rely on medical recommendations to support requests from getting out of gym class to granting special education designations. When medical professionals do not have answers, a school's applecart is upset and when that occurs, repercussions to the student and his/her family may result in academic maltreatment. Added to the mix are high financial burdens associated with special needs children for families *and* school districts.

Putting the finishing touches on this book inspired reflection. I took the Mom route and realized Littleton schools' AIP storm conditions echoed Melissa Ann's inutero beginning—a porphyric gene knitted into the fabric of her liver; extreme stress, emotional and physical abuse; exposure to and forced ingestion of toxins she had no cognitive awareness of or ability to control.

Jill's position was to commiserate with a fabricated, newly diagnosed AIPorphryic: *At just 11 years old, I was struggling with this disease. What I know is that it takes a toll physically, emotionally and mentally on the person with AIP and also that person's family and friends. Not only may the person have a sharp, stabbing pain through the stomach, but also a sharp, stabbing pain through the heart because it hurts to know you can't live like a 'normal' person. You can't go into certain places. You can't cope with certain situations. You may fall down at any time, possibly crying out in pain, possibly going on to lose your life. People label you a nut case. They just don't understand that you get depressed, stressed beyond stress or might even have a breakdown because of this illness. Living with AIP is going to hurt. People won't understand. They'll treat you differently and you will have to learn how to deal with having this disease as part of your life.*[268]

But fate was not finished with Jill—yet. Because of her physical growth and the assaults she was subjected to in middle school, her port had shifted and was causing significant daily pain that worsened with infusions and required replacement surgery. Instead of helping, neuropathic pain increased dramatically after surgery so she received frequent doses of morphine. Though she hated the "weird" feeling morphine gave her, it did offer relief. Upon discharge from the hospital, the overwhelming pain continued to emanate. When the take-home prescription for Hydromorphone, which is three to five times stronger than morphine, ended Jill found she had become addicted to morphine. Thru research, she learned that morphine and heroin share a similar chemical base. When the suffocating pain would not relent, she succumbed to the relief that heroin, offered by then-boyfriend Aaron to help ease her pain, provided.

Then, at the age of seventeen, on the cusp of adulthood and *five and a half years after* Tri-State Labs had diagnosed her with AIP, a decision was made within that organization to "revisit" Jill's 2008 DNA results. Dr. Alaimo was perplexed when she received a letter from the Tri-State Labs director that stated "…splicing alteration, IVS10-31A>G (c.613-31A>G) [note: the second portion of the alteration had not been mentioned in the original report] which had been reported as pathogenic [this word was also not used in the original report]…suggest[s] that this alteration is a polymorphism; furthermore, the alteration is now listed in NCBI dbSNP as a single nucleotide variant (rs28990987)…."[269] The letter concluded, "Based on this information, we report that Jill Gould is most likely not affected with acute intermittent porphyria (AIP). To support this revised diagnosis, it would be important to obtain urinary porphobilinogen (PBG) and aminolevulinic acid (ALA) if the patient or a family member experiences symptoms of an acute porphyric attack such as abdominal pain, peripheral neuropathy, and/or central nervous system involvement…."[270]

As a result, based on a telephone conversation with the Tri-State Lab's doctor who had revised her 2008 AIP diagnosis to latent, the NCH hematologist assigned to Jill's care (Dr. O'Connor had left NCH for other employment), stopped AIP treatments. WHACK-A-Jill! She was devastated—and terrified about the inevitable return of AIP symptoms. The next two years were hell. Tri-State Labs acknowledged that Jill had an AIP variant gene yet refused to talk with us—about

---

268 Jill. June 2014.
269 Tri-State Genetic Laboratory.* Letter to Dr. Alaimo via Dr. Wade. June 12, 2014
270 Ibid.

anything—and certainly never suggested that she avoid AIP triggers, a typical warning made to "asymptomatic" AIP patients. As CNS symptoms slowly and steadily returned, apparently intimidated by Tri-State Lab's prestigious reputation, no medical professional offered help, claiming lack of knowledge and unfamiliarity with AIP and its treatment protocols. Nevertheless, in powering through that hell, dots connected—and answers did come.

Jill steeled herself as best she could and completed her senior year by juggling two academic venues: morning tutoring at the Littleton public library and afternoon sessions at SFTA. She experienced no AIP symptoms during the entire nine months she had spent in two different SFTA buildings. That school district used similar cleaning and marker products, though different brands than Littleton and, I suspect, had superior fresh air exchange ratios. She received her LHS diploma separated from her peers. Because of severe summer heat, the graduation ceremony was to be held in the school auditorium. Not having had the benefit of her monthly maintenance D10/Panhematin treatment, Jill was afraid to chance triggering a fainting/convulsive attack in front of the entire community so asked if she could receive her diploma outside. As her graduating classmates ambled by, a local television news station filmed the school superintendent handing Jill's diploma to her. A few classmates curiously stared at the goings on—most were focused on making it inside to the coolness of the auditorium. A local media reporter interviewed Jill. "Ghost Student to Graduate from Littleton High" was featured on the nightly news. The next day, a newspaper story printed the high school principal's quote extoling the graduating class as the kindest class she had known. Understandably, the principal's compliment to the class rang hollow for Jill.

Meanwhile Amelia,* contacted me via the Internet to share that her daughter Samantha,* same age as Jill, also suffers from an acute porphyria and has not produced the "requisite" heightened urinary porphyrin/precursor levels either. Medical treatment had been suspended in her case also. Amelia's youngest son, Liam,* also has acute porphyria however, his system *does* generate biochemical indicators during attack, so he receives treatment. Understandably, this presents challenging dynamics for Amelia's family which also includes Nathan,* who did not inherit the porphyria gene.

Jill entered and successfully completed a detox program in fall 2014 but within a few months was disabled yet again with crushing abdominal pains and other AIP symptoms. Back on the MAIP hamster wheel, we sent a urine sample to a highly acclaimed U.S. porphyria laboratory to be analyzed. Once again, the urinary results were frustrating but the report did note, "Erythrocyte porphobilinogen deaminase activity is low (the number had been taken from a six years earlier lab report) which is consistent with the finding that this patient has heterozygous mutation of the gene for this enzyme. Taken together (with the November 2014 urine sample), the results would be interpreted as consistent with latent acute intermittent porphyria."[271] Yet another U.S. porphyria expert had minimalized her condition. Jill's confidence shattered and heroin once again offered refuge. Thankfully, she

---

271 Tri-State Labs,* Southwest Extension. *Porphyria Test Results Report.* November 20, 2014

resumed substance abuse treatment—and I resumed researching, this time focused on the MAIP biochemical dilemma *and* heme deficiency.

Grasping for support, Jill joined a national porphyria support group's Facebook forum and connected with other AIPorphyrics. A bigger picture began to materialize when she discovered that she was not the only one who did not produce the "critical for diagnosis" urinary biochemical results. The number of people suffering with severe acute porphyric-type symptoms, including some who had been clinically diagnosed years earlier, reported that sometimes there was no change whatsoever in their urinary content during attacks struck me as prescient. My Mom-gut said something was amiss with the establishment's steadfast urinary high level biochemical-results position. Not happy with their non-supportive position, we responded to the experts.

In answer, an executive from that national group posted an undated, unattributed article on the group's social network page, and also sent it to Jill. It contained information about "DNA testing for acute hepatic porphyria indicating that certain mutations [such as Jill had] were called polymorphisms [not disease causing]."[272] "Sometimes," the article stated, "these polymorphisms appear in patients who do not have any acute hepatic porphyric symptoms [asymptomatic] and so are re-categorized as being latent in spite of the patient's responding well to treatment for AIP."[273] The article went on to reiterate the two ways AIP diagnosis is established: very high urine PBG levels during attack and genetic testing that results in identification of the disease causing gene.[274]

I wondered, "Why, if someone is *asymptomatic*, would they seek treatment? Besides, Jill *does* have acute symptoms." It did not make sense.

Jill had the AIP gene *and* had had observable, measurable symptoms for years. To say she was asymptomatic or latent when none of these experts had ever observed her in full blown AIP crisis with significant central, peripheral and autonomic nervous system involvement—all resolved with supplemental oxygen, Ativan, D10 drip and/or Panhematin—was ludicrous to me. But Jill was not alone. There were others. In addition to Amelia's daughter reporting horrific symptoms, we heard from patients and read the reports of others who had suffered terribly, sometimes for years, with severe symptoms. Many had been told their test results were "inconclusive" and no relief was forthcoming. Others had received the AIP diagnosis only years later when they produced the requisite urine biochemical markers. What was the "switch?" What made these patients suffer symptoms for years but not generate pink, purple, brown, ruby red or other spectrum colored urine?

Continuing to follow the AIP trail as the Haven Hospital doctor recommended we do so long ago, we located a "new" hematologist who, not being knowledgeable about AIP, promptly referred us to an out-of-state specialist. Dr. Boston* and I communicated by phone and letter until, most likely perturbed by my persistence, he sent a letter stating because her urinary biochemical test results were normal

---

272 U.S. Porpyhyria Group.* Letter to Jill. Circa Jan 2015.
273 Ibid.
274 Ibid.

(he ignored the report I had sent from years back when the urine was reported to be brown but had not been tested), Jill DID NOT have any porphyria. The "new" hematologist, relying on the expert's opinion, would not administer D10/Panhematin treatments. WHACK-A-Jill!

As Jill once again plummeted into darkness, I hit the search engines and re-examined documentation that stated U.S. experts have deemed urinary diagnostics to be problematic. This was confirmed by the Swedes, "…increased urinary excretion of the porphyrin PBG and ALA…despite decades of research…in the pathophysiology of AIP symptoms still has not been clarified."[275] Yet, the U.S., the U.K., and experts from many other countries continue to contend that extremely elevated porphyrin/precursor accumulation via urinary excretion is mandatory to diagnose AIP.

Hoping to resolve the issue, I reached out to Dr. Thorell to ask about the "problematic" AIP diagnostic and treatment dilemma. I was pleasantly surprised when he responded that my question was valid and had been discussed among AIP experts there, too. And I was elated when I read that, in Sweden, lack of "red urine" or the presence of normal U-PBG test results does not exclude a patient who presents with other obvious symptoms from receiving treatment for AIP. Dr. Thorell went on to discuss the possibility of "phases" of ALA and PBG ratios during attacks, but said the matter was still being researched. He also indicated that the treating physician's differential diagnostic skill played a significant role in treating cases and advised doctors faced with cases that could not easily be determined to be AIP to take a better safe than sorry approach in order to prevent potential unfortunate outcomes.

Preliminary anecdotal reports from around the world and expert experience from the AIP Swedish heartland, with generations of in-depth AIP knowledge and experience confirmed it was indeed possible that not all AIPorphyrics excrete darkened and/or ALA/PBG-laden urine during attacks. Another dot had been connected. My thoughts returned to Dr. Morton and the fact that testimony by U.S. porphyria experts from UMass Medical Center had warned that the urinary test "…was not reliable, had never been validated and should not be used"[276] made me wonder if that was so, why this same porphyrin/precursor measurement method continues to be fiercely championed by U.S. experts.

As the weeks turned to months, it became increasingly obvious to me and Jill that without monthly maintenance D10/Heme treatments, her physical and mental health steadily deteriorated. We both knew what was needed for her to improve—supplemental heme—but were stymied by ambivalent doctors who would not treat her. Jill had crossed into the world of the adult AIPorphyric.

That treatment was being withheld simply because her pee didn't turn a pink, red, brown or purplish shade when she was in obvious AIP distress did not make

275 Johansson, Möller, Fogh, Harper. *Biochemical Characterization of Porphobilinogen Deaminase-Deficient Mice During Phenobarbital Induction of Heme Synthesis and the Effect of Enzyme.* http://www.ncbi.nlm.nih.gov/pmc/articles/PMC1430985/. Published online by "Molecular Medicine." September 2003.
276 No author given. *"MCS" and Porphyria.* http://www.quackwatch.com.search/webglimpse.cgi?ID=1&query=Porphyria.

sense to me. I had seen with my own eyes—for five and a half years—that Drs. Piersen's and O'Connor's treatment protocol had pulled Jill out of devastating circumstances. I revisited the Tri-State Labs article that had been sent to Jill months earlier and noted the author had given himself an "out:" "If someone who does not have a confirmed diagnosis of acute porphyria documented by very high PBG levels, is having symptoms that seem consistent with an acute porphyria attack, Panhematin is administered at the discretion of the treating physician."[277] I had shared that document with Jill's "new" hematologist to no avail. And because I had also provided him with mountains of information that included documentation of the 140 treatments Jill had received, I wondered what Dr. Boston might had told him aside from that written statement.

The stars began to align when Facebook friends forwarded me a link to "Purple Pigments: The pathophysiology of acute porphyric neuropathy"[278] that showed how energy "dysfunction" and porphyric neuropathy results from a deficiency in heme biosynthetic pathway enzymes. Though I'd read versions of it before, this time it sunk in. I dove more fully into researching heme deficiency. I also read several relatively recent (2004-2011) articles written by researchers from Australia, Taiwan, Israel, Spain, Sweden and the United Kingdom. Each presented a link between PBGD and heme deficiency in mice trials with the ultimate goal being AIP gene therapy.

I realized that with all the research I had done about porphyria, I could not remember coming across anything significant about heme deficiency or gene therapy studies produced by *U.S.* experts. I wondered why the United States remained silent about these issues. So, starting with heme deficiency, I Googled, "U.S. articles mentioning heme deficiency?" Oddly, an Eniss Pharmaceuticals* Roundtable transcript appeared on the computer screen. Puzzled, I wondered about the connection and began to read.

I learned that Eniss Pharmaceuticals is the manufacturer of the new medication purported to be stronger and more rapid than the standard glucose and/or hematin treatment with the ability to "stop AIP attacks in their tracks." The drug suppresses ALAs and is in clinical trials through a U.S. national porphyria support group. I noted that Tri-State Labs' Dr. Shiffer* was a participant in the roundtable session. As I read his responses to Eniss executives questions, my initial intrigue about a U.S. porphyria expert partaking in the session not only turned into full head bells ringing but the wheels began whirring—this time at the highest velocity ever. The serendipitous points that made that happen:

- Panhemantin, used in the U.S. and Normosang used throughout Europe and South Africa, both referred to as "hemin," "hematin" or "heme" are accepted

---

277 The Porphyria Consortium banner. *Diagnostic Testing for the Acute Porphyrias - Clarification of Test Results.* www.porphyriafoundation.com/content/diagnostic-testing-acute-porphyrias-clarification-testing-results. Published online by the American Porphyria Foundation, Testing for Porphyria page, Important Update link. Undated.
278 Lin, Lee, Park, Kiernan. *Purple Pigments: The pathophysiology of acute porphyric neuropathy.* www.ncbi. nlm.nih.gov/pubmed/21855406. Published online at "Clinical Neurologist" via PubMed. December 2011.

therapies for treating acute porphyrias. Dr. Shiffer said that there was not a wealth of clinical information available about Panhematin because of a lack of high quality studies. "Really?" I thought, "Thirty years as *the* U.S. treatment for AIP and there is a lack of high quality studies about this orphan drug? Why? 'Enough' heme not only resolved Jill's many attacks, it had allowed her to resume a relatively stable quality of life for months at a time."

- Asked about diagnosing AIP, Dr. Shiffer indicated that it is a difficult disease to diagnose in terms of symptoms but is easily diagnosed biochemically by measuring urine porphobilinogen. "Over a half a century in the U.S. and AIP symptoms are *still* a mystery?" I mused, "If purple urine is considered a hallmark signal of AIP activity, why isn't it found in the *symptoms* category? And as far as the biochemical diagnostic method that U.S. and other experts continually tout—I, and many others, note that while the scientific evidence of what happens in the hepatic biosynthetic pathway to cause AIP activity to flare up is well documented, why has nothing turned up about how, why and when excess precursors/porphyrins migrate to an acute porphyric's urine and actually *turn color* during attacks? What is the trigger for that to happen?"

- Dr. Shiffer described Tri-State Lab's use of mice to test the effect of this new drug on the AIP gene, thereby demonstrating a connection to Eniss Pharmaceuticals. "So Tri-State Labs, Dr. Shiffer and Eniss are spending time, energy and money researching ALA suppression in regard to this particular drug that is currently being endorsed by a U.S. national porphyria support organization that Dr. Shiffer is a part of," I ruminated. Things were beginning to make sense.

- Eniss president/COO asked for an update about gene therapy research programs in development and whether gene therapy might eliminate the need for a drug like the one Eniss is developing. Dr. Shiffer replied he knew of a gene therapy trial happening in Europe, but doubted whether such therapy would eliminate the need for the new drug. "Really downplays all the ongoing research happening *outside* the USA," I thought. Given the preceding point, I began to understand why AIP gene research was not being conducted in the U.S.

The connection between Eniss Pharmaceuticals and a U.S. porphyria expert prompted my search for other possible links between U.S. porphyria experts and pharmaceutical companies. I found articles with mention or authorship attribution to certain individuals and focused on the accompanying disclosure and conflict of interest statements. Head bells chimed when I noted several familiar names with relationships to different companies that manufacture and/or market various porphyria drugs. But one in particular caught my attention. Dr. Shiffer was identified as a stock shareholder of Eniss Pharmaceuticals and a patent holder for Eniss' AIP "wonder" drug.

I came across an Eniss investor report that stated the pharmaceutical company is collaborating with American and European porphyria organizations to offer an "alternative therapy" for a group of ultra-rare genetic diseases (hepatic porphyrias) including AIP. *That* got my attention. "AIP is *ultra-rare? Really?* How, when and why did AIP go from rare to ultra-rare status? And by whom could that be quantified? For years, AIP incidence and prevalence numbers have shown inconsistency.

Then an eye-opening clue jumped out. The same investor report noted that high- or hyper-excreter [of urinary biochemical markers] AIPorphyrics are specifically recruited for the "wonder" drug's clinical trials. That clearly left Jill and other patients whose urinary excretions are "not up to scientific snuff" yet whose CNS symptoms are no less severe, out. My research intensified.

Beginning with the 1600s, European immigrants came to, and some settled in, America. By the late nineteenth century, the Swedes were familiar with the illness that was ultimately called acute intermittent porphyria. Between the nineteenth and twentieth centuries, about 1.3 million Swedes emigrated from Sweden to the United States.[279] AIP's high prevalence in Sweden is attributed to the founder effect which essentially means many cases are derived from a single lineage.[280] Sweden's population base, while maintaining a somewhat steady upward trajectory, has for the most part remained cloistered with migration into the country largely attributed to familial connectedness.[281] Therefore the homogeneity of AIP genes in that region remains high.

It is understandable that other countries should benefit from the Swedes' experience and wisdom. And it stands to reason that patients who produce urinary biochemical markers during attacks could be considered to have "Swedish AIP."

However, the U.S. has long been the recipient of untold numbers of immigrants and transients. It is not unrealistic to surmise that AIP genes hitched rides in the livers of some of these people, resulting in genetic variations and mutations. So it seems to defy logic that experts from the U.S. or any other country whose population base is comprised of generations-long mixtures of immigrant and/or transient people would demand that the "founder effect" diagnostic model of AIP be unmovable. And it does not excuse the experts who, upon hearing from patients who suffer with, and whose physicians have documented, a range of CNS symptoms associated with AIP but do not generate urinary *proof*, for ignoring or disavowing their suffering.

Yet that is what has happened, at least in the U.S. where experts have pandered to those who meet the "Swedish porphyria red urinary holes in the snow" high- and hyper-excreting model AIPorphyrics. I have heard from many who have been deemed asymptomatic or latent because their urine does/did not meet biochemical margins and have come to consider these patients, *particularly* those identified, like Jill with the AIP gene, to be *atypical* AIP presenters or *hypo*-excreters—decidedly *not* latent.

Within a month or so after her diagnosis had been "revised," the "non-disease" causing gene began to spark physical, neurological and psychiatric problems for Jill as

---

279 Wikipedia. Swedish Emigration to the United States. http://en/wikipedia.org/wiki/Swedish emigration to the United States
280 Founder effect definition. Genetics Home Reference. http://ghr.nlm.nih.gov/glossary=foundereffect
281 http://focus-migration.hwwi.de/Sweden.6254.0.html?&L=1

she and I went from doctor to doctor seeking to resume Panhematin treatments. All the while, my gut and jangling head bells had me convinced that for all the marvelous, modern scientific advances being made, as far as AIP is concerned, there are holes in U.S. medical knowledge with life-threatening implications. Since reading Dr. Sassa's "Modern diagnosis and management of the porphyrias"[282] years back wherein he described three AIP *types* (Type I, Type II and Type III) depending on PBG-D activity in erythrocytes, I had wondered if AIP should be considered a spectrum disorder. I jumped on the PBG-D wagon and begged each doctor we saw to test Jill's PBG-D level. But the American experts continue to insist that high levels of urinary PBG and ALA is absolutely necessary for a definitive diagnosis of active AIP and ignore any mention of PBG-D.

As all of this was happening, a wonderfully brilliant researcher and friend, Barbara from Australia, was studying now deceased, venerable Rockefeller University Biochemical Hematologist Dr. Sassa's writings in depth and sent his 2000 article, *Molecular aspects of the inherited porphyrias* to my attention.

As I scrutinized the document, multiple lightbulbs lit, music began to play and my head bells quieted for the first time in a long, long time. More dots started to line up. In that article, Dr. Sassa discussed the three types of AIP and described the molecular aspects of porphyrins in the heme biosynthetic pathway—and offered an explanation as to *why* urine changes color in AIP: "the urine is often dark red in color due to the presence of an oxidation product of PBG."[283]

"Oxygen!" "Cellular level!" "The molecular AIP heme/oxygen binding glitch!" It all made sense. My memory zoomed back to 2008 when Dr. O'Connor said that Jill's "blood cells were oddly misshapen" but didn't know why. It became painfully obvious to this non-medical, non-scientific mom that the oxygen in Jill's blood cells was inadequate; the "fault" for her (and probably other hypo-excreters) not producing "colored" urine during attacks (or at all) likely lies in the *oxidation product of PBG* described by Sassa.

Simplistically stated, there are three important factors involved in AIP activity: 1) the gene, 2) the blood, 3) the liver. The biochemical hematology base that Dr. Sassa established and documented has apparently long been forgotten or disregarded, at least in U.S. porphyria circles where for over thirty years the gene and the liver have taken center stage in AIP diagnosis and treatment. To wit, as of May 2016, the APF's SAB is comprised of fifteen experts, seven of whom are gastroenterology or liver specialists (including the chair, a former Rockefeller University employee), two geneticists—and for a "rare" illness that is largely treated by hematologists in the U.S., only *one hematologist*. Whether by design or ignorance, the American AIP "equation" is clearly stilted to genetics and gastroenterology and woefully inadequate in blood/enzyme (PBG-D) expert representation. And, by adhering for decades only to research and documentation that its SAB members produce and disseminate,

---

282 Sassa, S. MD, PhD, Laboratory of Biochemical Hematology, The Rockefeller University, NY. *Modern diagnosis and management of the porphyrias. Published in British Journal of Hematology, 135,281-292.2006.*
283 Sassa, S. & Kappas, A. The Rockefeller University, NY. *Molecular aspects of the inherited porphyrias. Published in Journal of Internal Medicine 2000; 247: 169-178.*

it is quite obvious that when it comes to diagnostic delay and ineffective treatment methods, a grave disservice has been done to my daughter and perhaps others. Finally, the identified link between Dr. Shiffer and Eniss Pharmaceutical's endeavors gives fair reason why U.S. participation in possible AIP curative gene therapy, for all intents and purposes, is not laudable.

Before and following his demise, Dr. Sassa's Japanese colleagues continued to pursue his AIP/PBG-D findings. American porphyria "experts" did not. The Japanese found success. American genetic experts "revised" Jill's AIP diagnosis based on incomplete information (without including blood/enzyme/oxidation activity into the big picture) and U.S. porphyria cohorts rallied round, disregarding (or unaware of) the crux of the simplistic AIP "equation."

As a parent, watching one's child suffer with a chronic illness is grueling. When that illness is repeatedly dismissed by experts who not only continue to base a diagnoses on seemingly inadequate information but who refuse to tell (or ask permission of) the parents of a juvenile patient the reason for wanting to revisit her DNA results five and a half years after the original AIP diagnosis was made is inexcusable. Adding insensitive statements from professionals and doctors who dismiss, deny, and/or ignore a patient's plea for medical help with slap-down responses ("sorry, you're back to square one;" "DID NOT have any porphyria;" "one individual is widening the gap") is despicable.

The number of children with acute porphyric presentations appears to be on the rise. Today's parents are the most highly educated and medically interactive ever and take the role of their child's health care advocacy very seriously. The burden for providing *accurate* and *complete* AIP information, identification and treatment belongs to the experts—*not* the patients or their doctors.

For months on end, the undertow of Jill's AIP was just below the surface, evident only to her and me. One by one, medical professionals turned their backs and withheld the life-saving Panhematin her liver so desperately needed. The relentless physical, neurological and psychiatric manifestations gained momentum and drove a desperate Jill time and again to seek illegal relief to ease the debilitating symptomatic pains. Then, when the fainting/convulsive/abdominal pain episodes returned, Jill found herself in the MedCity ER yet again, facing the notoriously obnoxious Dr. Berkov. Her PBG-D level hovered at a low 5.8. Jill answered Berkov's tactlessness and the American "experts'" purposeful intent to withhold a legal, biologic life-saving treatment from an AIPorphyric who knows the difference between heme adequacy and heme deficiency with a suicide attempt that sent her into addiction rehab. There, her medical condition continued to deteriorate and, not surprisingly, the professionals could (or would) not treat what was clearly the genesis of Jill's addiction—a *medical* condition—AIP.

Whatever her future brings, what Jill has already been through regarding AIP is her greatest accomplishment. If one person is spared a portion of what she has endured, or finds clues in this book to help respond to his/her own or a loved one's health puzzle, whether porphyria or school chemical effects or bullying related, *Purple Canary* will have achieved its objective to start or expand conversations. It is highly unlikely that AIP will become the "fifth A" to plague contemporary school occupants but God willing, porphyria will more frequently become a differential diagnosis consideration. And as that happens, it should be no surprise when AIP moves from the ultra-rare to the uncommon disease category and is no longer under-diagnosed but recognized and effectively *treated*—for high- or hyper-excreters *and* atypical, hypo-excreting presenters alike.

A UCLA scientist published a paper that proved physical and social pains are processed in some of the same regions of the brain. The (dACC) brain section is "where the sting of social pain is processed… [and] is directly affected by opioid drugs including heroin."[284] That finding, Dr. Sassa's influential writings; the Swedish expert's answer about the intermittent absent biochemical makers during acute porphyric attack; the Eniss Pharmaceutical transcript contents and the support of so many AIPorphyrics and/or their caregivers offered me final Purple Canary dot connections. If U.S. porphyria experts expect to retain that status, in this mom's opinion, there is work to do. As for me, I will attend to my daughter's precarious health position because, as PO Zlotowski encouraged, "Do whatever you have to do to protect your daughter" and because, as Jonathan Morrow said, "That's a mother's job."

I wanna feel the love
I wanna feel the way it used to be
I wanna be the one
The one I used to see
In the mirror
Where everything's clearer.
I could finally breathe
But the mirror is broken
And my scars are open
For everyone to see.
I wanna feel the strength,
The strength I used to have
And I wanna feel which way
Just which way the wind blows.
And then I'll know
That I can let go
Spread my wings and fly away.
But my wings are broken
And my scars are open
For everyone to see
And the memories, they still come to me[285]

zalavitz, M. *In the Brain: Broken Hearts Hurt Like Broken Bones.* http://healthland.time. 012/02/27/in-the-brain-broken-hearts-hurt-like-broken-bones/. Published by Time.com. Body d. February 27, 2012.
Gould. Lyrics to "Falling Away from Me."

The End

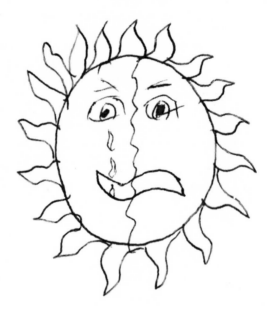

"A Purple Sun"

Illustration by Jill Gould

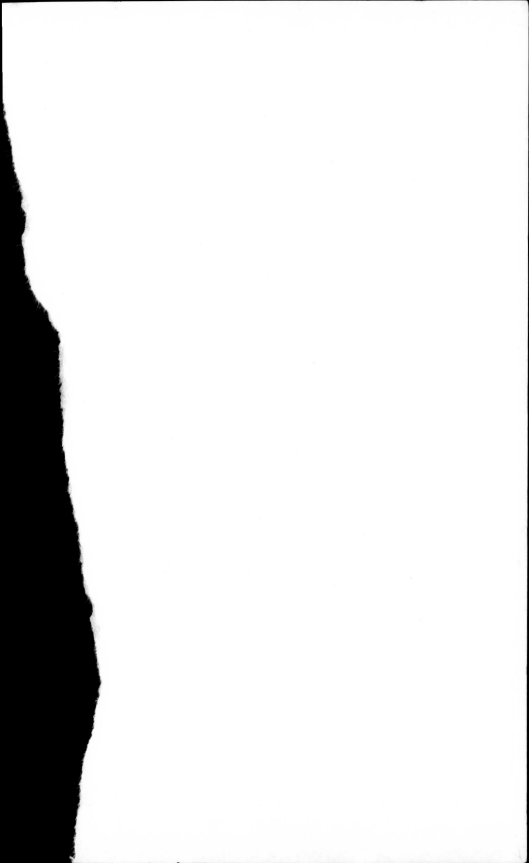

CPSIA information can be obtained
at www.ICGtesting.com
Printed in the USA
LVOW07s0002300117
522566LV00001B/111/P